MADHAVA NIDANA I.A.S.T

ENGLISH TRANSLATION WITH I.A.S.T TRANSLITERATION OF SANSKRIT VERSES

JANARDHANA V HEBBAR
RAGHURAM Y S

Made with ♥ on the Notion Press Platform
www.notionpress.com

|| Jai Guruji ||

I, Dr. Janardhana V. Hebbar, dedicate this book at the holy feet of Sri Guruji – Swami Vivekananda and my spiritual Guru, Dr. A. Chandrashekhara Udupa MBBS, FAGE, Managing Director, Divine Park Trust (R), Saligrama, Udupi. (www.divinepark.org)

He guides, He energizes, He shows the path,
He holds my hand and makes me walk!

Contents

Chief Editor *ix*

Preface *xi*

Acknowledgements *xiii*

1. PAÑCA NIDĀNA LAKṢAṆAM 1
2. JWARA NIDĀNAM 7
3. ATHĀTĪSĀRANIDĀNAM 26
4. GRAHAṆĪROGANIDĀNAM 34
5. ARŠAS NIDĀNAM 40
6. VILAMBIKĀ NIDĀNAM 50
7. KRIMI NIDĀNAM 58
8. PĀṆḌUROGA KĀMALĀ KUMBHAKĀMALĀ HALĪMAKA NIDĀNAM 62
9. RAKTAPITTA NIDĀNAM 69
10. RĀJAYAKṢMĀ-KṢATAKṢINA NIDĀNAM 73
11. KĀSA NIDĀNAM 81
12. HIKKĀ ŚWĀSA NIDĀNAM 87
13. SWARA BHEDA NIDĀNAM 98
14. AROCAKA NIDĀNAM 101
15. CHARDI NIDANAM 104
16. TRṢṆĀ NIDĀANAM 109
17. MŪRCHĀ, BHRAMA, NIDRĀ, TANDRĀ, SANNYASA NIDĀNAM 114
18. PĀNĀTYAYA, PARAMADA, PĀNĀJIRNA-PĀNAVIBHRAMA NIDANAM 121
19. DĀHA NIDĀNAM 128
20. UNMADA NIDANAM 131
21. APASMĀRA NIDĀNAM 143

Contents

22. VĀTA VYĀDHI NIDĀNAM 147

23. VĀTA RAKTA NIDĀNAM 168

24. URUSTAMBHA NIDĀNAM 174

25. ĀMAVĀTA NIDĀNAM 177

26. ŚŪLA PARIṆĀMAŚŪLA ANNADRAVAŚŪLA NIDĀNAM 181

27. UDĀVARTA ĀNĀHA NIDĀNAM 189

28. GULMA NIDĀNAM 197

29. HRDROGA NIDĀNAM 204

30. MUTRAKRICHANTAK NIDANAM 207

31. MŪTRĀGHĀTA NIDĀNAM 211

32. AŚMARĪ NIDĀNAM 217

33. PRAMEHA, PRAMEHA PIPAKĀ NIDĀNAM 222

34. MEDA ROGA NIDĀNAM 232

35. UDARA NIDĀNAM 235

36. ŚOTHA NIDĀNAM 243

37. VRDDHI NIDĀNAM 249

38. GALAGANDA-GANDAMALA-APACI-GRANTHI-ARBUDA NIDANAM 252

39. ŚLIPADA NIDĀNAM 260

40. VIDRADHI NIDĀNAM 262

41. VRAṆAŚOTHA NIDĀNAM 268

42. ŚĀRĪRA VRAṆA NIDĀNAM 272

43. SADYOVRAṆA NIDĀNAM 277

44. BHAGNA NIDĀNAM 284

45. NĀDĪ VRANA NIDĀNAM 288

46. BHAGANDARA NIDĀNAM 291

47. UPADAMSA NIDĀNAM 294

Contents

48. SUKA DOṢA NIDĀNAM 297

49. KUṢTHA NIDĀNAM 302

50. SITAPITTA UDARDA KOTHA NIDANAM 312

51. AMLAPITTA NIDĀNAM 314

52. VISARPA NIDANAM 317

53. VISPHOTA NIDĀNAM 323

54. MASURIKA NIDĀNAM 326

55. KṢUDRA ROGA NIDĀNAM 333

56. MUKHA ROGA NIDĀNAM 346

57. KARṆAROGANIDĀNAM 363

58. NĀSĀROGANIDĀNAM 369

59. NETRAROGANIDĀNAM 377

60. ŚIROROGANIDĀNAM 403

61. ASṚGDARA NIDĀNAM 409

62. YONIVYĀPAT NIDĀNAM 412

63. YONIKANDA NIDĀNAM 416

64. MŪḌHAGARBHA NIDĀNAM 418

65. SŪTIKĀROGA NIDĀNAM 423

66. STANAROGA NIDĀNAM 425

67. STANYADUṢṬI NIDĀNAM 426

68. BĀLAROGA NIDĀNAM 429

69. VIṢAROGANIDĀNAM 438

70. VIṢAYĀNUKRAMAṆIKĀ 454

Chief Editor

Dr Raghuram YS BAMS, MD(Ayu)

Preface

Madhava Nidana is written by Acharya Madhavakara. Madhavakara was the author of 'Rugvinishchaya'. The work Rugvinishchaya later came to be known as and become popular in the name 'Madhava Nidana'
Madhava nidana is mainly a compilation from the earlier works of Ayurveda such as Charaka Samhita, Sushruta Samhita, Ashtanga Samgraha, Ashtanga Hridaya and Ravigupta's Shuddhasara.
In spite of Madhava Nidana being a compilation of various previous works, Madhava Nidana enjoys an independent and respected status of being an important treatise. Verses on 'Nidana' available in various sections of Charaka Samhita, Sushruta Samhita and Ashtanga Sangraha etc. are compiled and quoted in Madhava Nidana. The verses are arranged in systematic manner.

Speciality – The major contribution and speciality of Madhavakara in his work Madhava Nidana is the order of arranging the names of diseases in his own style.
It is the first and one of the rare books or treatise which has been compiled in a systematic way, subject wise and covering the topics related to causes, premonitory symptoms, symptoms, pathogenesis, complications and prognosis of diseases.

Specialities of Madhava Nidana –
In his treatise Madhava Nidana, Madhavakara has composed the pathological aspects of a number of diseases pertaining to various branches of Ayurveda. The compilation is in below said order -
Chapter 1 – deals with basics of Nidana Panchaka (5 tools of examining a disease
Chapters 2-19, 22-37 and 49-54 – deals with topics related to Kaya Chikitsa (General systemic diseases like Jwara i.e. fever, Atisara i.e. diarrhoea etc)
Chapters 20-21 – deals with Graha or Bhuta vidya (toxicology, worm infestations)
Chapters 38 and 55 – deals with Shalya Chikitsa or surgical aspects
Chapters 56-60 – deals with Shalakya chikitsa (diseases pertaining to eye, ear, nose, throat, head, tongue, teeth etc)
Chapters 61-68 – deals with Kaumarabhritya (paediatrics, diseases

occurring in children)
Chapter 69 – deals with Agadatantra (toxicology)
In total, 79 diseases have been described in Madhavanidana

Systematic compilation – In Madhava Nidana the Nidana (causative factors), Purva Rupas (premonitory symptoms), Rupa (signs and symptoms), Samprapti (pathogenesis), Upadrava (complications) and Sadhya-Asadhyata (prognosis of the disease) are described in a systematic manner
Shula and Visphota – Madhava, for the first time recognized Shula (colic) and Visphota (vesicles and blisters) as independent entities, initially they were considered as symptoms of diseases
Names of new diseases – like Amavata, Parinamashoola, Annadrava shula, Medoroga, Shitapitta, Amlapitta, Masurika, Pakshmashata and Yonikanda were mentioned and described for the first time in Madhava Nidana
Madhava Chikitsa and Ratnamala – These two are the books probably written by 'Madhavakara' in which treatment of the diseases explained in Madhava Nidana have been explained and discussed
The new alignment of the diseases, which were arranged in the work of Madhavakara was followed by his successors like Vrinda Madhava, Chakrapanidatta, Govindadas in their treatises

Commentaries

Teeka or Commentaries on Madhava Nidana –

Madhukosha – written by Vijayarakshita and Srikanthadatta
Atankadarpana – written by Vachaspati

Acknowledgements

Special thanks to Dr Raghuram YS for painstakingly editing the entire book. Special thanks to my family members who have been supporting me unconditionally throughout this journey of Easy Ayurveda. Thank you for tolerating all the pains.
Smt. Padmakshamma (mother), Karthyayini (wife and staff), Smt. Vanamala (mother-in-law).
Daughters – Sadhvi & Chinmayi

Sister Sharada, brother-in-law Mr ShashiKumar, Tushar, Ms Sharada.
All my staff who make Easy Ayurveda possible, everyday.
Dr Sudarshan CH, Dr Shilpa Ramdas, Dr Renita D'Souza.
Mr Sachidananda Bhat, Smt. Nayana, Mr Nikhil and Smt. Sumangala.
My mentors - Dr MB Gururaja, Dr MS Krishnamurthy and Dr Prashanth BK

CHAPTER ONE

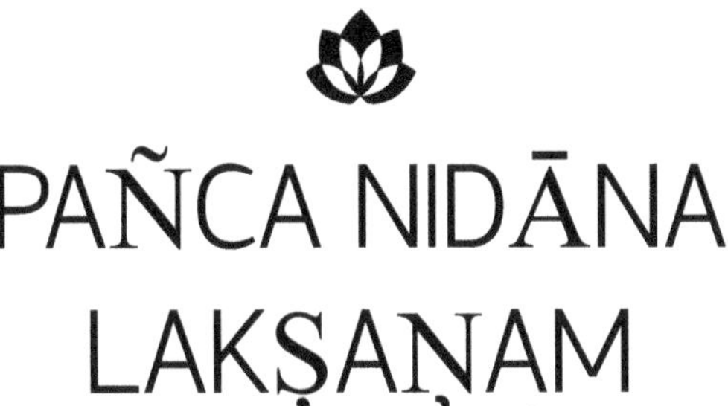

PAÑCA NIDĀNA LAKṢAṆAM

praṇamya jagadutpattisthitisaṃhārakāraṇam |
svargāpavargayordvāraṃ trailokyaśaraṇaṃ śivam ||1||
nānāmunīnāṃ vacanairidānīṃ samāsataḥ sadbhiṣajāṃ niyogāt |
sopadravāriṣṭanidānaliṅgo nibadhyate rogaviniścayo'yam ||2||
nānātantravihīnānāṃ bhiṣajāmalpamedhasām |
sukhaṃ vijñātumātaṅkamayameva bhaviṣyati ||3||

I have composed this 'Roga Viniscaya' treatise after offering my salutations and worship (prayers) to the holy feet of Lord Siva who is the chief cause for the creation, maintenance and destruction of the entire universe, one who bestows heaven and salvation and the protector of all the three worlds. I have composed this treatise based on the advice and motivation given to me by the revered physicians. The treatise also comprises the sayings of various sages on the complications, prognosis, causes, signs and symptoms of the diseases in brief.

This will help the physicians having low intellect, not having precise knowledge of various shastras – treatises (and hence unable to study and understand them). This treatise named 'roga viniscaya' has been composed with an idea of helping such physicians to gain the knowledge of various diseases and also to understand them. (1-3)

Note – Here the author of this treatise claims and announces the objectives with which he has composed this treatise and the purpose and kinds of physicians it would serve.

Nidana Panchaka - Five means of understanding the diseases

nidānaṃ pūrvarūpāṇi rūpāṇyupaśayastathā |
samprāptiśceti vijñānaṃ rogāṇāṃ pañcadhā smṛtam ||4||

(vā| ni| a| 1)

The five means or tools of understanding the diseases are –

1. Nidāna - causes, aetiology, aetiological factors of the disease,
2. Pūrvarūpa - premonitory symptoms, prodromata of the disease
3. Rūpa - signs and symptoms; clinical features, symptomatology of the disease,
4. Upasaya – diagnostic tests, pacification and aggravating factors which can be used for diagnosing the diseases through trial-and-error methods and also to differentiate one disease and the other through differential diagnosis and also to determine the prognosis of the diseases and
5. Samprāpti – pathogenesis of a disease, the process and pathway of formation of the disease (story of development of a disease, step by step)

These five means of understanding the diseases are called as Nidana Panchaka. (4)

Synonyms of Nidana

nimittahetvāyatanapratyayotthānakāraṇaiḥ |
nidānamāhuḥ paryāyaiḥ||| |5|
(vā| ni| a| 1) |

The synonyms of Nidāna (causative factors or aetiological factors of the disease) are –

Nimitta
Hetu
Ayatana
Pratyaya
Utthāna and
Kāraṇa (5)

Purvarupa – Premonitory symptoms of the disease

...prāgrūpaṃ yena lakṣyate ||5||

utpitsurāmayo doṣaviśeṣeṇānadhiṣṭhitaḥ |
liṅgamavyaktamalpatvādvyādhīnāṃ tadyathāyatham ||6||
(vā| ni| a| 1) |
Pūrvarūpa means 'premonitory symptoms of the diseases. These are those signs and symptoms which appear earlier to the actual disease i.e., the purvarupas appear before the manifestation of the actual disease. These purvarupas are not specifically assignable to the doshas as they are mild in nature (not clearly recognisable) and few in numbers. (6)

Rupa – signs and symptoms of the disease

tadeva vyaktatāṃ yātaṃ rūpamityabhidhīyate |
saṃsthānaṃ vyañjanaṃ liḍgaṃ lakṣaṇaṃ cihnamākṛtiḥ ||7||
(vā| ni| a| 1) |
The same premonitory signs and symptoms manifesting clearly in the later time are known as rupa i.e., 'signs and symptoms proper' or specific features of the disease. They synonyms of rupa are - vyanjana, linga, laksana, cinha and akrti. (7)

Upashaya – factors (medicine, food, activity) subsiding the disease and thereby helping in diagnosing (or differentially diagnosing) a disease

hetuvyādhiviparyastaviparyastārthakāriṇām |
auṣadhānnavihārāṇāmupayogaṃ sukhāvaham ||8||
vidyādupaśayaṃ vyādheḥ sa hi sātmyamiti smṛtaḥ |
viparīto'nupaśayo vyādhyasātmyābhisañjñitaḥ ||9||
(vā| ni| a| 1) |
Upaśaya is the administration of medicine, food or activity which bring about sukha (comfort, relief of symptoms) to the patient; (thereby helping in diagnosis). They are of the following kinds viz:

1. Viparīta (opposite) of hetu (cause), vyādhi (disease) or both,
2. Viparīthārthakārī (producing the opposite effect though not actually opposite) to either the hetu (cause), vyādhi (disease) of both.

This (upasaya) is also known as sātmya (compatible).
The opposite of upaśaya is anupasaya (increasing the discomfort) or

asātmya (incompatible) to the disease. (8-9)

Samprapti – pathogenesis of the disease

yathāduṣṭena doṣeṇa yathā cānuvirsapatā |
nirvṛttirāmayasyāsau samprāptirjātirāgatiḥ ||10||
(vā| ni| a| 1) |
The process of manifestation of the disease, by the morbid doshas which are circulating all over the body is known as samprāpti. Jāti or āgati are the synonyms of samprapti. (10)

Types of Samprapti
saṅkhyāvikalpaprādhānyabalakālaviśeṣataḥ |
sā bhidyate yathā'traiva vakṣyante'ṣṭau jvarā iti ||11||
doṣāṇāṃ samavetānāṃ vikalpoṃ'śāṃśakalpanā |
svātantryapāratantryābhyāṃ vyādheḥ prādhānyamādiśet ||12||
hetvādikārtsnyāvayavairbalābalaviśeṣaṇam |
naktandinartubhuktāṃśairvyādhikālo yathāmalam ||13||
(vā| ni| a| 1) |
iti prokto nidānārthaḥ sa vyāsenopadekṣyate |14|
(vā| ni| a| 1) |
Sankhyā, Vikalpa, Prādhánya, Bala and Kāla are the five types of samprapti.

Examples for Different Types ofSamprapti

1. Sankhyā Samprāpti
Eg: Counting jwaras (fevers) as eight in number etc (types and subtypes of diseases)
2. Vikalpa Samprāpti
Eg; To point out a symptom or a disease as arising from a specific property of a particular dosha (fractional understanding)
3. Prādhānya Samprāpti,
Eg: To signify a disease as primary (or secondary)
4. Bala Samprāpti
Eg: To qualify a disease as severe or mild depending upon the cause etc. (to determine the strength and severity of a disease)
5. Kāla Samprāpti

To signify that a disease is severe during a particular period of time such as night, day, season, time of digestion of food, etc.

These will be elaborated later. (11-13)

sarveṣāmeva rogāṇāṃ nidānaṃ kupitā malāḥ ||14||
tatprakopasya tu proktaṃ vividhāhitasevanam |15|
(vā| ni| a| 1) |
nidānārthakaro rogo rogasyāpyupajāyate ||15||
tadyathā jvarasantāpādraktapittamudīryate |
raktapittājjvarastābhyāṃ śoṣasyāpyupajāyate ||16||
plīhābhivṛddhyā jaṭharaṃ jaṭharācchotha eva ca |
arśobhyo jāṭharaṃ duḥkhaṃ gulmaścāpyupajāyate ||17||
(divāsvāpādidoṣaiśca pratiśyāyaśca jāyate) |
pratiśyāyādatho kāsaḥ kāsāt sañjāyate kṣayaḥ |
kṣayo rogasya hetutve śoṣasyāpyupajāyate ||18||
(ci| ni| a| 8) |
te pūrvaṃ kevalā rogāḥ paścāddhetvarthakāriṇaḥ |19|
(ca| ni| a| 8) |
kaściddhi rogo rogasya heturbhūtvā praśāmyati ||19||
na praśāmyati cāpyanyo hetutvaṃ kurute'pi ca |
evaṃ kṛcchratamā nṝṇāṃ dṛśyante vyādhisaṅkarāḥ ||20||
(ca| ni| a| 8) |
tasmādyatnena sadvaidyairicchadbhiḥ siddhimuddhatām |
jñātavyo vakṣyate yo'yaṃ jvarādīnāṃ viniścayaḥ ||21||
iti śrīmādhavakaraviracite mādhavanidāne pañcanidānalakṣaṇaṃ samāptam ||1||
The morbid (increased) doshas are considered to be the cause for all kinds of diseases. On the other hand, indulgence in different kinds of unhealthy foods or activities is considered to be the cause for morbid (abnormal) increase of the doshas. (14)

Nidanarthakara Roga - Sometimes one disease might become a cause for another disease. Examples include,

- Increased temperature of jwara (fever) may result in Raktapitta (bleeding disorders, purpura)

- Raktapitta may cause manifestation of fever
- Both jwara and raktapitta together may cause sosa (consumption, tuberculosis)
- Pliha vrddhi (enlargement of spleen) may cause jathara roga (enlargement of abdomen)
- Jathara (abdominal enlargement) may cause Sotha (oedema)
- Arsas (piles) may become the cause for troublesome jathara dukha (abdominal pain) and also gulma (abdominal tumour)
- Divasvapna etc doshas i.e., Sleeping at day time etc. (causative factors) might result into Pratisyaya (common cold)
- Pratisyaya may lead to kasa i.e., cough
- Kasa would lead to ksaya (emaciation) and
- Ksaya might cause sosa roga (tuberculosis, consumption)

At the beginning the causative disease is just a mild symptom complex. In due course of time, it might become a major disease. Some of them may disappear when the second disease manifests. On the other hand, some others continue to persist even as the second disease exists (during the course of the second disease). This would lead to a condition called vyadhi sankara i.e., coexistence of two or more diseases (like a syndrome) which is very troublesome. (15-20)

So, the physician who desires to become successful should strive hard to understand the diagnosis of diseases like jwara etc. which will be described further on. (21)
Thus ends the chapter called 'Pañcanidana Laksana'

CHAPTER TWO

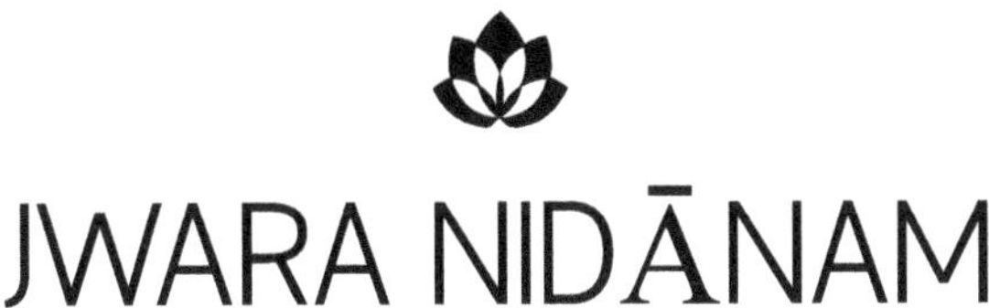

JWARA NIDĀNAM

Origin / History of Jwara (fevers)

dakṣāpamānasaṅkruddharudraniḥśvāsasambhavaḥ |
jvaro‘ṣṭadhā pṛthagdvandvasaṅghātāgantujaḥ smṛtaḥ ||1||
It was long ago that Jwara (fever) was born, from the wrath of Lord Rūdra who had been insulted by Daksa. It is of eight kinds; one from each dosa (vātaja, pittaja and kaphaja), one each from the combination of two dosas (vātapittaja,vātakaphaja, pittakaphaja), one from the combination of all the three doshas (sannipātaja, tridosaja) and one from āgantu (external causes). (1)

Note: The eight kinds of fever are as listed below –

Names of Fever according to Category:

A. Eka doshaja – caused by single dosha
1. Vataja
2. Pittaja
3. Kaphaja

B. Dwi dosaja / Dwandwa / Samsargaja – caused by two dosas
4. Vata-pittaja
5. Vata-kaphaja
6. Pitta-kaphaja

C. Tridosaja / Sannipataja – caused by three dosas
7. Vata-pitta-kaphaja

D. Agantuja – caused by external causes
8. Agantuja

Jwara Samprapti – pathogenesis of fever

mithyāhāravihārābhyāṃ doṣā hyāmāśayāśrayāḥ |
bahirnirasya koṣṭhāgniṃ jvaradāḥ syū rasānugāḥ ||2||
Due to the indulgence in improper foods and activities, the Dosas (vāta, pitta and kapha) undergo an increase (individually or in combination). These dosas reach the āmāśaya (stomach and intestines, gastrointestinal tract) and expel the kosthāgni (gastric fire, factors responsible for digestive activity) to the exterior (skin and other tissues) and circulating along with rasa (dhātu) (blood plasma) produces jwara (fever). (2)

Notes

The events leading to manifestation of jwara (fever) – pathogenesis of jwara

Indulgence in improper foods and activities

↓

Doshas undergo abnormal increase / aggravation either individually or in combination

↓

The increased doshas reach the stomach / intestines

↓

Causes expulsion of the gastric fire to the exterior

↓

The same doshas circulate along with the blood plasma

↓

Produce jwara – fever

Definition of Jwara

svedāvarodhaḥ santāpaḥ sarvāṅgagrahaṇaṃ tathā |
yugapadyatra roge ca sa jvaro vyapadiśyate ||3|| (su|u|taṃ|a| 39)
Jwara is defined as the disease in which there is obstruction to perspiration (sweating), increase of body temperature and pain all over the body. All

these symptoms occur and exist together. (3)

Purvarupa – Premonitory symptoms of Jwara

śramo'ratirvivarṇatvaṃ vairasyaṃ nayanaplavaḥ |
icchādveṣau muhuścāpi śītavātātapādiṣu ||4||
jṛmbhā'ṅgamardo gurutā romaharṣo'rucistamaḥ |
apraharṣaśca śītaṃ ca bhavatyutpatsyati jvare ||5||
(sāmānyato viśeṣāttu jṛmbhā'tyarthaṃ samīraṇāt |
pittānnayanayordāhaḥ kaphādannārucirbhavet ||6||
rūpairanyatarābhyāṃ tu saṃsṛṣṭairdvandvajaṃ viduḥ |
sarvaliṅgasamavāyaḥ sarvadoṣaprakopaje) ||7||
(su| u| taṃ| a| 39) |

Fatigue, restlessness, discolouration of the skin, bad taste in the mouth, eyes full of tears, alternate like and dislike for cold wind and warm sunlight, etc., yawning, body ache, feeling of heaviness of the body, horripilation (body hairs standing on ends), lack of appetite, stupor, lack of interest in anything and feeling of cold are the symptoms generally appearing earlier to the actual onset of fever (premonitory symptoms).

Even among these (premonitory symptoms),

- Yawning will be more, if vātaja jwara were to manifest later,
- Burning sensation will be found if pittaja jwara were to manifest later and
- Lack of appetite will be found if kaphaja jwara were to manifest in future.

Similarly, the symptoms of two or three došhas will appear in fevers caused due to a combination of two or three doshas respectively. (4-7)

Symptoms of Vataja Jwara

vepathurviṣamo vegaḥ kaṇṭhauṣṭhapariśoṣaṇam |
nidrānāśaḥ kṣavastambho gātrāṇāṃraukṣyameva ca ||8||
śirohṛdgātrarugvaktravairasyaṃ gāḍhaviṭkatā |
śūlādhmāne jṛmbhaṇaṃ ca bhavantyanilaje jvare ||9||

(su| u| taṃ| a| 39) |

The symptoms of Vātaja jwara (fever due to the increase of vāta doṣa) are - shivering (chill, rigours), non-corresponding time of onset and exacerbation, severe dryness of the throat and lips, loss of sleep, absence of sneezing, roughness of the skin (or decrease of moisture in the body) pain in head, chest and body, bad taste in the mouth, hard and dry faeces, pain in the abdomen, distension of abdomen and too many yawning. (8-9)

Symptoms of Pittaja Jwara

vegastīkṣṇo'tisāraśca nidrālpatvaṃ tathā vamiḥ |
kaṇṭhauṣṭhamukhanāsānāṃ pākaḥ svedaśca jāyate ||10||
pralāpo vaktrakaṭutā mūrchā dāho madastṛṣā |
pītaviṇmūtranetratvaṃ paittike bhrama eva ca ||11||
(su| u| taṃ| a| 39) |

The symptoms of Pittaja Jwara (fever due to the increase of pitta doṣa) are - very high temperature, diarrhoea, very little sleep, vomiting, ulcers in the throat, lips, mouth and nose, perspiration, delirium, bitter taste in the mouth, fainting, feeling of burning sensation all over the body, intoxication, thirst, yellow colouration of faeces, urine & eyes, etc., and giddiness. (10-11)

Symptoms of Kaphaja Jwara

staimityaṃ stimito vega ālasyaṃ madhurāsyatā |
śuklamūtrapurīṣatvaṃ stambhastṛptirathāpi ca ||12||
gauravaṃśītamutkledo romaharṣo'tinidratā |
(srotorodho rugalpatvaṃ praseko lavaṇāsyatā |
nātyuṣṇagātratā, cchardirlālāsrāvo'vipākatā) |
pratiśyāyo'ruciḥ kāsaḥ kaphaje'kṣṇośca śuklatā ||13||
(su| u| taṃ| a| 39) |

The symptoms of Kaphaja Jwara (fever due to the increase of kapha doṣa) are - feeling of stiffness / cold all over the body, mild increase of temperature, lack of enthusiasm (laziness), sweet taste in the mouth, whitish urine and faeces, stiffness of extremities, abnormal feeling of contentment, feeling of heaviness, cold, nausea, horripilation, excessive sleep; obstruction to the channels, mild pains, excessive salivation, salty taste in the mouth, temperature is not very high, vomiting, saliva flowing out, indigestion of food, running nose, lack of appetite, cough and whitish eyes. (12-13)

Symptoms of Vatapitta Jwara

tṛṣṇā mūrchā bhramo dāhaḥ svapnanāśaḥśirorujā |
kaṇṭhāsyaśoṣo vamathū romaharṣo'rucistamaḥ ||14||
parvabhedaśca jṛmbhā ca vātapittajvarākṛtiḥ |15|
(su| u| taṃ| a| 39)
The symptoms of Vata-pittaja jwara (fever caused by combination of increased vata and pitta doshas) are - thirst, fainting, giddiness, burning sensation, loss of sleep, headache, dryness of throat and mouth, vomiting, horripilations, loss of taste (tastelessness), feeling of darkness before the eyes, pain in the small joints of hands and feet and yawning. - (14-15)

Symptoms of Vata-kapha Jwara

staimityaṃ parvaṇāṃ bhedo nidrā gauravameva ca ||15||
śirograhaḥ pratiśyāyaḥ kāsaḥ svedāpravartanam |
santāpo madhyavegaśca vātaśleṣmajvarākṛtiḥ ||16||
(su| u| taṃ| a| 39) |
The symptoms of Vata-kaphaja jwara (fever caused by combination of increased vata and kapha doshas) are - feeling of stiffness / cold in the body, pain in the small joints of hands and feet, too much of sleep, feeling of heaviness of the body, headache common cold / running nose, cough, lack of perspiration (sweating) and moderate increase of body temperature. (15-16)

Symptoms of Kapha-pitta Jwara

liptatiktāsyatā tandrā mohaḥ kāso'rucistṛṣā |
muhurdāho muhuḥśītaṃśleṣmapittajvarākṛtiḥ ||17||
(su| u| taṃ| a| 39) |
The symptoms of Kapha-pittaja jwara (fever caused by combination of increased kapha and pitta doshas) are - coating of the tongue, manifestation of bitter taste in the mouth, drowsiness, delusion, cough, loss of taste, thirst,

alternate feeling of heat and cold. (17)

Symptoms of Sannipata Jwara

kṣaṇe dāhaḥ kṣaṇe śītamasthisandhiśiroruja |
sāsrāve kaluṣe rakte nirbhugne cāpi locane ||18||
sasvanau sarujau karṇau kaṇṭhaḥśūkairivāvṛtaḥ |
tandrā mohaḥ pralāpaśca kāsaḥśvāso'rucirbhramaḥ ||19||
paridagdhā kharasparśā jihvā srastāṅgatā param |
ṣṭhīvanaṃ raktapittasya kaphenonmiśritasya ca ||20||
śiraso loṭhanaṃ tṛṣṇā nidrānāśo hṛdi vyathā |
svedamūtrapurīṣāṇāṃ cirāddarśanamalpaśaḥ ||21||
kṛśatvaṃ nātigātrāṇāṃ pratataṃ kaṇṭhakūjanam |
koṭhānāṃśyāvaraktānāṃ maṇḍalānāṃ ca darśanam ||22||
mūkatvaṃ srotasāṃ pāko gurutvamudarasya ca |
cirātpākaśca doṣāṇāṃ sannipātajvarākṛtiḥ ||23||
(ca| ci| a| 3) |

The symptoms of Sannipatajwara (fever caused by combination of all the three doshas increased together) are - feeling of heat and cold alternately, pain in the bones and joints, headache, eyes full of tears, dirty, reddish and bulging out; ringing and pain in the ears, feeling of thorns pricking inside the throat, drowsiness, delusion, delirium, cough, difficulty in breathing (dyspnoea), loss of taste, giddiness, tongue angry red at its edges and rough, weakness of the limbs, excessive expectoration of sputum mixed with blood and bile, rolling of the head on the pillow, thirst, loss of sleep, pain in the heart (or region of the heart), elimination of small quantities of sweat, urine and faeces at long intervals, not much of wasting of the body, continuous moaning (feeble sound in the throat), appearance of dark red spots and patches on the skin, dumbness (unable to speak), ulceration of the orifices of the body, feeling of heaviness of the abdomen, doshas undergoing paka (return to normalcy) very slowly. (1-23)

Prognosis of Sannipata Jwara

doṣe vibaddhe naṣṭe'gnau sarvasampūrṇalakṣaṇaḥ |
sannipātajvaro'sādhyaḥ, kṛcchrasādhyastato'nyathā ||24||
(ca| ci| a| 3) |

Sannipata jwara becomes incurable if the dosas are stagnated (profound and deep seated), if the digestive capacity of the patient is completely diminished and if all the symptoms are simultaneously manifested. Otherwise it is curable with difficulty. (24)

sannipātajvarasyānte karṇamūle sudāruṇaḥ |
śothaḥ sañjāyate tena kaścideva pramucyate ||25||
(ca| ci| a| 3) |
Sometimes there appears a profound swelling at the root of the ear at the end of the course of sannipata jwara and hardly anybody can get rid of it (it almost causes death). (25)

Agantuja Jwara

abhighātābhicārābhyāmabhiśāpābhiṣaṅgataḥ |
āganturjāyate doṣairyathāsvaṃ taṃ vibhāvayet ||26||
Agantu Jwara is caused by - abhighata (assault by weapons), abhichra (sorcery and witchcraft), abhishpa (curse by godly men) and abhyanga (possession by evil spirits, infection by microorganisms). Even in such fevers the symptoms of doshas have to be recognised. (26)

Symptoms of different types of Agantuja Jwara

śyāvāsyatā viṣakṛte tathā'tīsāra eva ca |
bhaktārouciḥ pipāsā ca todaśca saha mūrchayā ||27||
oṣadhigandhaje mūrchāśirorugvamathuḥ kṣavaḥ |
kāmaje cittavibhraṃśastandrā''lasyamabhojanam ||28||
(hṛdaye vedanā cāsya gātraṃ ca pariśuṣyati) |
bhayātpralāpaḥśokācca bhavet kopācca vepathuḥ |
abhicārābhiśāpābhyāṃ mohastṛṣṇā ca jāyate ||29||
bhūtābhiṣaṅgādudvego hāsyarodanakampanam |30|
(su| u| taṃ| a| 39) |
In agantu jwara caused by poison - bluish discolouration of the mouth, diarrhoea, loss of appetite, thirst, pain and fainting are seen.
In fever caused by smell of plants (pollen of flowers, etc.) - fainting, headache, vomiting and sneezing are seen.
In fever caused due to love or passion - mental aberration, stupor, inactivity

or laziness and lack of interest in food, pain in the heart and emaciation of the body are the symptoms.
In fever caused due to fear and grief - the patient will be having delirium.
In fever caused due to anger - he will have tremors.
In fever caused due to sorcery and curse - the patient will be having delusion and thirst.
In fever caused due to possession by evil spirits - the patient will be highly emotional (irritable) and indulges in excess of laughing, weeping and shivering. (27-29)

kāmaśokabhayādvāyuḥ, krodhāt pittaṃ, trayo malāḥ ||30||
bhūtābhiṣaṅgātkupyanti bhūtasāmānyalakṣaṇāḥ |31|
Vata gets increased by lust, grief and fear. Pitta gets increased by anger. All the three doshas get increased from possession by evil spirits (or bacterial infection) and show their specific features. (30)

Visama Jwara – meaning and pathogenesis

doṣo'lpo'hitasambhūto jvarotsṛṣṭasya vā punaḥ ||31||
dhātumanyatamaṃ prāpya karoti viṣamajvaram |32|
(su| u| taṃ| a| 39) |
Doṣhas which have undergone slight / mild increase right from the beginning or the small quantities of doshas which have remained after the fever has gone away get aggravated once again due to consumption of unsuitable foods and activities, get lodged in one or the other dhātus (tissues) and produce Visama jwara (irregular or intermittent fevers). (31).

Types of Visama Jwara and their relationship with tissues

santataṃ rasaraktasthaḥ, so'nyedyuḥ piśitāśritaḥ ||32||
medogatastṛtīye'hni tvasthimajjagataḥ punaḥ |
kuryāccaturthakaṃ ghoramantakaṃ rogasaṅkaram ||33||
(su| u| taṃ| a| 31) |

Of such fevers, santata jwara involves rasa and rakta dhatus, anyedyuska jwara involves mamsa dhatu, tritiyaka jwara involves medas, caturthaka jwara involves asthi and majja dhatus, which is a dreadful disease-complex and is even fatal. (32-33)

Symptoms of Santata and other types of Visama Jwaras

saptāhaṃ vā daśāhaṃ vā dvādaśāhamathāpi vā |
santatyā yo'visargī syāt santataḥ sa nigadyate ||34||
ahorātre satatako dvau kālāvanuvartate |
anyedyuṣkastvahorātra ekakālaṃ pravartate ||35||
tṛtīyakastṛtīye'hni, caturthe'hni caturthakaḥ |36|
(su| u| taṃ| a| 31) |

Santata jwara is so named because the fever continues without remission for seven, ten, twelve or even more days.

Satataka jwara manifests twice in twenty-four hours.
Anyedyuska jwara manifests once in twenty-four hours.
Tritiyaka jwara manifests on alternative days.
Caturthaka jwara manifests on every fourth day. (34-35)

kecidbhūtābhiṣaṅgotthaṃ bruvate viṣamajvaram ||36||
(su| u| taṃ| a| 39) |
Some scholars opine that visama jwaras (intermittent fevers) are caused due to bhutabhisanga (bacterial infection). (36)

Types of manifestation of Tritiyaka Jwara

kaphapittāttrikagrāhī pṛṣṭhādvātakaphātmakaḥ |
vātapittācchirogrāhī trividhaḥ syāttṛtīyakaḥ ||37||
Tritiyaka jwara manifests in three ways viz,

a. if kapha and pitta are increased, fever starts with catching pain in the lower portion of the back,
b. if vāta and kapha are increased, the fever starts with pain in the upper portion of the back and
if vāta and pitta are increased, the fever starts with pain in the head. (37)

Types of manifestation of Caturthaka Jwara

caturthako darśayati prabhāvaṃ dvividhaṃ jvaraḥ |
jaṅghābhyāṃślaiṣmikaḥ pūrvaṃśirasto'nilasambhavaḥ ||38||
(ca| ci| a| 3) |

Chaturthaka also manifests in two ways,

a. if kapha is increased, fever starts with pain in the calf muscles and
b. if vata is increased it starts with pain in the head. (38)

Chaturthaka Viparyaya Jwara

viṣamajvara evānyaścaturthakaviparyayaḥ |
tryahād dvayahaṃ jvarayati hyādāvante ca muñcati ||39||
(ca| ci| a| 3) |
There is yet another kind of visama jwara known as chaturthaka viparyāya jwara. In this condition, fever is not found on the first and fourth day but found on two days in the middle. (39)

Vatabalasaka Jwara

nityaṃ mandajvaro rūkṣaḥśūnakastena sīdati |
stabdhāṅgaḥśleṣmabhūyiṣṭho bhavedvātabalāsakī ||40||
(a| saṃ| ni| a| 2) |
Vatabalasaka jwara is produced by increase of kapha and manifests as mild fever daily with dryness, oedema, debility and feeling of stiffness of the body. (40)

Pralepaka Jwara

pralimpanniva gātrāṇi gharmeṇa gauraveṇa ca |
mandajvaravilepī ca saśītaḥ syātpralepakaḥ ||41||
saṃ| ni| a| 2) |
Pralepaka jwara manifests with mild fever as though the skin is given a thin coating of heat, accompanied with a feeling of heaviness and cold. (41)

Ardhanga Santapayukta Jwara

vidagdhe'nnarase dehe śleṣmapitte vyavasthite |
tenārdhaṃśītalaṃ dehamardhamuṣṇaṃ prajāyate ||42||
kāye duṣṭaṃ yadā pittaṃśleṣmā cānte vyavasthitaḥ |
tenoṣṇatvaṃśarīrasya śītatvaṃ hastapādayoḥ ||43||
kāye śleṣmā yadā duṣṭaḥ pittaṃ cānte vyavasthitam |
śītatvaṃ tena gātrāṇāmuṣṇatvaṃ hastapādayoḥ ||44||
saṃ| ni| a| 2) |
If the annarasa (nutrient portion of the food) gets vidagdha (overcooked due to increase of pitta during the process of digestion), there manifests a fever with half the body being hot and the other half being cold. When pitta gets increased in the trunk followed by kapha in the extremities, then the fever manifests with the trunk being hot and with hands and feet (extremities) cold. When kapha is increased in the trunk and pitta in the extremities, fever manifests with the trunk being cold and the hands and feet (extremities) hot.

Note: These fevers are called Ardhanga Santapa Jwara wherein the rise of heat is evident in half of the body (with coldness prevailing in the other half of the body). They are special types of Visama Jwara.

Shitapurva and Dahapurva Jwara

tvaksthau śleṣmānilau śītamādau janayato jvare |
tayoḥ praśāntayoḥ pittamante dāhaṃ karoti ca ||45||
karotyādau tathā pittaṃ tvaksthaṃ dāhamatīva ca |
tasmin praśānte tvitarau kurutaḥśītamantataḥ ||46||
dvāvetau dāhaśītādijvarau saṃsargajau smṛtau |
dāhapūrvastayoḥ kaṣṭaḥ kṛcchrasādhyatamaśca saḥ ||47||
(su| u| taṃ| a| 39) |
When the aggravated kapha and vāta lodged in the skin, there is a manifestation of cold (rigours) at the beginning of fever. Later when its bouts reduce, the patient experiences burning sensation (heat) due to pitta at the end of the fever.
Similarly, when the aggravated pitta is lodged in the skin, there is a manifestation of burning sensation (heat) at the beginning of the fever. Later when its bouts reduce, the patient experiences cold (rigours) due to

vata and kapha at the end of the fever.

These two types of fevers dāhapūrva (preceded by heat) and śītapūrva (preceded by cold) are samsargaja i.e. produced by the combination of two dosas. Among these fevers dāhapūrva is difficult to treat and is almost incurable. (42-47)

Dhatugata Jwara – fevers localised in the tissues

Rasa dhatu gata jwara – fever residing in rasa tissue
gurutā hṛdayotkleśaḥ sadanaṃ chardyarocakau |
rasasthe tu jvare liṅgaṃ dainyaṃ cāsyopajāyate ||48||
The symptoms seen when jwara (fever) invades / resides in rasa dhatu (blood plasma) is - feeling of heaviness of the body, nausea, debility, vomiting, loss of appetite and timidity (feeling of helplessness). (48)

Rakta dhatu gata jwara – fever residing in blood tissue

raktaniṣṭhīvanaṃ dāho mohaśchardanavibhramau |
pralāpaḥ piḍakā tṛṣṇā raktaprāpte jvare nṛṇām ||49||
The symptoms evident when fever invades / resides in rakta dhatu (blood) is - haemoptysis, burning sensation, delusion, vomiting, dizziness, delirium, appearances of rashes (or small boils) on the skin and thirst. (49)

Mamsa dhatu gata jwara – fever residing in muscle tissue

piṇḍikodveṣṭanaṃ tṛṣṇā sṛṣṭamūtrapurīṣatā |
ūṣmā'ntardāhavikṣepau glāniḥ syānmāṃsage jvare ||50||
The symptoms found when fever invades / resides in mamsa dhatu (muscle tissue) is - pain in the calves, thirst, increased elimination of urine and faeces, high temperature, burning sensation inside, involuntary movements of the hands and feet and exhaustion manifest. (50)

Medo dhatu gata jwara – fever residing in fat tissue / adipose tissue

bhṛśaṃ svedastṛṣā mūrchā pralāpaśchardireva ca |
daurgandhyārocakau glānirmedaḥsthe cāsahiṣṇutā ||51||
The symptoms found when fever invades / resides in medo dhatu (fat /

adipose tissue) is - profuse sweating, thirst, fainting, delirium, vomiting, bad smell from the body, loss of taste (anorexia), exhaustion and intolerance (irritability). (51)

Asthi dhatu gata jwara – fever residing in bone tissue

bhedo'sthnāṃ kūjanaṃśvāso virekaśchardireva ca |
vikṣepaṇaṃ ca gātrāṇāmetadasthigate jvare ||52||
The symptoms found when fever invades / resides in asthi dhatu (bone tissue) is - splitting pain in the bones, low and indistinct sound from the throat (moaning), dyspnoea (increased respiration), diarrhoea, vomiting and throwing / involuntary movements of hands and feet. (52)

Majja dhatu gata jwara – fever residing in bone marrow tissue

tamaḥpraveśanaṃ hikkā kāsaḥśaityaṃ vamistathā |
antarndāho mahāśvāso marmacchedaśca majjage ||53||
The symptoms found when fever invades / resides in majja dhatu (bone marrow tissue) is - appearance of darkness before the eyes (feeling as if immersed in a zone of darkness), hiccough, cough, cold feeling, vomiting, burning sensation within the body, severe dyspnoea (greatly increased respiration) and cutting type of pain in the heart and other vital spots of the body. (53)

Shukra dhatu gata jwara – fever residing in semen / reproductive tissue

maraṇaṃ prāpnuyāttatra śukrasthānagate jvare |
śephasaḥ stabdhatā mokṣaḥśukrasya tu viśeṣataḥ ||54||
(su| u| taṃ| a| 39) |
The symptoms found when fever invades / resides in shukra dhatu (semen tissue / reproductive tissue) is - constant erection of the penis and profuse discharge of semen followed by death. (54)

Prognosis of fevers residing in the tissues

(rasaraktāśritaḥ sādhyo māṃsamedogataśca yaḥ |
asthimajjagataḥ kṛcchro śukrasthastu na sidhyati) ||1||

(ca| ci| a| 3) |

(Fever invading / residing in rasa and rakta (blood plasma and blood) tissues can be cured easily.

Similarly, the fevers residing in mamsa and medo dhatus (muscle and adipose / fat) tissues are also easily curable.

The fevers residing in asthi and majja (bones and bone marrow) tissues are difficult to cure.

The fever residing in shukra (semen, reproductive tissue) tissue does not respond to the treatment i.e. it is incurable). (54-1)

Prakrta (normal) and Vaikrta (abnormal) fevers explained on the basis of the seasonal relationship with the fevers

varṣāśaradvasanteṣu vātādyaiḥ prākṛtaḥ kramāt |
vaikṛto'nyaḥ sa duḥsādhyaḥ prākṛtaścānilodbhavaḥ ||55||
(vā| ni| a| 2) |

Fevers which manifest in varsa rtu (rainy season), Sarad rtu (autumn) and vasanta rtu (spring season) caused by vata, pitta and kapha respectively are considered as prakrta (normal / corresponding to the season). Apart from these fevers, the other fevers shall be considered as vaikrta (abnormal / not corresponding to the season). Prakrta fevers are easily curable. But vatika fever (fever caused by predominance of vata), though is prakrta (occurring in its normal season i.e., varsa rtu) cannot be easily treated. The fevers produced by vata are difficult to treat. Likewise, the Vaikrta fevers are also difficult to treat. (55)

Doshas and seasonal fevers

varṣāsu māruto duṣṭaḥ pittaśleṣmānvito jvaram |
kuryāt pittaṃ ca śaradi tasya cānubalaḥ kaphaḥ ||56||
tatprakṛtyā visargācca tatra nānaśanādbhayam |
kapho vasante tamapi vātapittaṃ bhavedanu ||57||
(vā| ni| a| 2) |

In Varsa Ritu (rainy season) – the vitiated vata produces fever being associated with pitta and kapha.

In Sarad Ritu (autumn season) - pitta produces fever being associated with kapha.

Fasting or therapeutic starvation doesn't do harm in both these conditions because of the nature of associated doshas and nature of the season (visarga – cold predominant season).

***Notes** - Logic and conditions behind administering fasting in rainy and autumn seasons* - The reason is – by nature pitta and kapha have fluid nature and can tolerate fasting. So, fasting can be readily recommended in Prakrata Vata fever occurring in the rainy season, especially when it is associated with pitta and kapha. The same rule is applicable in pitta fever associated with kapha occurring in Sharad Ritu also. Also – both these seasons (rainy and autumn) fall in visarga kala (cold predominant seasons) and hence fasting is recommended (the strength of the patients in these seasons is comparably good in comparison to heat predominant seasons).
In Vasanta Ritu (spring season) – the fever produced by vitiated kapha will probably have association and support of vata and pitta. (56-57)

Upashaya (subsiding factors) and Anupashaya (aggravating factors) for fevers in relation to the causative dosas
kāle yathāsvaṃ sarveṣāṃ pravṛttirvṛddhireva vā |58|
(vā| ni| a| 2) |
nidānoktānupaśayo viparītopaśāyitā ||58||
(vā| ni| a| 2) |
It is only at that specified time / season during which the causative dosa is aggravated (powerful), we usually get to see the onset or exacerbation of the fevers.
Also, the factors (etiological factors) responsible for increasing a particular dosha also bring about an increase (onset or exacerbation) of the fever (caused by that particular dosha). On the other hand, the opposites (anything which is opposite to those mentioned amongst the etiological factors for that particular dosha) will be helpful and would mitigate the fever also.

Note: This means to tell that all fevers (usually) have their onset or exacerbation in accordance to their respective dosha aggravating time or season.

Upasaya and Anupasaya mentioned here can also be used as tools for identifying the dosha involved in the causation of a given fever. (58)

Antarvega and Bahirvega Jwaras

antardāho'dhikastṛṣṇā pralāpaḥśvasanaṃ bhramaḥ |
sandhyasthiśūlamasvedo doṣavarcovinigrahaḥ ||59||
antarvegasya liṅgāni jvarasyaitāni lakṣayet |
santāpo hyadhiko bāhyastṛṣṇādīnāṃ ca mārdavam ||60||
bahirvegasya liṅgāni sukhasādhyatvameva ca |61|
(ca| ci| a| 3) |

Antarvega Jwara (fevers predominantly manifesting from within or residing inside the body) – is diagnosed by the presence of symptoms including - feeling of burning sensation inside (the body), excessive thirst, delirium, dyspnoea (increased / difficult respiration), giddiness, pain in the joints and bones, absence of perspiration and non-elimination of doshas and faeces.
Bahirvega Jwara (fevers predominantly manifesting from without or residing / manifesting outside, on the surface of the body) – is diagnosed by the presence of very high temperature externally, but thirst and the other symptoms (mentioned in antarvega jwara) being mild. This condition is said to be easily curable. (59-60)

Ama Jwara Symptoms

lālāpraseko hṛllāsahṛdayāśuddhyarocakāḥ ||61||
tandrālasyāvipākāsyavairasyaṃ gurugātratā |
kṣunnāśo bahumūtratvaṃ stabdhatā balavān jvaraḥ ||62||
āmajvarasya liṅgāni na dadyāttatra bheṣajam |
bheṣajaṃ hyāmadoṣasya bhūyo jvalayati jvaram ||63||
(śodhanaṃśamanīyaṃ ca karoti viṣamajvaram) |

The symptoms of ama jwara (unripe, early / first or initial stage of fever) are - profuse salivation, nausea, heaviness and oppression in the region of the heart (a strange discomfort in the cardiac region), loss of taste / appetite, drowsiness, laziness / lack of enthusiasm, indigestion, bad taste in the mouth (manifestation of abnormal tastes / opposite tastes in the mouth), feeling of heaviness of the body, loss of hunger, profuse urination, stiffness and high temperature.
During this stage of fever, medicines (treatment) should not be given. If

given, the medicines will cause an increase (in the severity) of fever. Also if sodhana (purificatory) and samana (palliative) therapies are administered in ama jwara, they will lead to Visama Jwara (irregular fevers). (61-63)

Pacyamana Jwara Symptoms

jvaravego'dhikastṛṣṇā pralāpaḥśvasanaṃ bhramaḥ |
malapravṛttirutkleśaḥ pacyamānasya lakṣaṇam ||64||
The symptoms of Pacyamana Jwara (intermediate / middle stage or stage of ripening of the fever) are – severity in fever or bouts of fever (increase of temperature), severe thirst, delirium, dyspnoea (increased / difficult respiration), giddiness, frequent elimination of faeces and nausea. (64)

Nirama Jwara Symptoms

kṣut kṣāmatā laghutvaṃ ca gātrāṇāṃ jvaramārdavam |
doṣapravṛttiraṣṭāho nirāmajvaralakṣaṇam ||65||
(ca| ci| a| 3) |
The symptoms of Nirama Jwara (terminal / late / last stage of the fever / ripe stage of fever / fever having absence of ama) are - appearance of hunger, slight emaciation and feeling of lightness of the body, decrease in intensity / temperature of the fever, elimination of dosas (and also faeces, urine etc.) and fever entering into the eighth day are the symptoms of Nirama jwara (fully ripe or terminal stage of fever). (65)

Signs of curability of fevers

balavatsvalpadoṣeṣu jvaraḥ sādhyo'nupadravaḥ |66|
(ca| ci| a| 3) |
Fever affecting strong persons (those having strong physique), produced by less dosas (dosas which are not severely aggravated) and having no complications are easily curable.

Signs of incurability of fevers

hetubhirbahubhirjāto balibhirbahulakṣaṇaḥ ||66||
jvaraḥ prāṇāntakṛdyaśca śīghramindriyanāśanaḥ |

jvaraḥ kṣīṇasya śūnasya gambhīro dairgharātrikaḥ ||67||
asādhyo balavān yaśca keśasīmantakṛjjvaraḥ |
(ca| ci| a| 3) |
Fevers caused by many and powerful causes, manifesting with many and powerful symptoms, those which destroy the sense faculties (power of perception of sense organs) in quick time will be life threatening (might lead to death) and incurable. Similarly, strong (severe) fevers affecting persons who are very weak and afflicting those having oedema all over the body, which are deep seated (in the tissues), continuing for long periods (has become chronic) and those causing furrows in between the hairs of the head all of a sudden -are also difficult to treat or incurable. (66-67)

Gambhira Jwara

gambhīrastu jvaro jñeyo hyantardāhena tṛṣṇayā ||68||
ānaddhatvena cātyarthaṃśvāsakāsodgamena ca |
(su| u| taṃ| a| 39) |
The fever which manifests with burning sensation inside the body, thirst, severe distension of the abdomen, dyspnoea (increased respiration) and cough is called as Gambhira Jwara. (68)

ārambhādviṣamo yastu yaśca vā dairgharātrikaḥ ||69||
kṣīṇasya cātirūkṣasya gambhīro yasya hanti tam |
visañjñastāmyate yastu śete nipatito'pi vā ||70||
śītārdito'ntaruṣṇaśca jvareṇa mriyate naraḥ |
yo hṛṣṭaromā raktākṣo hṛdi saṅghātaśūlavān ||71||
vaktreṇa caivocchvasiti taṃ jvaro hanti mānavam |
hikkāśvāsatṛṣāyuktaṃ mūḍhaṃ vibhrāntalocanam ||72||
santatocchvāsinaṃ kṣīṇaṃ naraṃ kṣapayati jvaraḥ |
hataprabhendriyaṃ kṣīṇamarocakanipīḍitam ||73||
gambhīratīkṣṇavegārtaṃ jvaritaṃ parivarjayet |
(su| u| taṃ| a| 39) |
Fever which is irregular even from its commencement, is chronic (continuing for long periods) is incurable. Likewise, gambhira (and antardaha jwara) fever affecting persons who are weak or having dryness of the body is also incurable.
The patient will face death if the fever presents with loss of consciousness,

darkness before the eyes, fainting – here the patient keeps laying down as he is not capable of getting up from that position, feeling cold externally and very hot internally (inside the body).

The fever is considered incurable and also tends to kill the person when it presents with frequent horripilation, redness of the eyes and pain as if injured by stone and similar other things in the region of the heart, patients breathing only through their mouth.
Fever associated with hiccough, increased respiration, thirst, delusion, unsteady gaze, interrupted respirations (more expiration and fewer inspirations), severe emaciation will destroy the person (is incurable).
The patients of fever having loss of complexion and sensory activities, extreme debility, loss of appetite, deep seated fever, and having very high temperatures are to be refused treatment (because such a fever is incurable). (39-73)

Premonitory symptoms of 'fever which is subsiding'

dāhaḥ svedo bhramastṛṣṇā kampaviḍbhidasañjñatā |
kūjanaṃ cāsyavaigandhyamākṛtirjvaramokṣaṇe ||74||
The symptoms of fever which is subsiding are - burning sensation, perspiration, giddiness, thirst, tremors, elimination of faeces (diarrhoea), loss of consciousness, making indistinct sounds (moaning) and bad smell from the mouth. (74)

Symptoms of 'relief from fever'

svedo laghutvaṃśirasaḥ kaṇḍūḥ pāko mukhasya ca |
kṣavathuścānnalipsā ca jvaramuktasya lakṣaṇam ||75||
(su| u| taṃ| a| 39) |
The symptoms of the person who has been relieved from fever are - perspiration, feeling of lightness of the body, itching of the head, appearance of ulcers in the mouth, sneezing and desire for food. (75)

iti śrīmādhavakaraviracite mādhavanidāne jvaranidānaṃ samāptam ||2||
Thus ends the chapter on Jwaras

CHAPTER THREE

ATHĀTĪSĀRANIDĀNAM

Etiological Factors of Atisara

gurvatisnigdharūkṣoṣṇadravasthūlātiśītalaiḥ |
viruddhādhyaśanājīrṇairviṣamaiścāpi bhojanaiḥ ||1||
snehādyairatiyuktaiśca mithyāyuktairviṣairbhayaiḥ |
śokādduṣṭāmbumadyātipānaiḥ sātmyartuparyayaiḥ ||2||
jalābhiramaṇairvegavighātaiḥ krimidoṣataḥ |
nṛṇāṃ bhavatyatīsāro lakṣṇaṃ tasya vakṣyate ||3||
(su| u| taṃ| a| 40) |

Over-indulgence in foods which are very heavy (hard to digest), very unctuous (fatty), very dry, very hot, very watery, very hard or very cold; foods which are mutually incompatible (antagonistic), taking foods in large quantities very frequently; foods which are not cooked or processed properly and taken at unusual times; excess or improper usage of therapies like oleation etc., consumption of poisons, fear, grief, drinking of polluted / contaminated water, consumption of excess of alcoholic drinks, changes in accustomed habits and abnormal changes in seasonal features (abnormal seasonal behaviours), over-indulgence in water sports, suppression of natural urges of the body and infestation by worms (intestinal parasites) – are the causative factors responsible for production of the disease atīsāra (diarrhoea). The symptoms of atisara are described herein. (1-3)

Samprapti – pathogenesis of Atisara

saṃśamyāpāndhāturagniṃ pravṛddhaḥ śakṛnmiśro vāyunā'dhaḥ praṇunnaḥ |
saratyatīvātisāraṃ tamāhurvyādhiṃ ghoraṃ ṣaḍvidhaṃ taṃ vadanti |
ekaikaśaḥ sarvaśaścāpi doṣaiḥ śokenānyaḥ ṣaṣṭha āmena coktaḥ ||4||
(su| u| taṃ| a| 40) |

Watery elements of the body undergo increase (following consumption of etiological factors). They then diminish / inactivate the gastric fire (digestive activities), get mixed with faeces, move downwards (out of the body through the rectum) by the action of vāta, in large quantities and very frequently producing the dreadful disease called Atīsāra. It is of six kinds, one from each dosha, one from the combination of the three doṣas together, fifth from grief and the sixth from āma (undigested food).(4)

Cycle of pathogenesis of Atisara – diarrhoea

Consumption of etiological factors of diarrhoea

↓

Abnormal increase in watery elements in the body

↓

Cause diminution / depletion of gastric fire (and weaken the digestion)

Gets mixed with faeces (increased watery elements get mixed with faeces)

Gets stimulated and propelled downwards by the action of vata (vata pushes water mixed faeces in the downward direction, towards the colon)

Excessive and frequent discharge of watery faeces (loose stools)

This disease is called as atisara – diarrhoea – it manifests in 6 different types

Notes – In Atisara types we can find that apart from those types formed by predominant aggravation of doshas there are 2 special forms. One is caused by ama. Ama is a by-product of sluggish digestion (caused by weak digestive fire – weak capacity of the stomach and intestine to digest the food). If not dealt with properly, this ama can cause different kinds of diseases including atisara. This also reflects that weak digestive power and subsequent formation of ama is one of the main causes for manifestation of atisara. This is called amatisara. The other type i.e., shokatisara is caused by excessive and constant grief. This reflects the psychological component of diarrhoea. We also learn that a weak or imbalanced mind or emotional turmoil can cause or trigger the diseases or symptoms of the gastrointestinal system. Nervous diarrhoea is an example of this condition.

Purvarupa – premonitory symptoms of atisara

hṛnnābhipāyūdarakukṣitodagātrāvasādānilasannirodhāḥ |
viṭsaṅga ādhmānamathāvipākā bhaviṣyatastasya puraḥsarāṇi ||5||
(su| u| taṃ| a| 40) |
The premonitory symptoms of diarrhoea include - pricking type of pain in the region of the heart, umbilicus, rectum, lower abdomen and flanks; weakness of the body, non-elimination of flatus, constipation, distension of the abdomen and indigestion of food. (5)

Symptoms of Vataja Atisara

aruṇaṃ phenilaṃ rūkṣamalpamalpaṃ muhurmuhuḥ |
śakṛdāmaṃ sarukśabdaṃ mārutenātisāryate ||6||
Elimination of faeces which is slightly brown in colour, frothy, viscid, less in quantity but expelled very frequently and is accompanied with pain and noise are the symptoms of vātaja atīsāra (diarrhoea due to increase of vāta dosa).(6)

Symptoms of Pittaja Atisara

pittāt pītaṃ nīlamālohitaṃ vā tṛṣṇāmūrchādāhapākopapannam |7|
(su| u| taṃ| a| 40) |
Faeces which are deep yellow, blue or red in colour; the patient having thirst, fainting, burning sensation and ulcerations (of the alimentary tract) are the symptoms of pittaja atīsāra (diarrhoea due to increase of pitta). (7)

Symptoms of Kaphaja Atisara

śuklaṃ sāndraṃ śleṣmaṇā śleṣmayuktaṃ visraṃ śītaṃ hṛṣṭaromā manuṣyaḥ ||7||
(su| u| taṃ| a| 40) |
Faeces which is white, semi-solid, mixed with mucus and fat, cold and the patient having frequent horripilations (hairs standing on ends) are seen in kaphaja atīsāra (diarrhoea due to increase of kapha).(7)

Symptoms of Tridosaja Atisara

varāhasnehamāṃsāmbusadṛśaṃ sarvarūpiṇam |
kṛcchrasādhyamatīsāraṃ vidyāddoṣatrayodbhavam ||8||

In tridoshaja atisāra (diarrhoea caused due to increase of all the three dosas together) there will be elimination of faeces resembling the fat of wild boar or water in which mutton is washed. The patient will also have the symptoms of all the three doṣas. This condition is difficult to cure. (8)

Symptoms of Shokaja Atisara

taistairbhāvaiḥ śocato'lpāśanasya bāṣpoṣmā vai vahnimāviśya jantoḥ |
koṣṭhaṃ gatvā kṣobhayettasya raktaṃ taccādhastāt kākaṇantīprakāśam ||9||
nirgacchedvai viḍvimiśraṃ hyaviḍvā nirgandhaṃ vā gandhavadvā'tisāraḥ |
śokotpanno duścikitsyo'timātraṃ rogo vaidyaiḥ kaṣṭa eṣa pradiṣṭaḥ ||10||
(su| u| taṃ| a| 40) |

In persons who are very much afflicted with grief (due to loss of wealth, kith and kin, etc.,), who consume little food or no food at all, the heat of the tears (and also of the fluids of the nose, mouth, throat) increase in quantity. This enters into the alimentary tract and inactivates the digestive fire (digestive activity) and causes vitiation of the rakta dhātu (blood). This vitiated blood resembling the seed of kākaṇanti (guñjā – Abrus precatorius) gets expelled out of the body either mixed with faeces or alone (not mixed with faeces), with or without bad smell. This type of atisara – diarrhoea is known as śokātisāra. It is considered by physicians as difficult to cure.(9-10)

Symptoms of Amaja Atisara

annājīrṇāt pradrutāḥ kṣobhayantaḥ koṣṭhaṃ doṣā dhātusaṅghānmalāṃśca |
nānāvarṇaṃ naikaśaḥ sārayanti śūlopetaṃ ṣaṣṭhamenaṃ vadanti ||11||
(su| u| taṃ| a| 40) |

In persons in whom the food is not properly digested, the dosas get increased by combining with undigested food. They travel in wrong channels and cause vitiation of koshta (abdominal cavity giving occupancy to many visceral organs, mainly stomach and colon), the dhātus (tissues) and malas (waste products) and cause elimination of faeces of many colours, frequently accompanied with pain in the abdomen. This is the sixth kind of atisara known as āmātisāra (diarrhoea due to indigestion).(11)

Ama & Pakva Atisara

saṃsṛṣṭamebhirdoṣaistu nyastamapsvavasīdati |
purīṣaṃ bhṛśadurgandhi picchilaṃ cāmasañjñitam ||12||
etānyeva tu liṅgāni viparītāni yasya vai |
lāghavaṃ ca viśeṣeṇa tasya pakvaṃ vinirdiśet ||13||
(su| u| taṃ| a| 40) |

If the faeces associated with the vitiated doshas (and symptoms of aggravated dosas) has foul smell and is very sticky and if it sinks in the water, it (faeces) is said to be ama-mala i.e., faeces associated with ama (uncooked, inadequately processed hence abnormal). On the other hand, if the faeces have opposite features of those mentioned above i.e. if it is not associated with foul smell and stickiness and floats on the water, it is said to be pakva mala (well formed, well processed and hence normal). (12-13)

Signs of incurability of atisara

pakvajāmbavasaṅkāśaṃ yakṛtkhaṇḍanibhaṃ tanu |
ghṛtatailavasāmajjaveśavārapayodadhi ||14||
māṃsadhāvanatoyābhaṃ kṛṣṇaṃ nīlāruṇaprabham |
mecakaṃ snigdhakarbūraṃ candrakopagataṃ ghanam ||15||
kuṇapaṃ mastuluṅgābhaṃ sugandhi kuthitaṃ bahu |
tṛṣṇādāhatamaḥśvāsahikkāpārśvāsthiśūlinam ||16||
sammūrchāratisammohayuktaṃ pakvavalīgudam |
pralāpayuktaṃ ca bhiṣagvarjayedatisāriṇam ||17||
asaṃvṛtagudaṃ kṣīṇaṃ dūrādhmātamupadrutam |
gude pakve gatoṣmāṇamatisārakiṇaṃ tyajet ||18||
(su| u| taṃ| a| 40) |
śvāsaśūlapipāsārtaṃ kṣīṇaṃ jvaranipīḍitam |
viśeṣeṇa naraṃ vṛddhamatīsāro vināśayet ||19||
(su| sū| a| 33) |
(śothaṃ śūlaṃ jvaraṃ tṛṣṇāṃ kāsaṃ śvāsamarocakam |
chardiṃ mūrchāṃ ca hikkāṃ ca dṛṣṭāvātīsāriṇaṃ tyajet) |

Diarrhoea is said to be incurable if the faeces is having the colour of ripened fruit of jambū (Eugenia jambolina), pieces of liver; which is very thin (like water), that which resembles ghee, oil, muscle-fat, marrow, mutton-broth, milk, curds, mutton-wash; which is black, blue, pink, brown or shining black in colour and appearance (like that of collyrium – black and dry); is unctuous (greasy, oily) and having many colors, containing shining particles (resembling the shining particles on the peacock feather), is heavy / scabelous, smells like that of a dead body, brain, putrefied matter or has even a sweet smell and large in quantity. When the diarrhoea is incurable the patient also has thirst, burning sensation, darkness before the eyes, dyspnoea (difficulty in breathing), hiccough, pain in the flanks and bones, fainting, restlessness, delusion, suppuration in the layers of the anus and rectum (ulcers in the rectum) and delirium. In the presence of these symptoms the physician should reject (not treat) the patient of diarrhoea (because the disease would be incurable). Treatment should be refused to the patients of diarrhoea whose anal sphincters are unable to close, who are emaciated, who have highly distended abdomen, suppuration (ulceration) of the rectum and have very low body temperature. Diarrhoea is going to kill patients who have increased / difficult respiration (dyspnoea), pain in the abdomen, thirst, emaciation, fever and who are of old age. Likewise, those who have oedema, pain in the abdomen, fever, thirst, cough, dyspnoea (breathing difficulty), loss of taste (appetite), vomiting, fainting and hiccoughs should also be rejected.(14-19)

Raktatisara

pittakṛnti yadā'tyarthaṃ dravyāṇyaśnāti paittike |
tadopajāyate'bhīkṣṇaṃ raktātīsāra ulbaṇaḥ ||20||

Patients suffering or have suffered from pittātisāra i.e., diarrhoea caused by predominant aggravation of pitta (or even others) who indulge in foods and activities causing increase of pitta, will develop quickly a dreaded disease-raktātisāra (diarrhoea in which heavy bleeding occurs). (20)

Pravahika

vāyuḥ pravṛddho nicitaṃ balāsaṃ nudatyadhastādahitāśanasya |
pravāhato'lpaṃ bahuśo malāktaṃ pravāhikāṃ tāṃ pravadanti tajjñāḥ ||21||
(su| u| taṃ| a| 40) |
pravāhikā vātakṛtā saśūlā pittāt sadāhā sakaphā kaphācca |
saśoṇitā śoṇitasambhavā ca tāḥ sneharūkṣaprabhavā matāstu |
tāsāmatīsāravadādiśecca liṅgaṃ kramaṃ cāmavipakvatāṃ ca ||22||
(सु. उ. तं. अ. ४०) |

In persons who indulge in unsuitable foods, vāta gets increased, and after getting associated with kapha produces the disease called by experts as pravāhikā. In this, the patient will eliminate little quantities of faeces mixed with mucus, frequently, only after straining.

Vātaja pravāhikā is characterized by elimination of faeces accompanied with pain.
Pittaja pravāhikā is characterized by elimination of faeces accompanied with burning sensation.
Kaphaja pravāhikā is characterized by elimination of faeces mixed with kapha (mucus).
Raktaja pravāhikā is characterized by elimination of faeces with admixture of blood with more moisture or little of it as the case may be.

The other symptoms of this disease and determination of āma (inadequately processed / unripe / unformed) and pakva (adequately processed / ripe / formed) state of faeces are the same as those of diarrhoea. (21-22)

Symptoms indicating that 'diarrhoea has been cured'
yasyoccāraṃ vinā mūtraṃ samyagvāyuśca gacchati |
dīptāgnerlaghukoṣṭhasya sthitastasyodarāmayaḥ ||23||
(su| u| taṃ| a| 40) |
iti śrīmādhavakaraviracite mādhavanidāne'tīsāranidānaṃ samāptam ||3||
Atīsāra (diarrhoea) is said to have been cured when the patient is able to eliminate flatus and urine independent of expulsion of faeces (i.e. faeces is not eliminated while passing urine or expelling fart), when his digestion capacity increases (he has developed hunger) and lightness of the abdomen. (23)

Symptoms of Jwaratisara
(jvarātīsārayoruktaṃ nidānaṃ yat pṛthak pṛthak |
tatsyājjvarātisārasya tena nātroditaṃ punaḥ) ||1||
Jwaratisara is caused by a combination of independent etiological factors of jwara (fever) and atisara (diarrhoea). Similarly, the premonitory symptoms, symptoms, aggravating and relieving factors and pathogenesis explained individually in relation to fever and diarrhoea are mixed up (combined) in the clinical picture of jwaratisara. This is the reason that this condition has not been detailed in this context.

iti śrīmādhavakaraviracite mādhavanidāne'tīsāranidānaṃ samāptam ||3||

Thus ends the chapter on Atīsāra.

CHAPTER FOUR

GRAHAṆĪROGANIDĀNAM

Samprapti – Pathogenesis of Grahani Roga

atīsāre nivṛtte'pi mandāgnerahitāśinaḥ |
bhūyaḥ sandūṣito vahnirgrahaṇīmabhidūṣayet ||1||
(su| u| taṃ| a| 40) |
Grahani disease occurs in persons who have been recently relieved of diarrhoea but still have poor digestion (even others having poor digestion right from the beginning). When such persons indulge in unsuitable foods and activities, the doshas undergo increase. These doshas in turn affect the agni. This agni (digestive fire / activity) which has been contaminated by the doshas undergoes aggravation and affects the grahani (duodenum). (1)

ekaikaśaḥ sarvaśaśca doṣairatyarthamūrchitaiḥ |
sā duṣṭā bahuśo bhuktamāmameva vimuñcati ||2||
pakvaṃ vā sarujaṃ pūti muhurbaddhaṃ muhurdravam |
grahaṇīrogamāhustamāyurvedavido janāḥ ||3||
(su| u| taṃ| a| 40) |
Thus, the grahani (duodenum) gets excessively affected by the doshas either individually or in combination (individual dosha or combination of doshas). Such affected duodenum causes expulsion of most of the consumed food in an undigested or digested form. In this condition the faeces is foul smelling, sometimes hard (solid, constipated) and sometimes fluid (diarrhoea) in nature and is accompanied with pain in the abdomen. Scholars of Ayurveda call this disease as Grahani Roga.(2-3)

Grahani – chain of pathogenesis

Person who has just (recently) been relieved from atisara (diarrhoea) but still has weak digestion (poor digestive fire – capacity)

↓

Takes unsuitable foods and activities

↓

Abnormal increase in dosas

↓

Aggravated dosas afflict the agni (digestive fire / capacity)

↓

Agni disturbed due to contamination / affliction by dosas will further contaminate (afflict) the grahani (duodenum)

↓

Further the duodenum gets excessively affected by individual or combination of aggravated dosas

↓

The affected duodenum expels the food either in an undigested form or digested form

↓

The faeces smell foul and sometimes there is constipation and sometimes diarrhoea along with pain in the abdomen

↓

This disease is called as Grahani

Note – These chains of events happen in a similar way even in those who haven't recovered from diarrhoea. These people have weak digestion from the beginning and in them the chronology of events of pathogenesis takes place in the same way explained here.

Purvarupa – premonitory symptoms of Grahani

pūrvarūpaṃ tu tasyedaṃ tṛṣṇā''lasyaṃ balakṣayaḥ |
vidāho'nnasya pākaśca cirāt kāyasya gauravam ||4||
(ca| ci| a| 15) |
Premonitory symptoms of Grahani disease are - thirst, lack of enthusiasm, debility, improper digestion of food due to the action of weak digestive fire, delayed digestion of food and feeling of heaviness of the body.(4)

Etiological factors, pathogenesis and symptoms of Vataja Grahani

kaṭutiktakaṣāyātirūkṣasanduṣṭabhojanaḥ |
pramitānaśanātyadhvaveganigrahamaithunaiḥ ||5||

mārutaḥ kupito vahniṃ sañchādya kurute gadān |
tasyānnaṃ pacyate duḥkhaṃ śuktapākaṃ kharāṅgatā ||6||
kaṇṭhāsyaśoṣo'kṣuttṛṣṇā timiraṃ karṇayoḥ svanaḥ |
pārśvoruvaṅkṣaṇagrīvārugabhīkṣṇaṃ visūcikā ||7||
hṛtpīḍākārśyadaurbalyaṃ vairasyaṃ parikartikā |
gṛddhiḥ sarvarasānāṃ ca manasaḥ sadanaṃ tathā ||8||
jīrṇe jīryati cādhmānaṃ bhukte svāsthyamupaiti ca |
sa vātagulmahṛdrogaplīhāśaṅkī ca mānavaḥ ||9||
cirādduḥkhaṃ dravaṃ śuṣkaṃ tanvāmaṃ śabdaphenavat |
punaḥ punaḥ sṛjedvarcaḥ kāsaśvāsārdito'nilāt ||10||
(ca| ci| a| 15) |
Vata gets abnormally increased due to indulgence in foods which are pungent, bitter, astringent, dry, contaminated, and scanty or no food at all; too much of walk, suppression of natural urges of the body, excess sexual activities.
The vata thus increased destroys the agni – digestive fire (digestive capacity) and produces Vātaja Grahaṇi Roga. Vataja Grahani Roga.

In this type of Grahani, the food gets digested with difficulty and undergoes fermentation. There also occurs hardness of the body parts, dryness of the throat and mouth, increased hunger and thirst, darkness before the eyes, noise in the ears, constant pain in the flanks, thighs, groins and neck; vomiting and diarrhoea occur together, pain in the region of the heart, emaciation, weakness, bad taste in the mouth, cutting pain in the rectum / anal region, desire for foods of all the tastes, mental depression, distension of the abdomen after the digestion of food and during the period of digestion and feeling of comfort on taking food.

The patient gets suspicious of getting (prone to or doubtful of possibly getting) vāta gulma (abdominal tumour), hrd roga (disease of the heart), plīhā (splenic disorder), in future. (Alternatively, we can tell that the symptoms very much resemble those of vāta gulma - abdominal tumour, hrd roga - disease of the heart, plīhā - splenic disorder, causing difficulty in diagnosis).

Such a patient having cough and breathing trouble (dyspnoea, difficulty in respiration) repeatedly voids faeces after a long time, which is watery or dry, thin, frothy, improperly processed, accompanied with pain and noise. (5-10)

Etiological factors, pathogenesis and symptoms of Pittaja Grahani

kaṭvajīrṇavidāhyamlakṣārādyaiḥ pittamulbaṇam |
āplāvayaddhantyanalaṃ jalaṃ taptamivānalam ||11||
so'jīrṇaṃ nīlapītābhaṃ pītābhaḥ sāryate dravam |
pūtyamlodgārahṛtkaṇṭhadāhārucitṛḍarditaḥ ||12||
(ca| ci| a| 15) |

Pitta undergoes abnormal increase due to indulgence in foods which are pungent and uncooked, causing heartburn, sour and alkaline in nature. This increased pitta would activate the gastric fire (digestive power or activity) just like the hot water poured over burning fire and produces pittaja grahaṇi roga.

In this condition the patient will be eliminating faeces which are inadequately processed, bluish yellow or deep yellow in colour, watery and fetid. The person will have bad, sour belching; burning sensation in the chest and throat, loss of taste (tastelessness) or appetite and thirst. (11-12)

Etiological factors, pathogenesis and symptoms of Kaphaja Grahani

gurvatisnigdhaśītādibhojanadatibhojanat |
bhuktamātrasya ca svapnāddhantyagniṃ kupitaḥ kaphaḥ ||13||
tasyānnaṃ pacyate duḥkhaṃ hṛllāsacchardyarocakāḥ |
āsyopadehamādhuryaṃ kāsaṣṭhīvanapīnasāḥ ||14||
hṛdayaṃ manyate styānamudaraṃ stimitaṃ guruḥ |
duṣṭo madhura udgāraḥ sadanaṃ strīṣvaharṣaṇam ||15||
bhinnāmaśleṣmasaṃsṛṣṭaguruvarcaḥpravartanam |
akṛśasyāpi daurbalyamālasyaṃ ca kaphātmake ||16||
(ca| ci| a| 15) |

Kapha gets abnormally increased due to indulgence in foods which are heavy (hard to digest), too unctuous (very fatty), cold and taken excessively (very frequently); and sleeping immediately after midday meal. This aggravated kapha destroys (inactivates) the digestive fire and causes kaphaja grahani disease.

In these patients the food gets digested with difficulty. He also would have nausea, vomiting, loss of taste (appetite), coating in the mouth (on the tongue), sweet taste in the mouth, cough, expectoration, running in the nose, heaviness of the heart, feeling as if the abdomen is filled with dense fluids, hardness (devoid of movements, tight), and heaviness of the abdomen, bad and sweet smelling belchings, debility & lack of interest in women (disinterest towards sex). The faeces is semi-solid (loose stools), inadequately processed (associated with ama), mucous mixed and heavy. The patient is debilitated though not emaciated and is non-enthusiastic. (13-16)

Etiological factors, pathogenesis and symptoms of Tridosaja Grahani

pṛthagvātādinirdiṣṭahetuliṅgasamāgame |
tridoṣaṃ nirdiśedevaṃ, teṣāṃ vakṣyāmi bheṣajam ||17||
(ca| ci| a| 15) |

The presence of causes and symptoms of all the three dosas together is found in case of tridosha grahani roga. (17)

This means to say that tridoshaja grahani is caused in those who consume the etiological factors responsible for aggravation of all vata, pitta and kapha together. In this condition, the symptoms mentioned in vataja, pittaja and kaphaja grahani are present in combination (mixed up).

Sangrahani & Ghatiyantra Grahani

antrakūjanamālasyaṃ daurbalyaṃ sadanaṃ tathā |
dravaṃ śītaṃ ghanaṃ snigdhaṃ sakaṭīvedanaṃ śakṛt |1|
āmaṃ bahu sapaicchilyaṃ saśabdaṃ mandavedanam |
pakṣānmāsāddaśāhādvā nityaṃ vā'pyatha muñcati ||2||
divā prakopo bhavati rātrau śāntiṃ vrajecca sā |
durvijñeyā duścikitsyā cirakālānubandhinī ||3||
sā bhavedāmavātena saṅgrahagrahaṇī matā |
svapataḥ pārśvayoḥ śūlaṃ galajjalaghaṭīdhvaniḥ |
taṃ vadanti ghaṭīyantramasādhyaṃ grahaṇīgadam ||4||

Sangrahani - Sangrahani is marked by presence of gurgling sound in the intestines, lethargy / laziness, weakness & malaise. In this condition the person excretes faeces which are liquid, cold, dense, and unctuous and associated with pain in the waist. The faeces which are inadequately processed (ama) is eliminated in large quantities, associated with slimy (sticky) material along with sounds and mild pain during excretion. These symptoms may appear once in 15, 30 or 10 days or even daily. The symptoms are pronounced during the day time and subside by night time.

The nature of the disease cannot be understood easily, cannot be easily treated and persists (continues) for a long time. This condition is caused by vata associated with ama and is called sangraha grahani or samgrahani.

Ghatiyantra Grahani – This is also a variant of grahani disease. The person in this condition suffers from pain in the flanks while lying down and sounds resembling 'that produced when a pot is dipped in the water' are heard from the abdomen. This condition is incurable. (1-4)

Determination of ama and pakva states and signs of incurability of grahani

doṣaṃ sāmaṃ nirāmaṃ ca vidyādatrātisāravat ||18||
liṅgairasādhyo grahaṇīvikāro yaistairatīsāragado na sidhyet |
vṛddhasya nūnaṃ grahaṇīvikāro hatvā tanūṃ naiva nivartate ca ||19||
The determination of āma and pakva states of dosas and faeces in grahani disease shall be understood on the same lines as explained in the context of atisara (diarrhoea). The symptoms (and signs) of incurability of grahani are the same as the symptoms (and signs) of incurability of atisara. Grahaṇī roga does not leave the old people without killing them. (18-19)

Prognosis of grahani roga – age wise

(bālake grahaṇī sādhyā yūni kṛcchrā samīritā |
vṛddhe tvasādhyā vijñeyā mataṃ dhanvantareridam) ||1||
iti śrīmādhavakaraviracite mādhavanidāne grahaṇīroganidānaṃ samāptam ||4||
(Grahaṇī roga is easily curable in children, cured with difficulty in the middle-aged persons and incurable in the senile - thus opines Dhanwantari). (1)

iti śrīmādhavakaraviracite mādhavanidāne grahaṇīroganidānaṃ samāptam ||4||
Thus ends the chapter on Grahaṇīroga.

CHAPTER FIVE

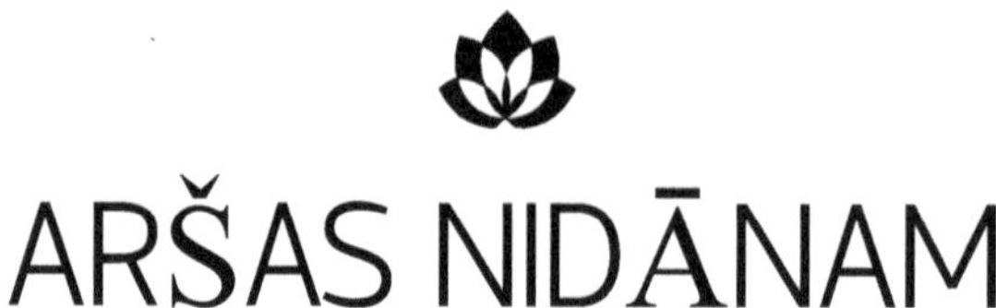

ARŠAS NIDĀNAM

Types of Arshas – Piles

pṛthagdoṣaiḥ samastaiśca śoṇitāt sahajāni ca |
arśāṃsi ṣaṭprakārāṇi vidyādgudavalitraye ||1||
Arśhas (piles, haemorrhoids) is of six types, viz., one from each doṣa (vataja, pittaja and kaphaja), fourth from the combination of all three doshas together (tridosaja, sannipataja), fifth from rakta – blood (raktaja) and the sixth which is sahaja (congenital / hereditary). Piles will appear in the three folds of the rectum. (1)

Definition of Arsas

doṣāstvaṅmāṃsamedāṃsi sandūṣya vividhākṛtīn |
māṃsāṅkurānapānādau kurvantyarśāṃsi tān jaguḥ ||2||
(vā| ni| a| 7) |
The aggravated doshas contaminate the skin, muscle and adipose tissue (fat) and cause sprouts of muscle of different shapes in the rectum (anal region) and other places. These sprouts are called as Arśhas. (2)

Causes of Vataja Arshas

kaṣāyakaṭutiktāni rūkṣaśītalaghūni ca |
pramitālpāśanaṃ tīkṣṇaṃ madyaṃ maithunasevanam ||3||
laṅghanaṃ deśakālau ca śītau vyāyāmakarma ca |
śoko vātātapasparśo heturvātārśasāṃ mataḥ ||4||
(ca| ci| a| 14) |
The causes for Vataja Arshas include over-indulgence in foods which are of

astringent, pungent or bitter tastes, which are dry, cold, light (very quickly digestible), very scanty and non-nutritive; strong alcoholic drinks, excessive indulgence in sex, fasting / starvation, exposure to cold season, living in cold places, excessive physical activity, grief, exposure to heavy breeze and sunlight.(3-4)

Causes of Pittaja Arshas

kaṭvamlalavaṇoṣṇāni vyāyāmāgnyātapaprabhāḥ |
deśakālāvaśiśirau krodho madyamasūyanam ||5||
vidāhi tīkṣṇamuṣṇaṃ ca sarvaṃ pānānnabheṣajam |
pittolbaṇānāṃ vijñeyaḥ prakope heturarśasām ||6||
(ca| ci| a| 14) |

The causes of Pittaja Arshas include - over-indulgence in foods which are pungent, sour, salt and hot; physical exertion, too much exposure to fire and sunlight, hot season, living in hot places; anger, excessive consumption of alcoholic drinks, jealousy, drinks, foods and medicines which cause heart-burn (corrosive), penetrating (into the tissues) nature and heat producing and other causative factors which lead to increase of pitta. (5-6)

Causes of Kaphaja Arshas

madhurasnigdhaśītāni lavaṇāmlagurūṇi ca |
avyāyāmo divāsvapnaḥ śayyāsanasukhe ratiḥ ||7||
prāgvātasevā śītau ca deśakālāvacintanam |
ślaiṣmikāṇāṃ samuddiṣṭametat kāraṇamarśasām ||8||
(ca| ci| a| 14) |

The causes of Kaphaja Arshas include - over-indulgence in foods which are sweet, fatty, cold, salty, sour and heavy (hard to digest); lack of physical activity, sleeping at daytime, very comfortably soft bed and seat, exposure to eastern breeze, cold season and places, not worrying and others causative factors which lead to increase of kapha. (7-8)

Dvandva and Tridosaja Arshas

hetulakṣaṇasaṃsargādvidyāddvandvolbaṇāni ca |
sarvo hetustridoṣāṇāṃ sahajairlakṣaṇaṃ samam ||9||
(ca| ci| a| 14) |

Dvandva arshas is produced by the causative factors of any two doshas (causative factors which aggravated two doshas simultaneously). These types of arshas will have combined symptoms of aggravation of both those doshas. Similarly, Tridoshaja arshas is produced by causative factors of all the three doshas. The symptoms of this type of arshas are similar to those of Sahaja arśhas (arshas present right from the birth – congenital). (9)

Symptoms of Vataja Arsas

gudāṅkurā bahvanilāḥ śuṣkāścimacimānvitāḥ |
mlānāḥ śyāvāruṇāḥ stabdhā viśadāḥ paruṣāḥ kharāḥ ||10||
mitho visadṛśā vakrāstīkṣṇā visphuṭitānanāḥ |
bimbīkharjūrakarkandhūkārpāsīphalasannibhāḥ ||11||
kecit kadambapuṣpābhāḥ kecit siddhārthakopamāḥ |
śiraḥpārśvāṃsakaṭyūruvaṅkṣaṇādyadhikavyathāḥ ||12||
kṣavathūdgāraviṣṭambhahṛdgrahārocakapradāḥ |
kāsaśvāsāgnivaiṣamyakarṇanādabhramāvahāḥ ||13||
tairārto grathitaṃ stokaṃ saśabdaṃ sapravāhikam |
rukphenapicchānugataṃ vibaddhamupaveśyate ||14||
kṛṣṇatvaṅnakhaviṇmūtranetravaktraśca jāyate |
gulmaplīhodarāṣṭhīlāsambhavastata eva ca ||15||
(vā| ni| a| 7) |

The symptoms of Vātaja arśhas are: -

Sprouts (pile masses) are dry (doesn't have exudates and do not bleed and hence dry), have itching (tingling sensation), are shrunk (small in size, not developed properly), blue or bluish pink in colour, stiff (hard), non-sticky (non-slimy), dry, rough, furrowed, each one of different shape, curved, pointed tip, cracked, resemble fruits of bimbī (Cephalandra indica), kharjūra (date palm), karkandhū (Zizyphus ceroplia) and kārpāsa (cotton seeds). Some masses appear like kadamba flowers (having many sprouts), and some others resemble mustard seeds (very small in size).

The person complains of excessive pain in the head, flanks, shoulders, waist, thighs, groins, sneezing, belching, constipation, pain near the heart, anorexia, cough, difficult respiration (dyspnoea), irregular digestion, ringing in the ears and giddiness. The patient eliminates faeces which is scrabulous, scanty, associated with noise, straining and pain; frothy and associated with slimy discharges (material) and semi-solid in consistency or is constipated. There is blackish discoloration of skin, nails, faeces, urine, eyes and face. Gulma (abdominal tumour), pliha (spleen enlargement), udara (enlargement of abdomen) and asthila (enlargement of prostate) may appear as its complications. (10-15)

Symptoms of Pittaja Arshas

pittottarā nīlamukhā raktapītāsitaprabhāḥ |
tanvasrasrāviṇo visrāstanavo mṛdavaḥ ślathāḥ ||16||
śukajihvāyakṛtkhaṇḍajalaukovaktrasannibhāḥ |
dāhapākajvarasvedatṛṇmūrchārucimohadāḥ ||17||
soṣmāṇo dravanīloṣṇapītaraktāmavarcasaḥ |
yavamadhyā haritpītahāridratvaṅnakhādayaḥ ||18||
(vā| ni| a| 7) |

The symptoms of Pittaja arshas are:-

Sprouts (pile masses) are blue, red, yellow or black in colour. They will discharge thin blood, fetid smell, less in number (small in size), smooth to touch and suspended (flaccid, loose, hanging). These masses resemble the parrot’s tongue, piece of liver or mouth part of a leech. The patient complains of burning sensation, suppuration (ulceration), fever, perspiration, thirst, fainting (loss of consciousness), anorexia and delusion. He eliminates faeces which are hot, watery, blue, yellow or red in colour and not properly processed (associated with ama). Some of these masses will resemble barley i.e. thick in the centre and thin / tapering towards the ends. The skin, nails, face, teeth, urine and faeces will get discoloured and will attain green, yellow or turmeric colour. (16-18)

Symptoms of Kaphaja Arsas

śleṣmolbaṇā mahāmūlā ghanā mandarujaḥ sitāḥ |
utsannopacitasnigdhastabdhavṛttagurusthirāḥ ||19||
picchilāḥ stimitāḥślakṣṇāḥ kaṇḍvāḍhyāḥ sparśanapriyāḥ |
karīrapanasāsthyābhāstathā gostanasannibhāḥ ||20||
vaṅkṣaṇānāhinaḥ pāyubastinābhivikarṣiṇaḥ |
saśvāsakāsahṛllāsaprasekārucipīnasāḥ ||21||
mehakṛcchraśirojāḍyaśiśirajvarakāriṇaḥ |
klaibyāgnimārdavacchardirāmaprāyavikāradāḥ ||22||

vasābhasakaphaprāyapurīṣāḥ sapravāhikāḥ |
na sravanti na bhidyante pāṇḍusnigdhatvagādayaḥ ||23||
(vā| ni| a| 7) |

The symptoms of Kaphaja arshas are:-
Sprouts (pile masses) are deep rooted, hard (dense), with mild pain, and white in colour. These masses are elongated and elevated, big in size and circumference, unctuous / oily (smooth), stiff (not flabby – do not pit or get depressed when pressed), round in shape, heavy and fixed / stable. The masses are slimy / slippery, immobile (or damp, wet), smooth / shining, associated with severe itching and feels comfortable on touching.
They resemble karira (bamboo shoot/sprout), seed of panasa (jackfruit), or teet of cow udder.
The patient may have swelling or distension in the groins (hernia?), dragging sensation in the rectum, bladder, and umbilicus; difficulty in respiration, cough, nausea, salivation, anorexia, running in the nose, dysuria, heaviness of the head, fever with cold; impotency, indigestion, vomiting and other diseases which are caused by ama (undigested material). The faeces will resemble fat, mixed with mucus and is accompanied with straining. There will be no exudation (of mucus or blood) from the pile mass. There will also be no cracks and splits in spite of being subjected to friction by faeces. (19-24)

Symptoms of Tridosaja Arsas

सर्वैः सर्वात्मकान्याहुर्लक्षणैः सहजानि च |२४|
sarvaiḥ sarvātmakānyāhurlakṣaṇaiḥ sahajāni ca |24|
In case of Tridosaja arshas the symptoms of all the three dosas will be found together. (23)

Symptoms of Raktarsas – bleeding piles

raktolbaṇā gudekīlāḥ pittākṛtisamanvitāḥ ||24||
vaṭaprarohasadṛśā guñjāvidrumasannibhāḥ |
te'tyarthaṃ duṣṭamuṣṇaṃ ca gāḍhaviṭkaprapīḍitāḥ ||25||
sravanti sahasā raktaṃ tasya cātipravṛttitaḥ |
bhekābhaḥ pīḍyate duḥkhaiḥ śoṇitakṣayasambhavaiḥ ||26||

hīnavarṇabalotsāho hataujāḥ kaluṣendriyaḥ |
(vā| ni| a| 7) |
In case of raktarshas, (haemorrhoids, bleeding piles) all symptoms are similar to pittaja arshas. The sprouts (pile mass) resemble the shape and size of pittaja arshas. The sprouts will resemble the buds of vata (Ficus bengalensis), seeds of guñja (Abrus precatorius) or vidruma (coral).
There is continuous, frequent and heavy loss (bleeding) of dirty (contaminated) and hot blood from these masses due to the friction of hardened faeces on these masses. Due to heavy and excessive loss of blood, the skin of the patient appears (resembles) that of a monsoon frog (yellowish or greenish brown colour of frogs as evident in the rainy season). The person will suffer from various disorders due to excessive bleeding. This leads to loss of colour, strength, enthusiasm and ojas (essence of all the tissues) or valour. The senses (sense organs) become weak and the patient may later develop other diseases due to loss of blood. (24-26)

Dosha association in Raktarshas and related symptoms

(tatrānubanyodvividhaḥśleṣmaṇomārutasyaca|)
viṭ śyāvaṃ kaṭhinaṃ rūkṣamadhovāyurna vartate ||27||
tanu cāruṇavarṇaṃ ca phenilaṃ cāsṛgarśasām |
kaṭyūrugudaśūlaṃ ca daurbalyaṃ yadi cādhikam ||28||
tatrānubandho vātasya heturyadi ca rūkṣaṇam |
śithilaṃ śvetapītaṃ ca viṭ snigdhaṃ guru śītalam ||29||
yadyarśasāṃ ghanaṃ cāsṛk tantumat pāṇḍu picchilam |
gudaṃ sapicchaṃ stimitaṃ guru snigdhaṃ ca kāraṇam |
śleṣmānubandho vijñeyastatra raktārśasāṃ budhaiḥ ||30||(ca| ci| a| 14) |
There are two kinds of dosa associations with Raktarshas i.e. that of vata and kapha.
In case of vata association, the faeces will be black in colour, hard and dry. The flatus is not expelled out. There occurs thin, red coloured, and frothy blood discharges from the pile mass. The patient would have pain in the waist, thighs and rectum and extreme weakness. Consumption of dry things (foods) are the causative factors of vata aggravation in bleeding piles.
In case of kapha association, the faeces will be broken (semi-solid), whitish yellow in colour, unctuous, heavy and cold.
There will be exudation of thick, sticky, whitish yellow (pale) blood having

thread like structures in it from the pile masses. The anal region of the patient will be sticky, and wet (as if covered by wet cloth). Consumption of heavy and unctuous things is the causative factor of kapha aggravation in bleeding piles. (27-30)

Purvarupa – premonitory symptoms of arshas

viṣṭambho'nnasya daurbalyaṃ kukṣerāṭopa eva ca |
kārśyamudgārabāhulyaṃ sakthisādo'lpaviṭkatā ||31||
grahaṇīdoṣapāṇḍvarterāśaṅkā codarasya ca |
pūrvarūpāṇi nirdiṣṭānyarśasāmabhivṛddhaye ||32||
(ca| ci| a| 14) |
The premonitory symptoms of arshas include - stasis of food in the stomach without digestion, debility / weakness, gurgling noise in the abdomen, emaciation, too many belchings, weakness of the thighs, scanty faeces, presence of symptoms resembling those of grahani dosha (sprue), pandu (anaemia) and udara (distension of abdomen) causing confusion in diagnosis. (31-32)

Involvement of dosa subtypes and folds of rectum in manifestation of arshas

pañcātmā mārutaḥ pittaṃ kapho gudavalitrayam |
sarva eva prakupyanti gudajānāṃ samudbhave ||33||
tasmādarśāṃsi duḥkhāni bahuvyādhikarāṇi ca |
sarvadehopatāpīni prāyaḥ kṛcchratamāni ca ||34||
(ca| ci| a| 14) |
In the manifestation of arsas vis-a-vis piles, all five subtypes (divisions) of vata, pitta and kapha and all three layers (folds) of rectum are vitiated (affected). All the five divisions of each of the dosas invade (vitiate) all the three layers (folds) of the rectum to produce arshas. So, arshas is a very painful disease and also gives rise to many other diseases. It affects and troubles the whole body and is difficult to cure. (33-34)
Note - The affliction of all the above-mentioned components in the pathogenesis of arshas is limited to gudaja arsas i.e., piles or masses occurring in the anal region. One should have a clear knowledge of the same because 'pile like masses' also occur in other areas of the body and they are

also called arshas. Example – Nasarsha – mass occurring in the nose which resembles the pile mass. Such types of arshas do not involve the subtypes of doshas and 3 layers of the rectum / anus.

Prognosis (curability and incurability) of arshas

bāhyāyāṃ tu valau jātānyekadoṣolbaṇāni ca |
arśāṃsi sukhasādhyāni na cirotpatitāni ca ||35||
dvandvajāni dvitīyāyāṃ valau yānyāśritāni ca |
kṛcchrasādhyāni tānyāhuḥ parisaṃvatsarāṇi ca ||36||
sahajāni tridoṣāṇi yāni cābhyantarāṃ valim |
jāyante'rśāṃsi saṃśritya tānyasādhyāni nirdiśet ||37||
(ca| ci| a| 14) |
Pile masses located in the external layer (fold) of the rectum, those manifested due to increase of any one dosha, and which are of recent onset are easily curable.
Arshas caused by increase of any two doshas together, located in the middle layer (fold) of the rectum and existing for more than a year, are difficult to cure.
The arshas which is congenital (hereditary), which is caused by simultaneous aggravation of all the three doshas, and located in the innermost layer (fold) of the rectum is incurable. (35-37)

Other signs of prognosis of arshas

śeṣatvādāyuṣastāni catuṣpādasamanvite |
yāpyante dīptakāyāgneḥ pratyākhyeyānyato'nyathā ||38||
(ca| ci| a| 14) |
Patients who are fortunate to have a balance of lifespan (have the fortune of having long life), good services of all the four limbs of treatment (physician, medicine, nurse and patient), having good digestive capacity can hope to live on with arshas. On the other hand, the persons in whom none of the above-mentioned features are present shall be refused treatment (should not be treated because they are incurable). (38)

Incurability of arshas based on the associated complications
haste pāde mukhe nābhyāṃ gude vṛṣaṇayostathā |

śotho hṛtpārśvaśūlaṃ ca yasyāsādhyo'rśaso hi saḥ ||39||
hṛtpārśvaśūlaṃ sammohaśchardiraṅgasya rugjvaraḥ |
tṛṣṇā gudasya pākaśca nihanyurgudajāturam ||40||
(ca| ci| a| 14) |
tṛṣṇā arocakaśūlārtamatiprasrutaśoṇitam |
śothātisārasaṃyuktamarśāṃsi kṣapayanti hi ||41||
(su| sū| a| 33) |
Appearance of oedema in the hands, feet, face, umbilicus, rectum and scrotum, pain in the region of the heart and flanks are symptoms of bad prognosis in arshas.
Pain in the region of the heart and flanks, delusion, vomiting, diffuse pain all over the body, fever, thirst, suppuration (ulceration) of the rectum -these symptoms kill the patients of arshas.
Thirst, anorexia, colic, heavy bleeding from the pile mass, generalized oedema and diarrhoea also kill the patient. (39-41)

Lingaja Arsas and other types of Arsas

meḍhrādiṣvapi vakṣyante yathāsvaṃ, nābhijāni ca |
gaṇḍūpadāsyarūpāṇi picchilāni mṛdūni ca ||42||
(vā| ni| a| 7) |
Arsas (sprouts) also develop on the penis and other regions of the body including nose, eyes and ears. The symptoms of these conditions are found along with the disease manifesting in these structures. The arshas manifesting near the umbilicus have the resemblance of the mouth part of earthworm; are slippery and soft. (42)

Carmakila

vyāno gṛhītvā śleṣmāṇaṃ karotyarśastvaco bahiḥ |
kīlopamaṃ sthirakharaṃ carmakīlaṃ tu tadviduḥ ||43||
(vā| ni| a| 7) |
Vyana (a division / subtype of vata) associated with kapha will invade the skin causing arshas on the skin. This arshas resembles a nail which is firm and rough (hard). This is also known as Carmakila (warts) (43)

Types and symptoms of Carmakila

vātena todapāruṣyaṃ pittādasitavaktratā |
śleṣmaṇā snigdhatā cāsya grathitatvaṃ savarṇatā ||44||
(vā| ni| a| 7) |
The carmakila in which vata is predominant is painful and rough. The carmakila in which pitta is predominant would have a black coloured opening. The carmakila in which kapha is predominant is of the same colour of the skin, is unctuous (smooth) and is knotted. (44)

iti śrīmādhavakaraviracite mādhavanidāne'rśonidānaṃ samāptam ||5||
Thus ends the chapter on Arsas.

CHAPTER SIX

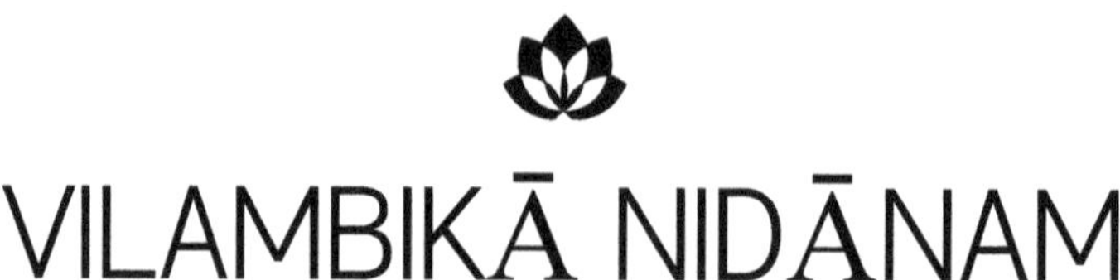

VILAMBIKĀ NIDĀNAM

Kinds of Jatharagni – digestive fire

mandastīkṣṇo'tha viṣamaḥ samaśceti caturvidhaḥ |
kaphapittāniladhikyāttatsāmyājjāṭharo'nalaḥ ||1||

The jatharāgni (gastric fire, digestive activity) is of four kinds, they are –

Mandagni (manda agni) – caused due to predominance of kapha
Tiksnagni (tiksna agni) – caused due to predominance of pitta
Visamagni (visama agni) – caused due to predominance of vata
Samagni (sama agni) – caused due to the normalcy of all the three doshas

Behaviour and functions of different kinds of agni

viṣamo vātajān rogān tīkṣṇaḥ pittanimittajān |
karotyagnistathā mando vikārān kaphasambhavān ||2||
samā samāgneraśitā mātrā samyagvipacyate |
svalpā'pi naiva mandāgnerviṣamāgnestu dehinaḥ ||3||
kadācit pacyate samyakkadācinna vipacyate |
mātrā'timātrā'pyaśitā sukhaṃ yasya vipacyate |
tīkṣṇāgniriti taṃ vidyāt samāgniḥ śreṣṭha ucyate ||4||

1. Mandāgni – This type of agni dominated by kapha either partially digests the food (to a small extent) or is incapable of digesting even a small quantity of food. This type of agni causes kapha diseases.
2. Tīkşngāni – This type of agni dominated by pitta digests the usual or even excess quantity of food without any difficulty. This agni is powerful and can

digest the food within a short span of time. This type of agni causes pitta diseases.
3. Visamāgni – This type of agni dominated by vata sometimes digests the food properly and sometimes improperly. This erratic and fluctuant behaviour of the agni is due to the influence of vata. This type of agni causes vata diseases.
4. Samāgni – This type of agni is due to normalcy and balance of all the three doshas i.e., vata, pitta and kapha. This is a healthy state of digestive activity. This kind of agni digests the normal quantity of food without causing any difficulty,

Among these 4 kinds of agni, only samāgni is said to be ideal (conducive to health). (2-4)

Types of Ajirna – indigestion

āmaṃ vidagdhaṃ viṣṭabdhaṃ kaphapittānilaistribhiḥ |
ajīrṇaṃ kecidicchanti caturthaṃ rasaśeṣataḥ ||5|| (su| sū| a| 46) |
ajīrṇaṃ pañcamaṃ kecinnirdoṣaṃ dinapāki ca |
vadanti ṣaṣṭhaṃ cājīrṇaṃ prākṛtaṃ prativāsaram ||6||
There are basically three kinds of ajirna (indigestion) caused due to the predominance of one or the other type of dosha in each type. They are –

Āma ajīrṇa – caused by kapha excess
Vidagdha ajīrṇa – caused by pitta excess
Vistabdha ajīrṇa – caused by vata excess

Other types of ajīrṇa

Rasasesa ajīrna - Others include a fourth one the rasasesa ajīrna as fourth type of ajīrṇa. This type of indigestion is related to āhāra rasa (indigestion on a nutrient portion of food).
Dinapāki ajīrṇa – According to some others the fifth type of ajīrṇa is dinapāki ajīrṇa. In this type of indigestion, the food is digested the next day but without causing any difficulty (delayed digestion).
Prativasara ajīrṇa - Yet others consider prativasara ajirna as the sixth type of ajīrṇa. This type of indigestion is found every day, normally, immediately

after taking the food i.e. until the taken food is digested. This is a normal state and the indigestion is temporary and not pathological. It goes away once the food is digested. (5-6)

Nidana – etiological factors of ajīrṇa (indigestion)

atyambupānādviṣamāśanācca sandhāraṇāt svapnaviparyayācca |
kāle'pi sātmyaṃ laghu cāpi bhuktamannaṃ na pākaṃ bhajate narasya ||7||
īrṣyābhayakrodhapariplutena lubdhena rugdainyanipīḍitena |
pradveṣayuktena ca sevyamānamannaṃ na samyakparipākameti ||8||
(su| sū| a| 46) |
mātrayā'pyabhyavahṛtaṃ pathyaṃ cānnaṃ na jīryati |
cintāśokabhayakrodhaduḥkhaśayyāprajāgaraiḥ ||9|| (ca| vi| a| 2) |

The general causes of indigestion include drinking water in large quantities, taking large or small quantitiesof food at unusual times, suppression of natural urges of the body, erratic sleep patterns i.e., not sleeping during night times and excessive sleeping during daytime. These factors cause indigestion of food in spite of the person taking - normal quantity of food, foods which have been accustomed and foods at proper time.
Food does not get digested properly in a person who is afflicted with jealousy, fear, anger, greed, grief, humility and hatred feelings. (One would not digest the food properly in spite of taking normal food at proper time when he or she is afflicted with worry, grief, fear, anger, misery, (pain) or loss of sleep).(7-9)

Symptoms of āmājīrṇa

tatrāme gurutotkledaḥ śotho gaṇḍākṣikūṭagaḥ |
udgāraśca yathābhuktamavidagdhaḥ pravartate ||10||
The symptoms of āmājīrṇa are – heaviness (of the abdomen and /or of the whole body), nausea, swelling of the cheeks and eyes, belchings similar to those occurring soon after meals (non-acidic, not having burning sensation). (10)

Symptoms of Vidagdhajirna

vidagdhe bhramatṛṇmūrchāḥ pittācca vividhā rujaḥ |
udgāraśca sadhūmāmlaḥ svedo dāhaśca jāyate ||11||
Symptoms of vidagdhajirna includes - giddiness, thirst, fainting, sour belching and belching with a feel of smoke being eliminated, perspiration, burning sensation inside and other symptoms of pitta (increase). (11)

Symptoms of Vistabdhājīrṇa and Rasasesajirna

viṣṭabdhe śūlamādhmānaṃ vividhā vātavedanāḥ |
malavātāpravṛttiśca stambho mohā'ṅgapīḍanam ||12||
rasaśeṣe'nnavidveṣo hṛdayāśuddhigaurave |13|
Symptoms of Vistabdhājīrṇa include - with pain in the abdomen (colic), tympanitis, non-movement of stools and flatus (stools and fart are not expelled naturally), stiffness, delusion (unconsciousness), pain in body parts and other symptoms of vāta (increase).

Symptoms of Rasasesajirna include - aversion to food, unpleasant feeling in the region of the heart (bad belching), and heaviness (in the region of the heart or the abdomen). (12)

Ajirna Upadrava – complications of indigestion

mūrchā pralāpo vamathuḥ prasekaḥ sadanaṃ bhramaḥ |
upadravā bhavantyete maraṇaṃ cāpyajīrṇataḥ ||13||
(su| sū| a| 46) |
The complications of ajirna / indigestion include – fainting (unconsciousness), delirium, vomiting, excessive salivation, debility, giddiness and even death. (13)

Eating indiscipline and ajirna

anātmavantaḥ paśuvadbhuñjate ye'pramāṇataḥ |
rogānīkasya te mūlamajīrṇaṃ prāpnuvanti hi ||14||

Persons who do not have self-control and eat large quantities (without even being concerned about the quantity of food they take) of food recklessly like cattle (eating with animal instinct), will develop this disease ajirna. This indigestion (ajirna) is the root cause of many other diseases. (14)

Origin of Visucika, Alasaka and Vilambika disorders

ajīrṇamāmaṃ viṣṭabdhaṃ vidagdhaṃ ca yadīritam |
visūcyalasakau tasmādbhaveccāpi vilambikā ||15||
(su| u| taṃ| a| 56) |
There are three diseases namely Visūcikā, Alasaka and Vilambikā. These diseases arise from three types of ajirna i.e., Amajirna, Vidagdhajirna and Vistabdhajirna. (These need not be respectively). (15)

Visuchika

sūcībhiriva gātrāṇi tudan santiṣṭhate'nilaḥ |
yasyājīrṇena sā vaidyairvisūcīti nigadyate ||16||
na tāṃ parimitāhārā labhante viditāgamāḥ |
mūḍhāstāmajitātmāno labhante'śanalolupāḥ ||17||
(su| u| taṃ| a| 56) |
mūrchā'tisāro vamathuḥ pipāsā śūlaṃ bhramodveṣṭanajṛmbhadāhāḥ |
vaivarṇyakampau hṛdaye rujaśca bhavanti tasyāṃ śirasaśca bhedaḥ ||18||
(su| u| taṃ| a| 56) |
The disease in which the patient suffers from pricking pain, as though pierced by needles, caused by vata aggravated due to ajirna (indigestion) is named as visūcikā by the physicians. The pain is also stable and localized. People who are well versed with Ayurveda and the principles related to consumption of food mentioned therein and also follow the dietetic rules and regulations promptly will not suffer from this condition. This condition in fact occurs due to ajīrṇa manifesting in persons, who have mad craving for food and also eat recklessly without any limitation (without following the eating rules, regulations and etiquettes).
Symptoms of Visucika include - fainting, diarrhoea, vomiting, severe thirst, abdominal pain, giddiness, cramps / twitching, yawning, burning sensation all over, discolouration, tremors, pain in the region of the heart and headache.(16-18)

Alasaka

kukṣirānahyate'tyarthaṃ pratāmyet parikūjati |
niruddho mārutaścaiva kukṣāvupari dhāvati ||19||
vātavarconirodhaśca yasyātyarthaṃ bhavedapi |

tasyālasakamācaṣṭe tṛṣṇodgārau ca yasya tu ||20||
(su| u| taṃ| a| 56) |
The symptoms of Alasaka include - severe distension of the abdomen, unconsciousness, makes some sounds from within the throat (crying helplessly), flatus gets blocked downwards (doesn't move downwards easily) and hence takes an abnormal route and start moving upwards (reaching the region of heart and throat), severe or complete obstruction (non expulsion) of flatus and faeces, thirst and belching. (19-20)

Vilambika

duṣṭaṃ tu bhuktaṃ kaphamārutābhyāṃ pravartate nordhvamadhaśca yasya |
vilambikāṃ tāṃ bhṛśaduścikitsyāmācakṣate śāstravidaḥ purāṇāḥ ||21||
(su| u| taṃ| a| 56) |
The disease in which the food contaminated by the vitiated kapha and vata does not move out of the body either in upward or downward direction is defined as vilambikā by the ancient Ayurveda scholars. This is either a very difficult condition to treat or is incurable. (21)

Disturbing effects of ama

yatrasthamāmaṃ virujettameva deśaṃ viśeṣeṇa vikārajātaiḥ |
doṣeṇa yenāvatataṃ śarīraṃ tallakṣaṇairāmasamudbhavaiśca ||22||
(su| u| taṃ| a| 56) |
Ama gives rise to pain in whichever part of the body it resides (or gets localized). The same place also becomes the site for manifestation of many diseases, which are caused due to the action of the dosas travelling all over the body associated with āma. (22)

Symptoms of incurability of visucika and alasaka

yaḥ śyāvadantauṣṭhanakho'lpasañjño vamyardito'bhyantarayātanetraḥ |
kṣāmasvaraḥ sarvavimuktasandhiryāyānnaraḥ so'punarāgamāya ||23||
(su| u| taṃ| a| 56) |
The fatal signs / signs of incurability of ajīrna and associated diseases include - blackish discolouration of teeth, lips and nails, loss of consciousness, severe vomiting, in drawing of the eyes, feeble voice and looseness of all the joints of the body. (23)

Jirna Ahara Lakshanas – signs of proper digestion of food

udgāraśuddhirutsāho vegotsargo yathocitaḥ |
laghutā kṣutpipāsā ca jīrṇāhārasya lakṣaṇam ||24||
The signs of proper digestion of food are - pure belching (without bad smell or taste), enthusiasm, proper and timely elimination of urges (of faeces, flatus and urine), lightness of the body, appearance of hunger and thirst (desire for water) are the symptoms of proper digestion of food.

Upadravas of Visucika

nidrānāśo'ratiḥ kampo mūtrāghāto visañjñatā |
amī hyupadravā ghorā visūcyāṃ pañca dāruṇāḥ ||25||
The five difficult and dreadful complications of visūcikā are –

- loss of sleep
- restlessness
- tremors
- suppression of urine
- loss of consciousness (24-25)

Ajirna – as the root of other diseases

prāyeṇāhāravaiṣamyādajīrṇaṃ jāyate nṛṇām |
tanmūlo rogasaṅghātastadvināśādvinaśyati ||26||
Probably Ajirṇa occurs due to irregularities of food. This Ajīrṇa in turn is the cause for other diseases. On the other hand, when ajirna is cured other diseases also get destroyed automatically. (26)

General symptoms of Ajirna

glānigauravaviṣṭambhabhramamārutamūḍhatāḥ |
vibandho vā pravṛttirvā sāmānyājīrṇalakṣaṇam ||27||
The general symptoms of ajirna (indigestion) are feeling of weakness (without physical exertion) heaviness of the body, absence of movement

of the abdomen, giddiness, non-elimination of flatus, constipation or diarrhoea. (27)

iti śrīmādhavakaraviracite mādhavanidāne'gnimāndyājīrṇavisūcikālasakavilambikānidānaṃ samāptam ||6||

Thus ends the chapter on Ajīrna etc.

CHAPTER SEVEN

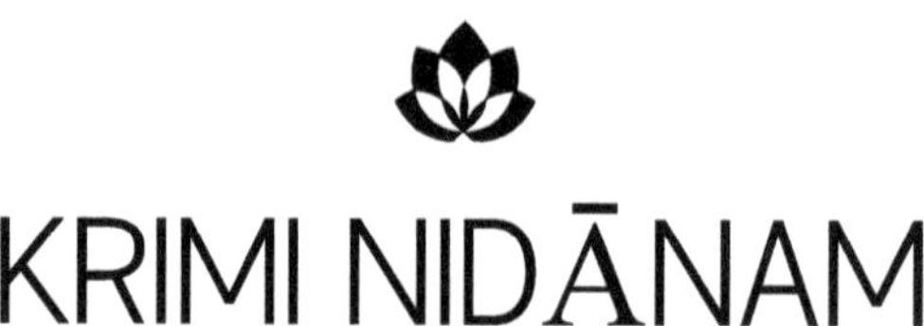

KRIMI NIDĀNAM

Krimi Bheda – types and origin of parasites

krimayaśca dvidhā proktā bāhyābhyantarabhedataḥ |
bahirmalakaphāsṛgviḍjanmabhedāccaturvidhāḥ ||1||
nāmato viṃśatividhā
Parasites are of two types - external and internal.
They are also counted as four kinds viz, arising from external dirt, kapha, rakta (blood) and purisa (faeces). They are totally twenty-four by name (and in number). (1)

Bahya Krimi – External parasites

bāhyāstatra malodbhavāḥ | (vā| ni| a| 14) |
tilapramāṇasaṃsthānavarṇāḥ keśāmbarāśrayāḥ ||2||
bahupādāśca sūkṣmāśca yūkā likṣāśca nāmataḥ |
dvidhā te koṭhapiḍakākaṇḍūgaṇḍān prakurvate ||3|| (vā| ni| a| 14) |
External parasites which take their origin from excreta (mala) resemble tila (sesame seed) in size, features and colour, reside in hairs and clothes, have many legs and are small. They are of two kinds namely yūka and likṣa. They produce rashes, small pimples, itching and vesicles. (2-3)

Abhyantara Krimi Nidana – Causes of internal parasites

ajīrṇabhojī madhurāmlanityo dravapriyaḥ piṣṭaguḍopabhoktā |
vyāyāmavarjī ca divāśayāno viruddhabhuk saṃlabhate krimīṃstu ||4||
Persons who indulge daily (regularly) with foods which are raw (uncooked) or consume foods when previously consumed foods are not properly

digested, sweet and sour, water and watery beverages or which are dry powders (flours) and jaggery: those who avoid physical exercise and those who sleep during day time and those who regularly consume incompatible (mutually antagonistic or unwholesome) foods become victims of krimiroga. (4)

Nidana – etiological factors of specific krimis

māṣapiṣṭāmlalavaṇaguḍaśākaiḥ purīṣajāḥ |
māṃsamatsyaguḍakṣīradadhiśuktaiḥ kaphodbhavāḥ ||5||
viruddhājīrṇaśākādyaiḥ śoṇitotthā bhavanti hi |
(su| u| taṃ| a| 54) |
Use of black gram, foods predominantly consisting of or prepared from flours, sour and salty foods, molasses and leafy vegetables give rise to growth of parasites in the faeces.
Use of mutton, fish, jaggery, milk, curds, fermented sugarcane juice, etc., gives rise to growth of parasites in kapha.
Indulgence in incompatible foods (mutually antagonistic foods), uncooked foods (or taking foods in the presence of indigestion of previously consumed foods) and leafy vegetables give rise to parasites in the blood. (5)

Abhyantara Krimi Lakshanas – general symptoms of presence of internal parasites

jvaro vivarṇatā śūlaṃ hṛdrogaḥ sadanaṃ bhramaḥ ||6||
bhaktadveṣo'tisāraśca sañjātakrimilakṣaṇam |
(su| u| taṃ| a| 54) |
Fever, discolouration, pain in the abdomen, disorders of (the region of) the heart, weakness, giddiness, aversion to food and diarrhoea are the symptoms of the presence of parasites inside the body. (6)

Kaphaja Krimi – size, shape, numbers, names and symptoms caused by these parasites

kaphādāmāśaye jātā vṛddhāḥ sarpanti sarvataḥ ||7||
pṛthubradhnanibhāḥ kecit kecidgaṇḍūpadopamāḥ |
rūḍhadhānyāṅkurākārāstanudīrghāstathā'ṇavaḥ ||8||

śvetāstāmrāvabhāsāśca nāmataḥ saptadhā tu te |
antrādā udārāveṣṭā hṛdayādā mahāgudāḥ ||9||
curavo darbhakusumāḥ sugandhāste ca kurvate |
hṛllāsamāsyasravaṇamavipākamarocakam ||10||
mūrchācchardijvarā nāhakārśyakṣavathupīnasān |
(vā| ni| a| 14) |
The Kaphaja Krimis take their origin from the stomach due to the excess of kapha (excess kapha in the stomach is an ideal environment for these krimis to manifest). The parasites arising from kapha reside in the stomach and move all over the alimentary tract (they move in the upward as well as downward direction). Some resemble a thick leather strip and some are long, resembling earthworms. Some others look like the fresh sprouts of grains; are thin, long, and small or round, white or coppery in colour. They are of seven kinds and are known as antrada, udaravesta, hrdayada, mahaguda, curava, darbhakusuma and sugandha.
They produce nausea, excess salivation, indigestion, anorexia, fainting, vomiting, fever, constipation or blocks in stomach due to ama or in colon due to faeces (enlargement of abdomen), emaciation, too many sneezes and running in the nose. (7-10)

Raktaja Krimi – size, shape, numbers, names and symptoms caused by these parasite

raktavāhisirāsthānaraktajā jantavo'ṇavaḥ ||11||
apādā vṛttatāmrāśca saukṣmyāt kecidadarśanāḥ |
keśādā romavidhvaṃsā romadvīpā udumbarāḥ |
ṣaṭ te kuṣṭhaikakarmāṇaḥ sahasaurasamātaraḥ ||12||
(vā| ni| a| 14) |
Parasites arising from rakta (blood) are found in all the organs / channels of blood i.e. raktavaha srotas (liver, spleen, arteries, veins and blood itself). They are very minute, devoid of legs, round in shape and have coppery colour. Among these many are very minute (microscopic) and hence cannot be visible (invisible) to the naked eyes. They are of six kinds and known as kesada, romavidhvamsa, romadvipa, udumbara, sourasa and matara. All these parasites cause kushta (leprosy, skin disorders) or many other diseases / symptoms which resemble kushta. (11-12)

Purishaja Krimi – size, shape, numbers, names and symptoms caused by these parasites

pakvāśaye purīṣotthā jāyante'dhovisarpiṇaḥ |
pravṛddhāḥ syurbhaveyuśca te yadā''māśayonmukhāḥ ||13||
tadā'syodgāraniḥśvāsā viḍgandhānuvidhāyinaḥ |
pṛthuvṛttatanusthūlāḥ śyāvapītasitāsitāḥ ||14||
te pañca nāmnā krimayaḥ kakerukamakerukāḥ |
sausurādāḥ saśūlākhyā lelihā janayanti hi ||15||
viḍbhedaśūlaviṣṭambhakārśyapāruṣyapāṇḍutāḥ |
romaharṣāgnisadanaṃ gudakaṇḍūrvimārgagāḥ ||16||
(vā| ni| a| 14) |

Parasites arising from purisa (faeces) are found in the large intestine. These parasites usually travel downwards. But when their numbers increase, they can even travel upwards towards the stomach. When they move upwards, they cause faecal smell in the mouth, belching and breath. They are big, round, thin or thick; blue, yellow, white or black in colour. They are of five kinds known as kakeruka makeruka, sausurada, sasula and leliha.

They produce diarrhoea, pain in the abdomen, constipation, emaciation, dryness, pallor (whitish-yellow discolouration), horripilations, poor digestion and itching in the anus. They even move into other places (organs nearby). (13-16)

iti śrīmādhavakaraviracite mādhavanidāne kriminidānaṃ samāptam ||7||
Thus ends the chapter on KrimiRoga.

CHAPTER EIGHT

PĀṆḌUROGA KĀMALĀ KUMBHAKĀMALĀ HALĪMAKA NIDĀNAM

Panduroga types

pāṇḍurogāḥ smṛtāḥ pañca vātapittakaphaistrayaḥ |
caturthaḥ sannipātena pañcamo bhakṣaṇānmṛdaḥ ||1||
(ca| ci| a| 16) |
Pānduroga (anaemia, disease characterized by pallor) is of five kinds - one each from (each dosa) vāta, pitta, kapha; fourth from the combination of all three doshas and fifth from eating mud.(1)

Nidana – etiological factors of Panduroga
vyāyāmamamlaṃ lavaṇāni madyaṃ mṛdaṃ divāsvapnamatīva tīkṣṇam |
niṣevamāṇasya pradūṣya raktaṃ doṣāstvacaṃ pāṇḍuratāṃ nayanti ||2||
(su| u| taṃ| a| 44) |
Over-exertion or strenuous physical exercises, sour and salty foods, alcoholic drinks, eating mud, sleeping during daytime, use of very irritating / strong / pungent substances (spices, etc.,) are the causative factors of Panduroga.
In persons who are excessively indulged in the above said causative factors, the dosas get excessively aggravated and produce whitish yellow discolouration of the skin by vitiating the rakta. This disease is called panduroga. (2)
Over-exertion or strenuous physical exercises, sour and salty foods,

alcoholic drinks, eating mud, sleeping during daytime, use of very irritating / strong / pungent substances (spices, etc.,) are the causative factors of Panduroga.
In persons who are excessively indulged in the above said causative factors, the dosas get excessively aggravated and produce whitish yellow discolouration of the skin by vitiating the rakta (blood). This disease is called panduroga. (2)

Purvarupa – premonitory symptoms of Panduroga

tvaksphoṭanaṣṭhīvanagātrasādamṛdbhakṣaṇaprekṣaṇakūṭaśothāḥ |
viṇmūtrapītatvamathāvipāko bhaviṣyatastasya puraḥsarāṇi ||3||
(su| u| taṃ| a| 44) |
Premonitory symptoms of Panduroga include - cracking of the skin, expectoration, debility, desire for eating earth (mud), oedema of the eye sockets (around the eyes), yellow discolouration of faeces and urine and indigestion. (3)

Vataja Pandu Symptoms
tvaṅmūtranayanādīnāṃ rūkṣakṛṣṇāruṇābhatāḥ |
vātapāṇḍvāmaye todakampānāhabhramādayaḥ ||4||
Symptoms of vataja pāṇdu (pandu disease caused by predominant vitiation of vata) are dryness, blackish-red discolouration of the skin, urine, eyes, etc., pricking / throbbing pain (of the body), tremors, enlargement of abdomen, giddiness, etc. (4)

Pittaja Pandu Symptoms
pītamūtraśakṛnnetro dāhatṛṣṇājvarānvitaḥ |
bhinnaviṭko'tipītābhaḥ pittapāṇḍvāmayī naraḥ ||5||
Symptoms of pittaja pāndu (pandu disease caused by predominant vitiation of pitta) – are yellowish discolouration of urine, faeces, eyes; burning sensation, thirst, fever and deep yellow discoloration of the body and watery faeces (diarrhoea). (5)

Kaphaja Pandu Symptoms
kaphaprasekaśvayathutandrālasyātigauravaiḥ |
pāṇḍurogī kaphācchuklaistvaṅmūtranayanānanaiḥ ||6||

Symptoms of kaphaja pandu (pandu disease caused by predominant vitiation of kapha) – are watery discharges (from mouth, nose, eyes etc.), oedema, drowsiness, lack of enthusiasm, excessive heaviness of the body and white discolouration of the skin, urine, eyes and face.(6)

Tridosaja Pandu Symptoms

jvarārocakahṛllāsaccharditṛṣṇāklamānvitaḥ |
pāṇḍurogī tribhirdoṣaistyājyaḥ kṣīṇo hatendriyaḥ ||7||
Symptoms of Tridosaja Pandu (pandu disease caused by predominant vitiation of kapha) – are fever, loss of taste (appetite), nausea, vomiting, thirst, tiredness / weakness. The person having the above-mentioned symptoms along with emaciation and loss of perception in the sense organs shall be considered as unfit for treatment and shall be refused treatment because this condition is incurable. (7)

Mrid Bhakshana Janya Pandu – Symptoms

mṛttikādanaśīlasya kupyatyanyatamo malaḥ |
kaṣāyā mārutaṃ, pittamūṣarā, madhurā kapham ||8||
kopayenmṛdrasādīṃścaraukṣyādbhuktaṃ ca rūkṣayet |
pūrayatyavipakvaiva srotāṃsi niruṇaddhyapi ||9||
indriyāṇāṃ balaṃ hatvā tejo vīryaujasī tathā |
pāṇḍurogaṃ karotyāśu balavarṇāgnināśanam ||10||
(ca| ci| a| 16) |
The doshas get increased in persons who have the habit of eating mud. Astringent mud increases vāta. Salty mud increases pitta. Sweet mud increases kapha.
The mud contaminates and vitiates the rasa and other tissues of the body. The mud is dry in nature and by its extreme dryness causes dryness of the food also. Mud doesn’t get digested in the body (gut). Being dry and indigestible, the mud fills up the passages of the body (mainly that of rasa dhatu) and blocks them. This leads to debility of sense organs, loss of physical strength, lustre (complexion), potency and ojas (essence of all the tissues - material responsible for natural resistance). They quickly cause pänduroga which brings about destruction of strength, normal colour and digestive fire (digestion capacity). Since this condition is caused by eating

mud, it is called mrd bhakshana janya pandu roga. (8-10)

Mrid bhakshana janya pandu lakshanas – Symptoms of pandu roga caused due to eating of mu

śūnākṣikūṭagaṇḍabhrūḥ śūnapānnābhimehanaḥ |
krimikoṣṭho'tisāryeta malaṃ sāsṛkkaphānvitam ||11||
(ca| ci| a| 16) |
Such persons (those suffering from pandu caused due to eating of mud) have oedema of the eye sockets, cheek bones, brows, feet (legs), umbilicus and genital organs; parasites develop inside their alimentary tract, eliminate watery faeces mixed with blood and mucus. (11)

Pandu Roga Asadhya Lakshanas – Signs of incurability of Pandu Roga

pāṇḍurogaścirotpannaḥ kharībhūto na sidhyati |
kālaprakarṣācchūnānāṃ yo vā pītāni paśyati ||12||
baddhālpaviṭ saharitaṃ sakaphaṃ yo'tisāryate |
dīnaḥ śvetātidigdhāṅgaśchardimūrchātṛḍarditaḥ ||13||
sa nāstyasṛkkṣayādyaśca pāṇḍuḥ śvetatvamāpnuyāt |
(ca| ci| a| 16) |
pāṇḍudantanakho yastu pāṇḍunetraśca yo bhavet |
pāṇḍusaṅghātadarśī ca pāṇḍurogī vinaśyati ||14||
(su| sū| a| 33) |
anteṣu śūnaṃ parihīṇamadhyaṃ mlānaṃ tathā'nteṣu ca madhyaśūnam |
gude ca śephasyatha muṣkayośca śūnaṃ pratāmyantamasañjñakalpam |
vivarjayetpāṇḍukinaṃ yaśo'rthī tathā'tisārajvarapīḍitaṃ ca ||15||
(su| u| taṃ| a| 44) |
Pandu roga is incurable if it is of long duration (has become chronic), and has existed for long enough to get deep seated.
It is also incurable in those people who have oedema for a long time (long standing), who sees all objects yellow (everything he sees appears yellow in colour), in those having constipation or less stools or diarrhoea with green coloured faeces mixed with mucus, who are very weak, whose body is very white / pale (due to loss of blood) i.e., the body appears as if coated in white, have vomiting, fainting and thirst. The person whose body becomes white due to excessive loss of blood will not survive.

Persons whose teeth, nails, eyes have become pale (yellowish white) and who sees everything around him as being pale (yellowish white) are going to die of panduroga.

Patients (of pandu roga) who have oedema of the extremities i.e. the limbs and head are swollen but the middle part of the body (trunk) is emaciated or patients who have swelling of the trunk while the limbs and head are not swollen should be considered as incurable.

Those who have swelling of rectum, penis and scrotum, who faint often and have loss of consciousness, who are having diarrhoea and fever are also to be refused treatment (because these conditions will be incurable). (12-15)

Nidana, Samprapti of Kamala Roga – Etiological factors and pathogenesis of Jaundice

pāṇḍurogī tu yo'tyarthaṃ pittalāni niṣevate |
tasya pittamasṛṅmāṃsaṃ dagdhvā rogāya kalpate ||16||

In such patients of pandu roga, who indulge in foods and habits which increase pitta, the pitta would get abnormally increased. This pitta on getting increased burns up the rakta (blood) and mamsa (muscle tissue) and produces the disease known as kamala. (16)

Symptoms of Kamala, Manifestation of Kumbha-kamala

hāridranetraḥsabhṛśaṃhāridratvaṅgakhānanaḥ|
raktapītaśakṛnmatrobhekavarṇohatendriyaḥ||17||
dāhāvipākadaurbalyasadanārucikarṣitaḥ|
kāmalābahupittaiṣākoṣṭhaśākhāśrayāmatā||18|| (ca| ci| a| 16)
kālāntarāt kharībhūtā kṛcchrā syāt kumbhakāmalā |19| (ca| ci| a| 16) |

The symptoms of kamala (jaundice) include - deep turmeric (yellow) colouration of the eyes, skin, nails and face, reddish-yellow faeces and urine, skin colour resembling that of frog (greenish, brown, or brownish yellow), weakness of sense organs, burning sensation, indigestion, weakness, debility, anorexia are the symptoms of kamala (jaundice). It involves both the kostha (alimentary tract) and also the shaka (rakta - blood and other tissues).

If left untreated kamala makes the organs rough (dry) / hard and turns into a difficult disease called kumbha-kamala. (17-18)

Signs of incurability of Kamala and Kumbha-kamala

kṛṣṇapītaśakṛnmūtro bhṛśaṃ śūnaśca mānavaḥ ||19||
saraktākṣimukhacchardiviṇmūtro yaśca tāmyati |
dāhārucitṛḍānāhatandrāmohasamanvitaḥ ||20||
naṣṭāgnisañjñaḥ kṣipraṃ hi kāmalāvān vipadyate |
(ca| ci| a| 16) |
chardyarocakahṛllāsajvaraklamanipīḍitaḥ ||21||
naśyati śvāsakāsārto viḍbhedī kumbhakāmalī |22|
The patient suffering from Kamala – jaundice will die soon if he has these symptoms – blackish-yellow faeces and urine, profound oedema, bleeding in the eyes and mouth; vomitus, faeces and urine also mixed with blood; loss of consciousness (fainting), burning sensation, anorexia, thirst, constipation or blockages caused in the stomach by ama or colon by impacted faeces, stupor, delusion, loss of digestion capacity and unconsciousness with.
The patient of kumbha kamala also dies if he has vomiting, anorexia, nausea, fever, debility, dyspnoea (increased / difficult respiration), cough or diarrhoea. (19-21)

Halimaka Symptoms

yadā tu pāṇḍorvarṇaḥ syāddharitaḥ śyāvapītakaḥ ||22||
balotsāhakṣayastandrā mandāgnitvaṃ mṛdujvaraḥ |
strīṣvaharṣo'ṅgamardaśca dāhastṛṣṇā'rucirbhramaḥ |
halīmakaṃ tadā tasya vidyādanilapittataḥ ||23||
When the colour of the skin (or nails, eyes, urine etc) of the patient of Pandu roga turns into yellow, green or blackish yellow colour, has loss of strength and enthusiasm, stupor, poor digestion, mild fever, disinterestedness in women (sex), pain in the body, burning sensation, thirst, anorexia, giddiness - the disease is to be known as halimaka (chlorosis) which is due to increased vata and pitta. (22-23)

Symptoms of Panaki

(santāpo bhinnavarcastvaṃ bahirantaśca pītatā |
pāṇḍutā netrayoryasya pānakīlakṣaṇaṃ bhavet) |
(ca| ci| a| 16) |
(Fever, diarrhoea, yellow colouration both externally and internally and pale eyes - these are the symptoms of the disease called 'Panaki'.)

iti śrīmādhavakaraviracite mādhavanidāne pāṇḍurogakāmalākumbhakāmalāhalīmakanidānaṃ samāptam ||8||||
Thus ends the chapter on Panduroga, Kamala, etc.

CHAPTER NINE

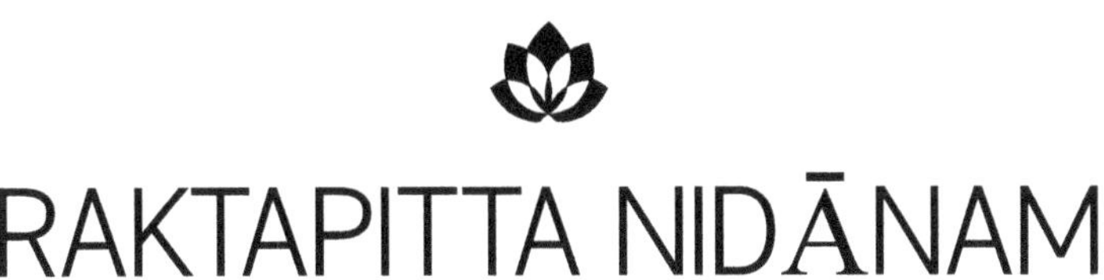

RAKTAPITTA NIDĀNAM

Nidana and Samprapti – Etiological factors and pathogenesis of Raktapitt

gharmavyāyāmaśokādhvavyavāyairatisevitaiḥ |
tīkṣṇoṣṇakṣāralavaṇairamlaiḥ kaṭubhireva ca ||1||
pittaṃ vidagdhaṃ svaguṇairvidahatyāśu śoṇitam |
tataḥ pravartate raktamūrdhvaṃ cādho dvidhā'pi vā ||2||
(su| u| taṃ| a| 45) |
ūrdhvaṃ nāsākṣikarṇāsyairmeḍhrayonigudairadhaḥ |
kupitaṃ romakūpaiśca samastaistatpravartate ||3||
Etiological factors of raktapitta include excessive exposure to sunlight, physical exercise, grief, walking long distances, excessive sexual intercourse; consumption of foods which are hot, alkaline, salty, sour and pungent.

Pathogenesis - All the above said causative factors when consumed lead to abnormal increase of pitta in its vidagdha state (by its uşna,tīksna properties). This aggravated pitta afflicts rakta – blood and quickly causes increase of blood and causes it to flow out of the body through upper or lower orifices or through both these orifices, viz, nostrils, eyes, ears and mouth being the upper passages and the urethra, vagina, rectum being the lower passages. In severe conditions, blood comes out of the hair follicles of the skin also.(1-3)

Purvarupa – premonitory symptoms of raktapitta

sadanaṃ śītakāmitvaṃ kaṇṭhadhūmāyanaṃ vamiḥ |
lohagandhiśca niḥśvāso bhavatyasmin bhaviṣyati ||4||
(su| u| taṃ| a| 45) |

Weakness, desire for cold things (food, drink, places, etc.,) feeling as though hot fumes are coming out of the throat, vomiting, smell of iron in the breath – are the premonitory symptoms of Raktapitta. (4)

Dosha association in Raktapitta

sāndraṃ sapāṇḍu sasnehaṃ picchilaṃ ca kaphānvitam |5| (ca| ci| a| 4) |
śyāvāruṇaṃ saphenaṃ ca tanu rūkṣaṃ ca vātikam ||5|| (ca| ci| a| 4) |
raktapittaṃ kaṣāyābhaṃ kṛṣṇaṃ gomūtrasannibham |
mecakāgāradhūmābhamañjanābhaṃ ca paittikam ||6|| (ca| ci| a| 4) |
saṃsṛṣṭaliṅgaṃ saṃsargāttriliṅgaṃ sānnipātikam | (ca| ci| a| 4) |
If kapha is associated, the blood coming out will be thick, yellowish, white, greasy and sticky.
If vāta is associated, the blood will be blackish red, frothy, thin and viscid.
If pitta alone is the cause, the blood coming out will be black resembling decoction of drugs, cow's urine, and black pigment of a cymbal, chimney soot or antimony.
If there is a combination of two or three doshas their specific symptoms are also found together. (5-6)

Dosha association in raktapitta having upward (urdhwaga) and downward (adhoga) course

ūrdhvagaṃ kaphasaṃsṛṣṭamadhogaṃ pavanānugam |
dvimārgaṃ kaphavātābhyāmubhābhyāmanuvartate ||7|| (ca| ci| a| 4) |
The upward one (i.e., rakta-pitta having upward course and bleeding occurring from upward orifices) is by association of kapha and the downward one (i.e., raktapitta having downward course and bleeding occurring from downward passages / orifices) is by association of vāta. Kapha and Väta together will cause for both the upward and downward movement (bleeding) of raktapitta.(7)

Sadhyadadhyata – prognosis of raktapitta

ūrdhvaṃ sādhyamadho yāpyamasādhyaṃ yugapadgatam |8| (su| u| taṃ| a| 45) |
ekamārgaṃ balavato nātivegaṃ navotthitam ||8||

raktapittaṃ sukhe kāle sādhyaṃ syānnirupadravam | (ca| ci| a| 4) |
Upward one (raktapitta having upward course) is easy to cure.
Downward one (raktapitta having downward course) is manageable i.e. persists all through life and can be handled with effective treatments and medicines from time to time.
Raktapitta having its course in both directions is incurable (impossible to cure).

Raktapitta is easy to treat, if bleeding occurs from any one passage, in persons who are strong, if bleeding is not large, if it is of recent origin, if seen in good season (favourable season for its cure) and if not associated with other complications.(8)

ekadoṣānugaṃ sādhyaṃ dvidoṣaṃ yāpyamucyate ||9||
yattridoṣamasādhyaṃ syānmandāgnerativegavat |
vyādhibhiḥ kṣīṇadehasya vṛddhasyānaśnataśca yat ||10||
(ca| ci| a| 4) |
Raktapitta is easy to treat if only one dosha is associated, is manageable (persists for life) if two doshas are associated and incurable if all the three doshas are involved. Likewise in persons having poor digestive functions where bleeding is copious; in persons debilitated by other diseases, who are of advanced age and who do not take any food, raktapitta is incurable.(9-10)

Upadrava – complications of raktapitta

daurbalyaśvāsakāsajvaravamathumadāḥ pāṇḍutādāhamūrchā,
bhukte ghoro vidāhastvadhṛtirapi sadā hṛdyatulyā ca pīḍā |
tṛṣṇā koṣṭhasya bhedaḥ śirasi ca tapanaṃ pūtiniṣṭhīvanatvaṃ,
bhaktadveṣāvipākau vikṛtirapi bhavedraktapittopasargāḥ ||11||
(su| u| taṃ| a| 45) |
Debility, dyspnoea (increased / difficult respiration), cough, fever, vomiting, intoxication, pallor (yellowish-white discolouration) ,burning sensation, fainting, severe heart-burn after consumption of food, constant anxiety, severe pain near the heart, thirst, tearing pain in the abdomen, headache, bad smelling sputum coming out, aversion to food and indigestion and abnormal colour of the blood, are the complications of raktapitta. (11)

Signs of incurability of Raktapitta

māṃsaprakṣālanābhaṃ kuthitamiva ca yat kardamāmbhonibhaṃ vā,
medaḥpūyāsrakalpaṃ yakṛdiva yadi vā pakvajambūphalābham |
yat kṛṣṇaṃ yacca nīlaṃ bhṛśamatikuṇapaṃ yatra coktā vikārā
stadvarjyaṃ raktapittaṃ surapatidhanuṣā yacca tulyaṃ vibhāti ||12||(su| u| taṃ| a| 45) |
Patients in whom the blood coming out resembles water in which mutton has been washed, a decoction, muddy water with lot of silt, fat, pus, pieces of liver, ripe fruit of jambu (Eugenia Jambolana),which is black or blue in color, which smells like a cadaver, or resembles a rainbow and who have one or more of the complications cited above - are to be refused treatment (i.e. in the presence of the above mentioned signs, raktapitta is considered as incurable and hence the physician shall refuse treating such patients). (12)

yena copahato raktaṃ raktapittena mānavaḥ | paśyeddṛśyaṃ viyaccāpi taccāsādhyamasaṃśayam ||13||
(ca| ni| a| 2) |
lohitaṃ chardayedyastu bahuśo lohitekṣaṇaḥ | lohitodgāradarśī ca mriyate raktapaittikaḥ ||14||
(su| sū| a| 33) |
If the patient (of raktapitta) sees everything visible (visible objects) and invisible (space, sky etc and those which doesn't have any colour) as red in colour, raktapitta should be considered as incurable.
If the patient of raktapitta vomits blood in large quantity, who sees everything as red, who gets belching accompanied with bleeding (or gets belching having the smell of iron) is going to die (i.e., such raktapitta conditions are definitely incurable and would lead to death). (13-14)

iti śrīmādhavakaraviracite mādhavanidāne raktapittanidānaṃ samāptam ||9||
Thus ends the chapter on Raktapitta.

CHAPTER TEN

RĀJAYAKṢMĀ-KṢATAKṢINA NIDĀNAM

4 main causes of Rajayakshma

vegarodhāt kṣayāccaiva sāhasādviṣamāśanāt |
tridoṣo jāyate yakṣmā gado hetucatuṣṭayāt ||1||
Yakṣmā is a disease caused by all the three doshas together. Below mentioned are the four important factors which would produce yakṣmā.

1. Suppression of natural urges
2. Loss or deficiency of tissues
3. Over-exertion and
4. Indulgence in unhealthy foods (1)

Samprapti – pathogenesis of yaksma

kaphapradhānairdoṣaistu ruddheṣu rasavartmasu |
ativyavāyino vā'pi kṣīṇe retasyanantarāḥ |
kṣīyante dhātavaḥ sarve tataḥ śuṣyati mānavaḥ ||2||
There are two pathways in which yaksma develops

1. When the rasavaha srotas (channels through which rasadhātu i.e., blood plasma circulates) become obstructed by the tridoshas among which kapha is predominant or
2. In persons who indulge in excessive sexual intercourse leading to the loss of semen

When these events occur, they cause deficiency of all the other dhātus – tissues of the body making the person too emaciated. Such a disease is called yaksma or rajayaksma. (2)

Purvarupa – premonitory symptoms of Rajayaksma

śvāsāṅgamardakaphasaṃsravatāluśoṣavamyagnisādamadapīnasakāsanidrāḥ |
śoṣe bhaviṣyati bhavanti sa cāpi jantuḥ śuklekṣaṇo bhavati māṃsaparo riraṃsuḥ ||3||
(su| u| taṃ| a| 41) |
svapneṣu kākaśukaśallakinīlakaṇṭhā gṛdhrāstathaiva kapayaḥ kṛkalāsakāśca |
taṃ vāhayanti sa nadīrvijalāśca paśyecchuṣkāṃstarūn pavanadhūmadavārditāṃśca ||4||
(su| u| taṃ| a| 41) |
The premonitory symptoms of rajayaksma include - dyspnoea (breathlessness, increased / difficult respiration), pain in the body, expectoration of sputum, dryness of the palate, vomiting, poor digestion, intoxication, running nose, cough, excessive sleep, eyes becoming bright white; person craves for meat and sexual intercourse. In his dreams he sees himself being carried away by the crow, parrot, porcupine, peacock vultures, monkey and chameleon, sees rivers without water, trees without leaves, breeze, smoke and forest fires. (3-4)

Lakshana – symptoms of Rajayaksma

aṃsapārśvābhitāpaśca santāpaḥ karapādayoḥ |
jvaraḥ sarvāṅgagaśceti lakṣaṇaṃ rājayakṣmaṇaḥ ||5|| (ca| ci| a| 8) |
(bhaktadveṣo jvaraḥ śvāsaḥ kāsaḥ śoṇitadarśanam |
svarabhedaśca jāyeta ṣaḍrūpaṃ rājayakṣmaṇi) |6|
Discomfort (pain) in the scapular region (shoulders) and flanks, feeling of warmth (mild burning sensation) in the hands and feet, fever all over the body are the symptoms of rājavaksmā.(5)
(According to other opinions - aversion to food, fever, dyspnoea or increased / difficult respiration, cough appearance of blood in the sputum and hoarseness of voice are the six symptoms of rajayakshma.)

Ekadasha Lakshanas – 11 symptoms of Rajayaksma

svarabhedo'nilācchūlaṃ saṅkocaścāṃsapārśvayoḥ |
jvaro dāho'tisāraśca pittādraktasya cāgamaḥ ||6|| (su| u| taṃ| a| 41) |
śirasaḥ paripūrṇatvamabhaktacchanda eva ca |
kāsaḥ kaṇṭhasya coddhvaṃso vijñeyaḥ kaphakopataḥ ||7|| (su| u| taṃ| a| 41) |
Symptoms caused by Vata predominance are 3 in number - Hoarseness of voice, pain in the shoulders, constriction (deformity) of shoulders and flanks
Symptoms caused by Pitta predominance are 4 in number - Fever, burning sensation, diarrhoea and blood in the sputum (haemoptysis)
Symptoms caused by Kapha predominance are 4 in number - Feeling of fullness of the head, aversion to food, cough and irritation in the throat
These are the (eleven) important symptoms of Rajayaksma. (6-7)

Six symptoms and Three symptoms, Prognosis of Rajayaksma

ekādaśabhirebhirvā ṣaḍbhirvā'pi samanvitam |
kāsātīsārapārśvārtisvarabhedārucijvaraiḥ ||8||
tribhirvā pīḍitaṃ liṅgaiḥ kāsaśvāsāsṛgāmayaiḥ |
jahyācchoṣārditaṃ jantumicchan suvimalaṃ yaśaḥ ||9|| (su| u| taṃ| a| 41) |
sarvairardhaistribhirvā'pi liṅgairmāṃsabalakṣaye | yukto varjyaścikitsyastu sarvarūpo'pyato'nyathā ||10||
mahāśanaṃ kṣīyamāṇamatīsāranipīḍitam | śūnamuṣkodaraṃ caiva yakṣmiṇaṃ parivarjayet ||11||
śuklākṣamannadveṣṭāramūrdhvaśvāsanipīḍitam | kṛcchreṇa bahumehantaṃ yakṣmā hantīha mānavam ||12||
Presence of all the eleven symptoms (enumerated above) or the six symptoms viz., cough diarrhoea, pain in the flanks, hoarseness of voice, anorexia and fever or even the three symptoms viz., cough, dyspnoea (increased / difficult respiration and appearance of blood in the sputum - calls for refusal of such patients by physicians desiring a good reputation.
This means to say that in the presence of all these symptoms together will indicate bad prognosis and hence the doctor can deny treating such conditions by the physicians who want to keep away from getting a bad name and reputation.

Appearance of all the symptoms (11 symptoms), or half of it (six – approximately half of eleven) or of even three, in persons who have loss of muscles (wasting of muscles) and strength are also indications of bad prognosis and hence should be refused by a wise physician.
Patients of yaksmā who eat large quantities of food but still undergo wasting; who are having diarrhoea, swelling of the scrotum and abdomen are also to be avoided (denied treatment).
Yaksma kills such persons who have whiteness of eyes, aversion to food, heavy and troublesome expirations and who eliminate large quantities of urine with difficulty. (8-12)

Conditions for treating the patients of Rajayaksma

jvarānubandharahitaṃ balavantaṃ kriyāsaham |
upakramedātmavantaṃ dīptāgnimakṛśaṃ naram ||13||
(su| u| taṃ| a| 41) |
Treatment can be given to patients of yakşmā who do not have fever, who are strong, able to withstand the discomforts of treatments, of strong will, good (strong) digestive capacity and who are not emaciated.(13)

Types of Sosa

vyavāyaśokavārdhakyavyāyāmādhvapraśoṣitān |
vraṇorahkṣatasañjñau ca śoṣiṇau lakṣaṇaiḥ śṛṇu ||14||
(su| u| taṃ| a| 41) |
Shosha (consumption, wasting, emaciation) is of 7 types. They are caused due to –

- sexual intercourse
- grief
- old age
- physical exertion,
- walking long distances,
- ulcers and
- injury to the chest

Henceforth the symptoms of the persons afflicted with above mentioned types of sosas are described. (14)

Vyavaya Sosa Lakshanas – Symptoms of wasting caused due to excessive indulgence in sexual intercourse

vyavāyaśoṣī śukrasya kṣayaliṅgairupadrutaḥ |
pāṇḍudeho yathāpūrvaṃ kṣīyante cāsya dhātavaḥ ||15||
(su| u| taṃ| a| 41) |

In persons who indulge in excessive sexual intercourse, symptoms of deficiency of semen and yellowish white discolouration of the body (pallor) and subsequent wasting of the other tissues of the body are seen. (15)

Soka Sosa & Jara Sosa Lakshanas – Symptoms of wasting caused due to grief & ageing

pradhyānaśīlaḥ srastāṅgaḥ śokaśoṣyapi tādṛśaḥ |16| (su| u| taṃ| a| 41) |
jarāśoṣī kṛśo mandavīryabuddhibalendriyaḥ ||16||
kampano'rucimān bhinnakāṃsyapātrahatasvaraḥ |
ṣṭhīvati śleṣmaṇā hīnaṃ gauravāratipīḍitaḥ ||17||
samprasrutāsyanāsākṣiḥ śuṣkarūkṣamalacchaviḥ |
(su| u| taṃ| a| 41) |

In people whose body is wasted due to excessive grief, too much of worry, looseness and weakness of the body are seen.

The symptoms of persons wasted due to senility (old age) include - emaciation, decrease of vigour, intellect, strength and capacity of sense organs; shaking of the body parts and anorexia. The voice of such a person would be husky, feeble and broken as that of a piece of broken bronze vessel. The patient tries hard to expectorate but brings out little sputum or no sputum. The other symptoms are heaviness of the body, restlessness, fluid oozing out of mouth, nose and eyes, loss of complexion and dryness (of faeces).(16-17)

Adhwa Sosa Lakshanas – Symptoms of wasting due to constant long-distance walking

adhvaśoṣī ca srastāṅgaḥ sambhṛṣṭaparuṣacchaviḥ ||18||
prasuptagātrāvayavaḥ śuṣkaklomagalānanaḥ |
(su| u| taṃ| a| 41) |

Persons wasted due to constant long-distance walking will be having weakness, hardness and loss of sensation of body parts, dryness of klomā, throat and mouth. (18)

Note – Kloma is an organ whose description has not been detailed in Ayurveda texts. As per this context and kloma being one of the roots of 'water transporting channels' in the body, it can be considered as pharynx or palate (roof of the inside of the mouth).

Vyayama Sosa – Symptoms of wasting caused due to excessive physical exertion

vyāyāmaśoṣī bhūyiṣṭhamebhireva samanvitaḥ |
liṅgairuraḥkṣatakṛtaiḥ saṃyuktaśca kṣataṃ vinā ||19||
(su| u| taṃ| a| 41) |

Persons wasted due to excess physical exertion will also have the same symptoms as above and symptoms of injury to the chest without of course an actual tear. (19)

Vrana Sosa – Symptoms of wasting caused due to ulcer / wound

raktakṣayādvedanābhistathaivāhārayantraṇāt |
vraṇitasya bhavecchoṣaḥ sa cāsādhyatamo mataḥ ||20||
(su| u| taṃ| a| 41) |

Wasting due to ulcer is caused by loss of blood, pain and control over food by the person. This condition is difficult to treat.(20)

Urah Kshata Nidana – Lakshanas – Causes and symptoms of 'chest injury'

dhanuṣā''yasyato'tyarthaṃ bhāramudvahato gurum |
yudhyamānasya balibhiḥ patato viṣamoccataḥ ||21||
vṛṣaṃ hayaṃ vā dhāvantaṃ damyaṃ vā'nyaṃ nigṛhṇataḥ |
śilākāṣṭhāśmanirghātān kṣipato nighnataḥ parān ||22||
adhīyānasya vā'tyuccairdūraṃ vā vrajato drutam |
mahānadīrvā tarato hayairvā saha dhāvataḥ ||23||
sahasotpatato dūraṃ tūrṇaṃ vā'pi pranṛtyataḥ |
tathā'nyaiḥ karmabhiḥ krūrairbhṛśamabhyāhatasya vā ||24||
vikṣate vakṣasi vyādhirbalavān samudīryate |
strīṣu cātiprasaktasya rūkṣālpapramitāśinaḥ ||25||
uro vibhajyate'tyarthaṃ bhidyate'tha virujyate |
prapīḍyate tataḥ pārśve śuṣyatyaṅgaṃ pravepate ||26||
kramādvīryaṃ balaṃ varṇo ruciragniśca hīyate |
jvaro vyathā manodainyaṃ viḍbhedāgnivadhāvapi ||27||
duṣṭaḥ śyāvaḥ sudurgandhaḥ pīto vigrathito bahuḥ |

kāsamānasya cābhīkṣṇaṃ kaphaḥ sāsṛk pravartate ||28||
sa kṣatī kṣīyate'tyarthaṃ tathā śukraujasoḥ kṣayāt |
(ca| ci| a| 16) |

Chest injury (tear inside the lungs) is caused due to one or more of - excessive indulgence in archery, carrying heavy loads on the head, combating / wrestling with strong persons, falling from a height recklessly, forcibly trying to stop a mighty bull or horse which is running, or taming wild animals, throwing heavy stones, wooden rafters or catapults, fighting with enemies (using weapons),reading loudly with high pitch, running fast for long distances, swimming mighty rivers, running along with horses, sudden jumping, strenuous dancing and such other acts of violence and excessive sexual intercourse, partaking of dry, scanty and non-nutritious foods.

As a result, the patient will have cut or pricking pain in the chest and flanks, followed by emaciation, tremors; loss of vigour, strength, complexion, interest and digestive capacity.

There also occurs the appearance of fever, grief, helplessness, diarrhoea, indigestion, cough with bad, black, fetid, yellowish pellets of sputum in large quantities coming out often mixed with blood. This condition is known as 'uraksata'. This condition causes quick loss of sukra (semen) and ojas (essence of all the tissues) and leads to severe emaciation.(20-28)

Purvarupa – premonitory symptoms

avyaktaṃ lakṣaṇaṃ tasya pūrvarūpamiti smṛtam ||29||

The very symptoms of this disease itself are seen in mild form during the premonitory period. (29)

Difference between Ksata and Ksina

uroruk śoṇitacchardiḥ kāso vaiśeṣikaḥ kṣate |
kṣīṇe saraktamūtratvaṃ pārśvapṛṣṭhakaṭīgrahaḥ ||30||
(ca| ci| a| 16) |

Pain in the chest, vomiting of blood, cough is prominent if ksata - trauma (tear) is present. On the other hand, if only emaciation is present, urine mixed with blood, catching pain in the flanks, back and waist (hips) are predominant. (30)

Prognosis of the disease

alpaliṅgasya dīptāgneḥ sādhyo balavato navaḥ |

parisaṃvatsaro yāpyaḥ sarvaliṅgaṃ tu varjayet ||31||
(ca| ci| a| 16) |

Uraksata which has mild symptoms, manifesting in strong persons, is of recent origin and occurring in whom the digestive capacity is good is curable.

Uraksata which has remained over one year (one year old), does persist throughout life, and that which has all the symptoms is incurable. (31)

इति श्रीमाधवकरविरचिते माधवनिदाने राजयक्ष्मक्षतक्षीणनिदानं समाप्तम् ||१०||

iti śrīmādhavakaraviracite mādhavanidāne rājayakṣmakṣatakṣīṇanidānaṃ samāptam ||10||

Thus ends the chapter on Rājayaksmā

CHAPTER ELEVEN

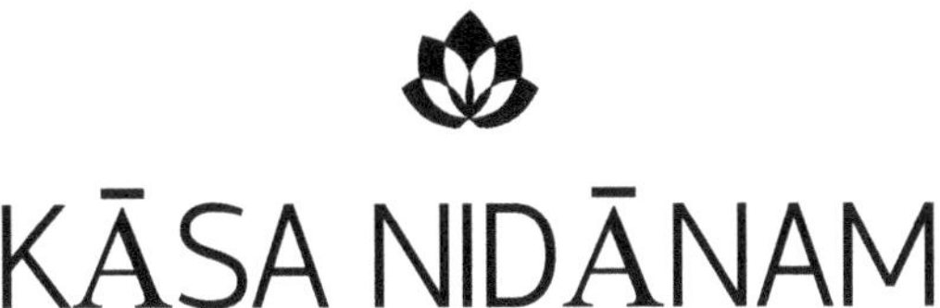

KĀSA NIDĀNAM

Kasa Nidana & Samprapti – etiological factors and pathogenesis of cough

dhūmopaghātādrasatastathaiva vyāyāmarūkṣānnaniṣevaṇācca |
vimārgagatvācca hi bhojanasya vegāvarodhāt kṣavathostathaiva ||1||
prāṇo hyudānānugataḥ praduṣṭaḥ sa bhinnakāṃsyasvanatulyaghoṣaḥ |
nireti vaktrāt sahasā sadoṣo manīṣibhiḥ kāsa iti pradiṣṭaḥ ||2||
(su| u| taṃ| a| 52) |
The etiological factors of Kasa – cough are as enlisted below –

- Smoke entering the nose, mouth and throat and harming these organs,
- Dust entering the nose, mouth and throat and harming these organs
- Excessive indulgence in exercises (strenuous physical activities)
- Excessive consumption of foods which are dry in nature
- Entry of the consumed food into wrong passages (respiratory passages – trachea etc)
- Suppression of natural urges of the body
- Suppression / forcibly controlling the sneezing urge

Pathogenesis of Kasa – cough:

The prana vata aggravated due to the above said etiological factors gets mixed (associated) with udana vata and comes out of the mouth suddenly, along with the other dosas (pitta and kapha), producing a sound resembling that made by obstructing (or hitting against) a broken piece of bronze. This disease is called kāsa (cough). (1-2)

Kasa Bheda – types of coughs

pañca kāsāḥ smṛtā vātapittaśleṣmakṣatakṣayaiḥ |
kṣayāyopekṣitāḥ sarve balinaścottarottaram ||3||
(a| hṛ| ni| a| 3) |

Kāsa is of five kinds –

- Vataja kasa – caused by predominant vitiation of vata
- Pittaja kasa – caused by predominant aggravation of pitta
- Kaphaja kasa – caused by predominant aggravation of kapha
- Ksataja kasa – caused due to the chest injury
- Ksayaja kasa – caused due to loss of tissues

The first four types of kasa if neglected will lead to ksaya (dhātuksaya-wasting of the tissues). These five types of kasa are stronger (dangerous, damaging, harmful) in the successive order. (3)

Note – going with strength of kasa as mentioned in the above said context –

Pittaja Kasa is stronger than Vataja Kasa.
Kaphaja Kasa is stronger than Pittaja Kasa.
Ksataja Kasa is stronger than Kaphaja Kasa.
Ksayaja Kasa is stronger than Ksataja Kasa.

Therefore, Ksayaja Kasa is more powerful and troublesome amongst all the kasa and Vataja Kasa is the least troublesome one. The prognosis of kasa also will follow the same chronology.

Purvarupa – premonitory symptoms of cough

pūrvarūpaṃ bhavetteṣāṃ śūkapūrṇagalāsyatā |
kaṇṭhe kaṇḍūśca bhojyānāmavarodhaśca jāyate ||4||
(ca| ci| a| 22) |
Premonitory symptoms (of cough) are - feeling as if the throat and mouth are filled with thorns / spikes and (pricking inside these organs), itching

sensation inside the throat and obstruction to inward movement of food (swallowing). (4)

Vataja Kasa – symptoms

hṛcchaṅkhamūrdhodarapārśvaśūlī kṣāmānanaḥ kṣīṇabalasvaraujāḥ |
prasaktavegastu samīraṇena bhinnasvaraḥ kāsati śuṣkameva ||5||
(su| u| taṃ| a| 52) |
In Vatika Kasa, the person suffers from - pain in the region of the heart, temples, head, abdomen and flanks; dry face (mouth), loss of strength, voice and ojas (essence of all the tissues, enthusiasm). The person will have continuous bouts of husky (small) and dry cough, and cracked voice due to aggravation of vata. (5)

Pittaja Kasa – symptoms

urovidāhajvaravaktraśoṣairabhyarditastiktamukhastṛṣārtaḥ |
pittena pītāni vamet kaṭūni kāset sapāṇḍuḥ paridahyamānaḥ ||6||
(su| u| taṃ| a| 52) |
In pittaja kasa, the person will have a burning sensation in the chest, fever, dryness of the mouth, bitter taste in the mouth, severe thirst, and bitter taste in the mouth, severe thirst, vomiting with the contents appearing yellow in colour and bitter in taste, anaemia and burning sensation inside the body. (6)

Kaphaja Kasa – symptoms

pralipyamānena mukhena sīdan śirorujārtaḥ kaphapūrṇadehaḥ |
abhaktaruggauravakaṇḍuyuktaḥ kāsedbhṛśaṃ sāndrakaphaḥ kaphena ||7||
(su| u| taṃ| a| 52) |
The symptoms of kaphaja kasa are – inside of the mouth is coated with thick secretions (saliva), weakness, headache, accumulation of kapha in the entire body, anorexia / tastelessness, heaviness, itching, heavy cough along with expectoration of thick sputum. (7)

Ksataja Kasa – causes, symptoms

ativyavāyabhārādhvayuddhāśvagajavigrahaiḥ |
rūkṣasyoraḥkṣataṃ vāyurgṛhītvā kāsamācaret ||8||
sa pūrvaṃ kāsate śuṣkaṃ tataḥ ṣṭhīvet saśoṇitam |
kaṇṭhena rujatā'tyarthaṃ virugṇeneva corasā ||9||
sūcībhiriva tīkṣṇābhistudyamānena śūlinā |
duḥkhasparśena śūlena bhedapīḍābhitāpinā ||10||
parvabhedajvaraśvāsatṛṣṇāvaisvaryapīḍitaḥ |
pārāvata ivākūjan kāsavegāt kṣatodbhavāt ||11||
(su| u| taṃ| a| 52) |

Etiological Factors – Excessive indulgence in sexual intercourse, carrying heavy weights, walking long distances, wrestling, taming or fighting with horses and elephants (forcibly trying to stop the running of horses and elephants) etc. are the causative factors of ksataja kasa.

Pathogenesis – The above-mentioned etiological factors cause injury in the chest (tear in the lungs) in a person who is dry (weak). The aggravated vata reaches the site of injury and produces cough.

Symptoms – Below mentioned are the symptoms of Ksataja Kasa –
Initially the person suffers from dry cough. Later this is followed by expectoration of blood mixed sputum.
The other symptoms include –

- Severe pain in the throat
- Severe pain in the chest
- The person feels as if he is pricked by sharp needles in the chest (and throat) / cutting or gnawing pain
- Intolerance to touch (the patient resists others from touching the afflicted area, painful area) / tenderness,
- Splitting pain and pain associated with burning sensation
- Splitting pain in the small joints of the hands and feet (interphalangeal joints),
- Fever
- Dyspnoea
- Severe thirst
- Hoarseness (change of) of voice
- Makes sounds from the throat resembling that of a pigeon (8-11)

Ksayaja Kasa – causes, symptoms

viṣamāsātmyabhojyātivyavāyādveganigrahāt |
ghṛṇināṃ śocatāṃ nṝṇāṃ vyāpanne'gnau trayo malāḥ |
kupitāḥ kṣayajaṃ kāsaṃ kuryurdehakṣayapradam ||12||
sa gātraśūlajvaradāhamohān prāṇakṣayaṃ copalabheta kāsī |
śuṣyan viniṣṭhīvati durbalastu prakṣīṇamāṃso rudhiraṃ sapūyam |
taṃ sarvaliṅgaṃ bhṛśaduścikitsyaṃ cikitsitajñāḥ kṣayajaṃ vadanti ||13||
(su| u| taṃ| a| 52) |
Etiological factors - Indulgence in irregular and untimely meals, unaccustomed foods, indulgence in excessive sex, suppression of bodily urges, too much jealousy, grief, etc.
Pathogenesis – Due to the above said etiological factors, the digestive fire gets contaminated. This fire in turn causes aggravation of all the three doshas. These aggravated dosas produce ksayaja kasa which would cause destruction of the body (wasting of body tissues).

Symptoms – Ksayaja Kasa would present with symptoms including pain in the body parts (all over the body), fever, burning sensation, delusion & threat to life. There occurs severe dryness / wasting of the body, extreme weakness, deterioration (destruction) of strength and muscles, and the patient expectorates blood with pus as he coughs. This form of cough having all the symptoms (symptoms caused by all three doshas) and is difficult to cure is called by the name Ksayaja Kasa by the clinical experts who are well versed in the knowledge of treatment principles (of Ayurveda). This cough would kill the weak ones. (12-14)

Prognosis

sādhyo balavatāṃ vā syādyāpyastvevaṃ kṣatotthitaḥ ||14||
navau kadācitsidhyetāmapi pādaguṇānvitau |
sthavirāṇāṃ jarākāsaḥ sarvo yāpyaḥ prakīrtitaḥ |
trīn pūrvān sādhayet sādhyān pathyairyāpyāṃstu yāpayet ||15||
(su| u| taṃ| a| 52) |
In strong people this cough (ksayaja) is sometimes curable and sometimes manageable.

Similarly, the ksataja kasa caused by chest injury is curable in weak and emaciated patients. It is sometimes curable and sometimes manageable in strong patients.
Ksayaja or Ksataja Kasa of recent origin are sometimes curable if the four limbs of treatment (physician, patient, medicines and attendants) are bestowed with good qualities and are operational towards cure of the disease.

All kinds of kasa caused due to ageing (and natural depletion of tissues occurring in the old age) are manageable in older persons if the four limbs of treatment are bestowed with good qualities.
The first three kinds of kasa (i.e., vataja, pittaja and kaphaja) are easily curable. Therefore, they shall be treated. The manageable kinds (chronic) of kasa shall be controlled by using a suitable diet etc. (15)

iti śrīmādhavakaraviracite mādhavanidāne kāsanidānaṃ samāptam ||11||
Thus ends the chapter of Kāsa.

CHAPTER TWELVE

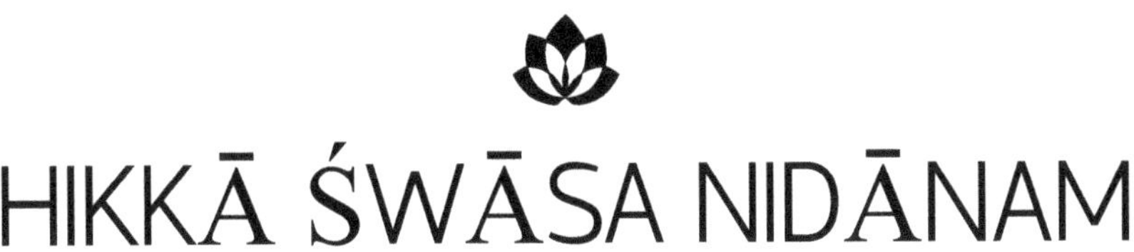

HIKKĀ ŚWĀSA NIDĀNAM

Hikka Swasa Nidanam – Etiological factors of hiccough and dyspnoe

vidāhiguruviṣṭambhirūkṣābhiṣyandibhojanaiḥ |
śītapānāśanasthānarajodhūmātapānilaiḥ ||1||
vyāyāmakarmabhārādhvavegāghātāpatarpaṇaiḥ |
hikkā śvāsaśca kāsaśca nṛṇāṃ samupajāyate ||2||
(su| u| taṃ| a| 50) |

Below mentioned are the etiological factors of hiccough and dyspnoea –

Excessive indulgence in foods which are corrosive (produce heartburn), heavy (difficult to digest), which could cause constipation, dry in nature and which cause blockages in the pores of the tissues or channels of transportation,
Excessive consumption of very cold water (or other beverages) and foods,
Starvation,
Living in cold places
Exposure to dust, smoke, sunlight and breeze,
Excessive physical exercise / exertion
Indulgence in activities beyond one's capacity,
Lifting or carrying heavy weights,
Walking long distances,
Suppression of natural urges and
Malnutrition

The person who indulges in the above-mentioned etiological factors becomes victim of hikkā (hiccough), śwāsa (dyspnoea / difficult respiration) and kasa (cough).(1-2)

Definition and meaning of Hikka

muhurmuhurvāyurudeti sasvano yakṛtplīhāntrāṇi mukhādivākṣipan |
sa ghoṣavānāśu hinastyasūn yatastatastu hikketyabhidhīyate budhaiḥ ||3||
(su| u| taṃ| a| 50) |
The aggravated Vāyu (udana along with prana vata) comes out of the mouth with immense velocity (speed), repeatedly, as if throwing the liver, spleen and intestines out of the mouth (the patient feels as if these organs are coming out of the mouth), it produces hik-hik sounds. Making the sounds in this way the vayu tends to cause harm to the life (life threatening) in quick time. Wise people (physicians) call this disease as hikka (compared to hiccough). (3)

Types of Hikka

annajāṃ yamalāṃ kṣudrāṃ gambhīrāṃ mahatīṃ tathā |
vāyuḥ kaphenānugataḥ pañca hikkāḥ karoti hi ||4||
(su| u| taṃ| a| 50) |
Vāta associated with kapha produces hikkā. This hikka is of 5 types, they are –

- Annajā hikka
- Yamalā hikka
- Ksudrā hikka
- Gambhīrā hikka and
- Mahatī hikka (4)

Hikka Purvarupa – Premonitory symptoms of Hikka

kaṇṭhorasorgurutvaṃ ca vadanasya kaṣāyatā |
hikkānāṃ pūrvarūpāṇi kukṣerāṭopa eva ca ||5||
(ca| ci| a| 21) |
Premonitory symptoms of hikkā are heaviness of throat and chest, astringent taste in the mouth and gurgling noise in the abdomen. (5)

Annaja Hikka

pānānnairatisaṃyuktaiḥ sahasā pīḍito'nilaḥ |
hikkayatyūrdhvago bhūtvā tāṃ vidyādannajāṃ bhiṣak ||6||
(su| u| taṃ| a| 50) |
This type of hikka is caused by excessive consumption of foods and drinks too quickly. Such foods and drinks taken in excess immediately impart pressure on vata. Thus, vata gets aggravated and moves in upward direction and causes hikka. Such a hikka caused by anna (foods and drinks) is called as Annajā hikkā. (6)

Yamala Hikka

cireṇa yamalairvegairyā hikkā sampravartate |
kampayantī śirogrīvaṃ yamalāṃ tāṃ vinirdiśet ||7||
(su| u| taṃ| a| 50) |
Yamala means two. Yamalā hikkā (its bouts) occur in pairs.
The hikka which occurs while causing shaking of head and neck, continues for a long time (repeatedly occurs, after breaks, intermittently) and occurs in pairs (produces two sounds of hik at a time, one after the other) is called Yamala hikka.(7)

Ksudra Hikka

prakṛṣṭakālairyā vegairmandaiḥ samabhivartate |
kṣudrikā nāma sā hikkā jatrumūlāt pradhāvitā ||8||
(su| u| taṃ| a| 50) |
Ksudrā hikkā is that which occurs occasionally (after long gaps), whose bouts are mild in intensity, and starts only from the base of the neck (junction of neck and chest). (8)

Gambhira Hikka

nābhipravṛttā yā hikkā ghorā gambhīranādinī |
anekopadravavatī gambhīrā nāma sā smṛtā ||9||
(su| u| taṃ| a| 50) |
Gambhirā hikkā, which starts from deep inside the umbilicus, is very

powerful, makes heavy sound and is accompanied with many complications. (9)

Maha Hikka

marmāṇyutpīḍayantīva satataṃ yā pravartate |
mahāhikketi sā jñeyā sarvagātravikampinī ||10||
(su| u| taṃ| a| 50) |
Mahāhikkā is that which produces powerful feeling as though all the vital organs are being pulled out of the body, continuously persists without giving a break, and causes tremors / shaking of the whole body. (10)

Symptoms of incurability of Hikka

āyamyate hikkato yasya deho dṛṣṭiścordhvaṃ nāmyate yasya nityam |
kṣīṇo'nnadviṭ kṣauti yaścātimātraṃ tau dvau cāntyau varjayeddhikkamānau ||11||
Patients of hikkā who have developed excessive stretching of the entire body, has gaze fixed in upward direction (or gets constricted) and the body always bent, is emaciated, has aversion towards food, has many bouts of sneezing and who has the last two types of hikka i.e., gambhira and mahati. These people shall be refused treatment (because this condition is incurable). (11)

atisañcitadoṣasya bhaktacchedakṛśasya ca |
vyādhibhiḥ kṣīṇadehasya vṛddhasyātivyavāyinaḥ ||12||
āsāṃ yā sā samutpannā hikkā hantyāśu jīvitam |
yamikā ca pralāpārtimohatṛṣṇāsamanvitā ||13||
The patient of hikka will succumb to death in quick time when there is excessive increase of all the doshas, he is unable to take food and hence has become emaciated, has become weak and debilitated as an effect of long-standing diseases, is aged, indulged in excessive sexual intercourse, who has yamala type of hikka, has delirium, pain, delusion and severe thirst. (12-13)

akṣīṇaścāpyadīnaśca sthiradhātvindriyaśca yaḥ |
tasya sādhayituṃ śakyā yamikā hantyato'nyathā ||14||
(ca| ci| a| 21) |

Yamalā hikkā is curable in those who are not emaciated (physically strong), who have strong mind, whose tissues and senses are good (and in a state of health), whereas it kills others (those who are weak physically and mentally, whose tissues and senses are not in a good state of health).(14)25!

Types of Swasa – dyspnoea

mahordhvacchinnatamakakṣudrabhedaistu pañcadhā |
bhidyate sa mahāvyādhiḥ śvāsa eko viśeṣataḥ ||15||
(su| u| taṃ| a| 51) |
Swasa which is counted as a mahāvyādhi (powerful disease) is a single entity (disease). But based on the different forms of its manifestation and on the basis of different kinds of etiological factors and symptoms swasa is mentioned to be of five kinds.

The five kinds of swasa are –

Mahatī Swasa
Urdhwa Swasa
Chinna Swasa
Tamaka Swasa and
Kşudra Swasa (15)

Dosha relationship with different kinds of swasa

(vātādhiko bhavet kṣudrastamakastu kaphodbhavaḥ |
kaphavātādhikaścaiva saṃsṛṣṭaśchinnasañjñakaḥ |
śvāso mārutasaṃsṛṣṭo mahānūrdhvastathā(to) mataḥ) |
(su| u| taṃ| a| 51) |
In Ksudra Swasa – vata is predominant (vataja)
In Tamaka Swasa – kapha is predominant (kaphaja)
In Chinna Swasa – Kapha and Vata are predominant (kapha-vataja)
In Mahat and Urdhva Swasa – Vata is predominant (vataja)
(Along with these, the other doshas are also associated – pitta)

Swasa Purvarupa – Premonitory symptoms of dyspnoea

prāgrūpaṃ tasya hṛtpīḍā śūlamādhmānameva ca |
ānāho vaktravairasyaṃ śaṅkhanistoda eva ca ||16||
The premonitory symptoms of Swasa are - pain in the region of the heart, abdominal colic and distension (tympanitis) and enlargement of abdomen / flatulence, bad taste in the mouth and pricking (throbbing) pain in the temples. (16)

Swasa Samprapti – pathogenesis of dyspnoea

yadā srotāṃsi saṃrudhya mārutaḥ kaphapūrvakaḥ |
viṣvagvrajati saṃruddhastadā śvāsān karoti saḥ ||17||
(su| u| taṃ| a| 51) |
The vata being obstructed by kapha, travelling in abnormal directions causes obstruction of the channels carrying prana - vital air (passages inside the lungs) and begins to move in all directions producing the disease swasa. (17)

Symptoms of Maha Swasa

uddhūyamānavato yaḥ śabdavadduḥkhito naraḥ |
uccaiḥ śvasiti saṃrudvo mattarṣabha ivāniśam ||18||
pranaṣṭajñānavijñānastathā vibhrāntalocanaḥ |
vivṛtākṣyānano baddhamūtravarcā viśīrṇavāk ||19||
dīnaḥ praśvasitaṃ cāsya dūrādvijñāyate bhṛśam |
mahāśvāsopasṛṣṭastu kṣiprameva vipadyate ||20||
(ca| ci| a| 21) |
Vata, having increased greatly moves upwards constantly and produces this condition called Maha swasa.
The patient afflicted by this condition would constantly breathe in producing heavy sounds resembling those produced by a mad or tired and intoxicated bull tied firmly to a peg, huffing and puffing along with pain.
The patient loses awareness and intellect; eyes begin to roll, with terrified looks and wide-open mouth. There will be obstruction to passage (excretion) of faeces and urine. The patient will have a broken voice (pronounces broken words with difficulty) and would feel helpless. The sounds of his breathing can be heard from a long distance. These are the symptoms of Maha Swasa. The person suffering from Maha Swasa will die

soon. (18-20)

Symptoms of Urdhva Swasa

ūrdhvaṃ śvasiti yo dīrghaṃ na ca pratyāharatyadhaḥ |
śleṣmāvṛtamukhasrotāḥ kruddhagandhavahārditaḥ ||21||
ūrdhvadṛṣṭirvipaśyaṃstu vibhrāntākṣa itastataḥ |
pramuhyan vedanārtaśca śuklāsyo'ratipīḍitaḥ ||22||
ūrdhvaśvāse prakupite hyadhaḥśvāso nirudhyate |
muhyatastāmyataścordhvaṃ śvāsastasyaiva hantyasūn ||23||
(ca| ci| a| 21) |
The person suffering from Urdhva Swasa will have long expiration (breathes out for a longer duration) but will be unable to breathe in (inspiration) easily.
The mouth and other passages will be filled up with sputum. The other symptoms will be produced by vata which has undergone severe aggravation.
The person looks with an upward gaze i.e., the eyes are fixed up. The eyeballs roll in different directions. He will faint (go unconscious) repeatedly and suffers from pain. There is whitish discoloration of the face and the patient will get restless.
The expiration gets deep and exacerbated while the inspiration gets obstructed. Due to this the person gets repeatedly restless and experiences loss of consciousness (faints). These are the features of Urdhva Swasa and this also kills the patient. (21-23)

Symptoms of Chinna Swasa

yastu śvasiti vicchinnaṃ sarvaprāṇena pīḍitaḥ |
na vā śvasiti duḥkhārto marmacchedarugarditaḥ ||24||
ānāhasvedamūrchārto dahyamānena bastinā |
viplutākṣaḥ parikṣīṇaḥ śvasan raktaikalocanaḥ ||25||
vicetāḥ pariśuṣkāsyo vivarṇaḥ pralapannaraḥ |
chinnaśvāsena vicchinnaḥ sa śīghraṃ vijahātyasūn ||26||
(ca| ci| a| 29) |
Chinna means interrupted or broken. In Chinna Swasa the respiration (breathing pattern) is often interrupted in the middle. It takes immense

effort for the person to breathe in this condition. In spite of all efforts the person is in distress because he breathes with interruptions. In this condition there will be severe pain in all the vital organs. Due to this pain the person will not be capable of breathing properly. Also, due to fear of the pain getting worsened, the person would not attempt at respiration.
The person also would suffer from abdominal distension (flatulence), perspiration and fainting (loss of consciousness), burning sensation in the urinary bladder, eyes filled with tears, emaciation, redness of one eye, loss of consciousness, dryness of the mouth, discolouration and delirium. These are the symptoms of Chinna Swasa. This condition also kills the patient in a quick time. (24-26)

Pathogenesis and Symptoms of Tamaka Swasa

pratilomaṃ yadā vāyuḥ srotāṃsi pratipadyate |
grīvāṃ śiraśca saṅgṛhya śleṣmāṇaṃ samudīrya ca ||27||
karoti pīnasaṃ tena ruddho ghurghurakaṃ tathā |
atīva tīvravegaṃ ca śvāsaṃ prāṇaprapīḍakam ||28||
pratāmyati sa vegena tṛṣyate sannirudhyate |
pramohaṃ kāsamānaśca sa gacchati muhurmuhuḥ ||29||
śleṣmaṇyamucyamāne tu bhṛśaṃ bhavati duḥkhitaḥ |
tasyaiva ca vimokṣānte muhūrtaṃ labhate sukham ||30||
tathā'syoddhvaṃsate kaṇṭhaḥ kṛcchrācchaknoti bhāṣitum |
na cāpi labhate nidrāṃ śayānaḥ śvāsapīḍitaḥ ||31||
pārśve tasyāvagṛhṇāti śayānasya samīraṇaḥ |
āsīno labhate saukhyamuṣṇaṃ caivābhinandati ||32||
ucchritākṣo lalāṭena svidyatā bhṛśamārtimān |
viśuṣkāsyo muhuḥ śvāso muhuścaivāvadhamyate ||33||
meghāmbuśītaprāgvātaiḥ śleṣmalaiśca vivardhate |
sa yāpyastamakaḥ śvāsaḥ sādhyo vā syānnavotthitaḥ ||34||
(ca| ci| a| 21) |

Pathogenesis – The aggravated vata moves in the opposite direction i.e., upwards and enters the channels of transportation of prana (vital air). On reaching these passages vata grasps the head and neck and further aggravates the kapha therein. On aggravating the kapha and finding its association, vata (along with kapha) causes pinasa (running nose). The movements of vata are also blocked by kapha. This vata which is obstructed by kapha (in the respiratory passages) will produce bubbling sounds in the throat. This ultimately produces severe bouts of increased respirations (in number and intensity) which pose a threat to life. This condition is called Tamaka Swasa.

Symptoms – The person suffers from darkness in front of the eyes (feels as if he is surrounded by darkness), severe thirst, and becomes motionless.
The person loses consciousness and faints as an effect of continuous bouts of cough.
The patient remains restless and worried until the sputum is expelled. He keeps trying hard to expel that sputum by coughing repeatedly. When due to repeated coughing the sputum gets expelled, the person finds momentary relief.
He would experience itching (obstruction) in the throat. He would be able to speak with great difficulty while putting constant effort. He will not be able to sleep when he lies down due to severe catching of breath (dyspnoea). This is also because the vayu (located in the flanks) creates severe pain in the flanks when he sleeps. He finds comfort when he comes back to sitting posture. (This is the only posture in which he finds relief).
He desires hot / warm comforts and when given he finds relief.
His eyes are wide open (swelling of eyes, upward gaze), there is sweating on the forehead and severe pain (in the chest).
There is dryness of the mouth.
He breathes in repeatedly and later breathes out putting all efforts and straining all his body parts with great difficulty and sounds.
The symptoms get increased during cloudy days, by use of cold water, getting exposed to the breeze flowing from the east and other kapha aggravating causative factors.
These are the symptoms of tamaka swasa. The disease is said to be yapya i.e., manageable (persists throughout life in spite of administering suitable treatment). This condition might also get cured if it is of very recent onset. (27-34)

Pratamaka Swasa

jvaramūrchāparītasya vidyāt pratamakaṃ tu tam |
udāvartarajo'jīrṇaklinnakāyanirodhajaḥ ||35||
When this disease i.e., tamaka swasa manifests along with fever and fainting

(loss of consciousness), it will be called as Pratamaka Swasa.

Causes – Pratamaka Swasa is caused by –

- Upward movement of vata in many channels (abdomen – alimentary tract) / reverse peristalsis,
- Inhalation / exposure to dust
- Indigestion (indigested foods, ama etc)
- Increase of wetness or dampness of the body / excessive consumption of foods soaked in water
- Suppression of urges of the body (35)

Santamaka Swasa

tamasā vardhate'tyarthaṃ śītaiścāśu praśāmyati |
majjatastamasīvāsya vidyāt santamakaṃ tu tam ||36||
(ca| ci| a| 21) |
When Tamaka Swasa is caused or gets increased (triggered) by tamas (darkness, contaminant of mind, inactivity, cloudy weather etc), makes the patient to go into a zone of darkness (the person feels as if he is entering into darkness or surrounded by darkness) and the symptoms get quickly subsided (patient gets comfort) by use of cold things, it is called as Santamaka Swasa. (36)

Symptoms of Kshudra Swasa

rūkṣāyāsodbhavaḥ koṣṭhe kṣudro vāta udīrayan |
kṣudraśvāso na so'tyarthaṃ duḥkhenāṅgaprabādhakaḥ ||37||
hinasti na sa gātrāṇi na ca duḥkho yathetare |
na ca bhojanapānānāṃ niruṇaddhyucitāṃ gatim ||38||
nendriyāṇāṃ vyathāṃ nāpi kāñcidāpādayedrujam |
sa sādhya ukto, balinaḥ sarve cāvyaktalakṣaṇāḥ ||39||
(ca| ci| a| 21) |
Causes - Ksudra Swasa is caused due to consumption of dry foods and physical exertion.
Vata getting aggravated by above said etiological factors moves upwards and

causes difficulty in respiration. Ksudra means less. Since this condition is caused by less causative factors and has less symptoms (symptoms of lesser strength and less severity) it is called as ksudra swasa.
Symptoms – The symptoms and bouts are mild in nature. The disease does not cause more trouble to the body or in any body part. It does not trouble the patient like other kinds of swasa (explained above). It doesn't pose a threat to the life of the patient.
This swasa doesn't cause any obstruction in the passage of food and respiration (the person can swallow food and water easily). It doesn't interfere with the functioning of the sense organs (the power of perception of sense organs remains intact, and is not disturbed). It doesn't produce any other disease or pain in the form of complications.
Ksudra Swasa is curable.
The other kinds of swasa are curable when they manifest in strong persons and when the symptoms manifest in an unclear / incomplete way (are mild or when in earlier stages of manifestation). (37-39)

Prognosis of Swasa

kṣudraḥ sādhyo matasteṣāṃ tamakaḥ kṛcchra ucyate |
trayaḥ śvāsā na sidhyanti tamako durbalasya ca ||40||
(su| u| taṃ| a| 51) |
Ksudra Swasa is curable. Tamaka Swasa is difficult to treat. The other three types of swasa are incurable. Tamaka Swasa occurring in weak persons is incurable. (40)

Dangerous nature of Swasa and Hikka

kāmaṃ prāṇaharā rogā bahavo na tu te tathā |
yathā śvāsaśca hikkā ca harataḥ prāṇamāśu ca ||41||
(ca| ci| a| 21) |
There are many dreadful diseases which take away life, but no disease is as quick as swasa and hikka in taking away the life of the patients. (41)

iti śrīmādhavakaraviracite mādhavanidāne hikkāśvāsanidānaṃ samāptam ||12||
Thus ends the chapter on Śwāsa-hikkā.

CHAPTER THIRTEEN

SWARA BHEDA NIDĀNAM

Swara Bheda Nidana, Samprapti, Bheda – Etiological factors, pathogenesis and types of hoarseness of voice

atyuccabhāṣaṇaviṣādhyayanābhighātasandūṣaṇaiḥ prakupitāḥ pavanādayastu |
srotaḥsu te svaravaheṣu gatāḥ pratiṣṭhāṃ hanyuḥ svaraṃ bhavati cāpi hi ṣaḍvidhaḥ saḥ ||1||
(su| u| taṃ| a| 53) |
(vātādibhiḥ pṛthak sarvairmedasā ca kṣayeṇa ca) |
Etiological factors - Speaking in high pitch, effect of (consumption of) poisons, studying or reading loudly, injury and such other causes are considered to be the etiological factors of swara bheda – hoarseness of vata.

Pathogenesis – The above-mentioned etiological factors cause abnormal increase of vata and other doshas. These doshas in turn get lodged in the channels and organs responsible for production of voice and destroy the voice producing hoarseness of voice.
Types – Swarabheda is of six kinds, one from each dosha (vata, pitta and kapha), one from combination of all the three doshas (tridoshaja / sannipataja), the fifth type caused by medas (adipose tissue) and the sixth form of swarabheda is caused by ksaya (depletion of body tissues).(1)

The six types of Swarabheda are –

1. Vataja Swarabheda
2. Pittaja Swarabheda
3. Kaphaja Swarabheda

4. Sannipataja Swarabheda
5. Ksayaja Swarabheda
6. Medoja Swarabheda

Symptoms of Vataja, Pittaja, Kaphaja and Sannipataja Swarabheda

vātena kṛṣṇanayanānanamūtravarcā bhinnaṃ śanairvadati gardabhavat kharaṃ ca |2|
(su| u| taṃ| a| 53) |
pittena pītanayanānanamūtravarcā brūyādgalena sa ca dāhasamanvitena ||2||
(su| u| taṃ| a| 53) |
brūyāt kaphena satataṃ kapharuddhakaṇṭhaḥ svalpaṃ śanairvadati cāpi divā viśeṣāt |3|
(su| u| taṃ| a| 53) |
sarvātmake bhavati sarvavikārasampat taṃ cāpyasādhyamṛṣayaḥ svarabhedamāhuḥ ||3||
(su| u| taṃ| a| 53) |

Vataja Swarabheda Symptoms – The patient would have blackish discolouration of eye, face, urine and faeces. His voice is broken and he speaks slowly, with a harsh voice resembling that of a donkey.

Pittaja Swarabheda Symptoms – The patient would have yellowish discoloration of the eyes, face, urine and faeces. He would experience a burning sensation in the throat.

Kaphaja Swarabheda Symptoms – In this condition the throat of the patient is always obstructed by kapha (sputum, thick fluid). Due to this, the patient speaks slowly (indistinct, in low pitch). He can speak a little clearly during day time (the speech and voice are slightly better).

Tridoshaja / Sannipataja Swarabheda Symptoms – In this condition, all the symptoms of all the doshas coexist. According to the opinion of the great sages, this condition is incurable. (2-3)

Symptoms of Ksayaja and Medoja Swarabheda

dhūpyeta vāk kṣayakṛte kṣayamāpnuyācca vāgeṣa cāpi hatavāk parivarjanīyaḥ |4|
(su| u| taṃ| a| 53) |
antargatasvaramalakṣyapadaṃ cireṇa medo'nvayādvadati digdhagalastṛṣārtaḥ ||4||

(su| u| taṃ| a| 53) |
Ksayaja Swarabheda Symptoms - In this type of hoarseness of voice, the patient feels as if hot fumes are coming out of the throat and nose, andas an impact of ksaya (depletion of tissues and destruction of nerves supplying the throat) the voice is completely destroyed. Such a patient who has completely lost his voice shall not be treated because it is incurable.
Medoja Swarabheda Symptoms – In this type of hoarseness of voice, the patient will have a coating of fat inside the throat or over the vocal nerves. As a result, the voice appears to be stuck within the throat (appears as though coming from great depth, from deep inside the throat). Whatever the person speaks is not clear. Some words (syllables) are clear and some are not clear and the person speaks slowly. The person will suffer from severe thirst in this condition. (4)

Prognosis of Swarabheda
kṣīṇasya vṛddhasya kṛśasya vā'pi cirotthito yaśca sahopajātaḥ |medasvinaḥ sarvasamudbhavaśca svarāmayo yo na sa siddhimeti ||5||(su| u| taṃ| a| 53) |
Swarabhedam is incurable in persons who are very weak, aged and emaciated. Also, swarabheda which is long standing or congenital, or that which occurs in persons who are obese and that which is produced by all the three dosas together (tridoshaja or sannipataja swarabheda) is incurable. (5)

iti śrīmādhavakaraviracite mādhavanidāne svarabhedanidānaṃ samāptam ||13||
Thus ends the chapter on Swarabheda.

CHAPTER FOURTEEN

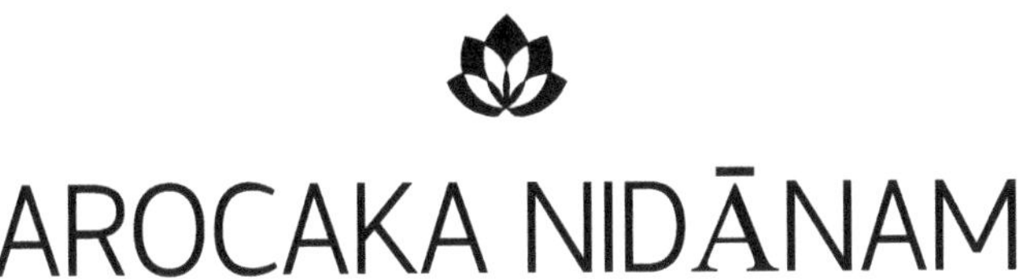

AROCAKA NIDĀNAM

Causes of Arocaka – Anorexia

vātādibhiḥ śokabhayātilobhakrodhairmanoghnāśanarūpagandhaiḥ|
arocakāḥ syuḥ ||| |1|
(ca| ci| a| 26) |
Arocaka (anorexia) is produced by the three doshas (vata, pita, kapha), excessive grief, fear, greed, anger and foods, the sight and smell of which are very unpleasant to the mind. (1)

Symptoms of doshaja (vataja, pittaja and kaphaja) arocaka
... parihṛṣṭadantaḥ kaṣāyavaktraśca mato'nilena ||1|| (ca| ci| a| 26) |
kaṭvamlamuṣṇaṃ virasaṃ ca pūti pittena vidyāt ||| |2| (ca| ci| a| 26) |
... lavaṇaṃ ca vaktram |
mādhuryapaicchilyagurutvaśaityavibaddhasambaddhayutaṃ kaphena ||2||
(ca| ci| a| 26) |
Vataja Arocaka – presents with tingling in the teeth (and gums) & manifestation of astringent taste in the mouth.
Pittaja Arocaka – presents with manifestation of bitter and sour taste, warmth and bad smell in the mouth.
Kaphaja Arocaka – presents with manifestation of salty or sweet taste, stickiness, heaviness, coldness, stiffness and thick coating of kapha inside the mouth. (2)

Arocaka caused by grief etc causes & Tridoshaja Arocaka

arocake śokabhayātilobhakrodhādyahṛdyāśucigandhaje syāt ||
svābhāvikaṃ cāsyamathāruciśca ||| |3| (ca| ci| a| 26) |

... tridoṣaje naikarasaṃ bhavettu ||3|| (ca| ci| a| 26) |
Agantuja Arocaka – is that which is caused due to grief, fear, excessive greed, excessive fear, anger and other mental affections, things unpleasant to mind (foods etc), unclean and dirty and foul-smelling things (foods). In this condition the taste of the mouth is normal. In spite of that, the person suffers from arocaka – anorexia.
Tridoshaja Arocaka – In tridosaja type of anorexia, the patient experiences many kinds of tastes (mixture of different tastes mentioned in doshaja types). (3)

Specific Dosha symptoms in Arocaka

hṛcchūlapīḍanayutaṃ pavanena, pittāttṛḍdāhacoṣabahulaṃ, sakaphaprasekam |
śleṣmātmakaṃ, bahurujaṃ bahubhiśca vidyādvaiguṇyamohajaḍatābhirathāparaṃ ca ||4|| (ca| ci| a| 26) |
Pain in the region of the heart is found in vātaja arocaka.
Thirst, burning sensation and local heat are found in pittaja arocaka.
In Kaphaja arocaka, excessive secretions / exudation from mouth, nose etc are found.
In tridoshaja type of arocaka many kinds of pain and discomforts are experienced.
Confused state of mind, delusion / fainting and dullness of the mind are the symptoms which are predominantly found in arocaka caused due to grief etc causes (agantuja arocaka). (4)

iti śrīmādhavakaraviracite mādhavanidāne arocakanidānaṃ samāptam ||14||
Thus ends the chapter of Arocaka.

Other terms related to Arocaka

1. Aruci / Arocaka) – tastelessness - inability to appreciate even a tasty food when it comes into contact with the tongue i.e., the person doesn't feel the taste of the food.
2. Annābhinandana – is a condition wherein there is inability to eat the food in spite of his or her favourite food being served (aversion to foods which were once liked).

3. Bhakta dwesa – is a condition wherein there is hatred towards food caused by touching, seeing, smell, hearing or remembering about the food.
4. Abhaktachchanda – is a condition where there is disinterest towards food due to anger, fear and other mental causes.
5. All these are included in the term arocaka by both Caraka and Suśruta (Madhukosh tīkā – Madukosha commentary).

CHAPTER FIFTEEN

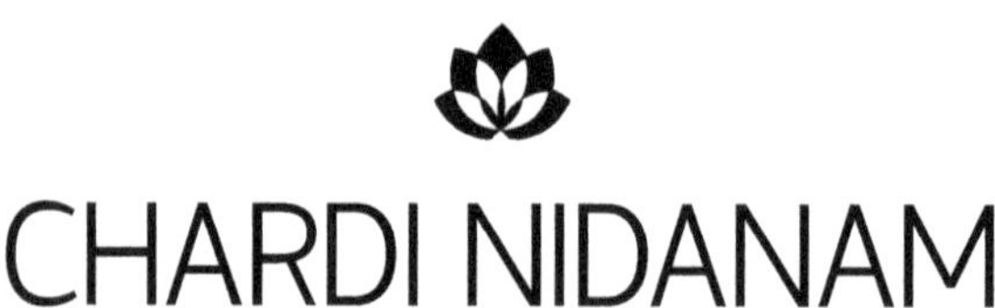

CHARDI NIDANAM

Types of Chardi – Vomiting

duṣṭairdoṣaiḥ pṛthak sarvairbībhatsālocanādibhiḥ |
chardayaḥ pañca vijñeyāstāsāṃ lakṣaṇamucyate ||1||
Chardi (vomiting) is of five types. They are - one from each dosha, fourth from the combination of all the three together and fifth from the sight of unpleasant things, etc. (1)

To sum up – The five kinds of chardi are –

1. Vataja Chardi
2. Pittaja Chardi
3. Kaphaja Chardi
4. Tridoshaja (sannipataja) Chardi
5. Agantuja Chardi (that occurring from sight of unpleasant things)

Chardi Nidana, Nirukti and Samprapti – Etiological actors, definition and pathogenesis of vomiting

atidravairatisnigdhairahṛdyairlavaṇairati |
akāle cātimātraiśca tathā'sātmyaiśca bhojanaiḥ ||2||
śramādbhayāttathodvegādajīrṇāt krimidoṣataḥ |
nāryāścāpannasattvāyāstathā'tidrutamaśnataḥ ||3||
bībhatsairhetubhiścānyairdrutamutkleśito balāt |
chādayannānanaṃ vegairardayennaṅgabhañjanaiḥ |
atyantamaparītasya cchardervai sambhavo dhruvam |

nirucyate chardiriti doṣo vaktraṃ pradhāvitaḥ ||4||
(su| u| taṃ| a| 49) |
Etiological Factors –

- Indulgence in foods which are very watery, very unctuous (fatty), unpleasant and very salty;
- Taking meals at odd time, in excess quantity and of unaccustomed food
- Excessive physical exertion
- Fear, sudden emotions / anxiety,
- Indigestion
- Infection by worms
- Pregnancy in women
- Eating foods very quickly
- Sight of terrific, fearsome, ugly and such other unpleasant things

Definition and Pathogenesis - The above said causes and similar others cause sudden increase of doshas. These doshas fill the mouth of the patient (with the contents of the stomach which have moved upwards) and come out forcibly through the mouth, causing immense discomfort (pain in different parts and organs of the body). This is called Chardi – vomiting. (2-4)

Chardi Purvarupa – Premonitory symptoms of vomiting

hṛllāsodgārarodhau ca praseko lavaṇastanuḥ |
dveṣo'nnapāne ca bhṛśaṃ vamīnāṃ pūrvalakṣaṇam ||5||
(su| u| taṃ| a| 49) |
The premonitory symptoms of vomiting are – nausea (oppression in the chest), obstruction of belching, thin (watery) and salty salivation and aversion to foods and drinks. (5)

Vataja Chardi Symptoms

hṛtpārśvapīḍāmukhaśoṣaśīrṣanābhyartikāsasvarabhedatodaiḥ |
udgāraśabdaprabalaṃ saphenaṃ vicchinnakṛṣṇaṃ tanukaṃ kaṣāyam |
kṛcchreṇa cālpaṃ mahatā ca vegenārto'nilācchardayatīha duḥkham ||6||

(ca| ci| a| 23) |
The symptoms of vataja chardi include - pain in the region of the heart and flanks, dryness of the mouth, pain / discomfort in head and umbilicus, cough, hoarseness of voice, and pricking sensation / pain all over the body. The vomiting occurs with great sounds during belching, mixed with froth, with less of fluids, composed of blackish material, thin, astringent in taste, brought out (vomited) with difficulty, scanty, severe bouts and severely troublesome (accompanied with pain all over the body). (6)

Pittaja Chardi Symptoms

mūrchāpipāsāmukhaśoṣamūrdhatālvakṣisantāpatamobhramārtaḥ |
pītaṃ bhṛśoṣṇaṃ haritaṃ satiktaṃ dhūmraṃ ca pittena vamet sadāham ||7||
(ca| ci| a| 23) |
The symptoms of pittaja chardi are – fainting (loss of consciousness), severe thirst, dryness of mouth, burning sensation in the head, palate and eyes: darkness before the eyes & dizziness. In the vomiting, yellowish, greenish or black with reddish tinge, very hot, bitter material is expelled along with burning sensation. (7)

Kaphaja Chardi Symptoms

tandrāsyamādhuryakaphaprasekasantoṣanidrārucigauravārtaḥ |
snigdhaṃ ghanaṃ svādu kaphādviśuddhaṃ saromaharṣo'lparujaṃ vamettu ||8||
(ca| ci| a| 23) |
The symptoms of Kaphaja Chardi are - stupor / drowsiness, sweet taste in the mouth, excessive salivation, a feeling of happiness (which is abnormal) or contentment (no desire to eat food anymore), feeling sleepy, anorexia, and feeling of heaviness of the body. While vomiting, the patient brings out unctuous (fatty), thick, sweet tasting, and white coloured material, accompanied with horripilations and little or no pain. (8)

Tridoshaja Chardi Symptoms

śūlāvipākārucidāhatṛṣṇāśvāsapramohaprabalā prasaktam |
chardistridoṣāllavaṇāmlanīlasāndroṣṇaraktaṃ vamatāṃ nṛṇāṃ syāt ||9||

(ca| ci| a| 23) |
The symptoms of tridoshaja chardi are - pain in the abdomen, indigestion, anorexia, burning sensation, thirst, dyspnoea (increased / difficult respirations), and delusions, being severe and constant. The vomited material would be salty or sour, blue or red in colour, semisolid and hot. (9)

Symptoms of incurability of Chardi

viṭsvedamūtrāmbuvahāni vāyuḥ srotāṃsi saṃrudhya yadordhvameti |
utsannadoṣasya samācitaṃ taṃ doṣaṃ samuddhūya narasya koṣṭhāt ||10||
viṇmūtrayostatsamagandhavarṇaṃ tṛṭśvāsahikkārtiyutaṃ prasaktam |
pracchardayedduṣṭamihātivegāttayā'rditaścāśu vināśameti ||11||
(ca| ci| a| 23) |
When the aggravated vayu moves in upward direction and blocks the channels of faeces, sweat, urine and water (body fluids) in a person in whom the other doshas (pitta and kapha) have already undergone severe aggravation, it brings with it the doshas accumulated in the koshta (visceral organs, stomach and intestines) in the upward direction. In this case the person vomits the material which would have the smell and colour similar to those of faeces and urine. Apart from this, the patient will also suffer from severe thirst, dyspnoea (increased or difficult respiration) and hiccough which are constant. The person would have vomiting with continuous bouts occurring with great force associated with severe discomfort. Such type of vomiting is incurable and the person will face death in quick time. (10-11)

Agantuja and Krimija Chardi Symptoms

bībhatsajā daurhṛdajā''majā ca hyasātmajā ca krimijā ca yā hi |
sā pañcamī tāṃ ca vibhāvayecca doṣocchrayeṇaiva yathoktamādau ||12||
(su| u| taṃ| a| 49) |
śūlahṛllāsabahulā krimijā ca viśeṣataḥ | krimihṛdrogatulyena lakṣaṇena ca lakṣitā ||13||
(su| u| taṃ| a| 49) |
Agantuja Chardi – The fifth kind of vomiting occurs due to sight and contact of things which are unpleasant, pregnancy, indigestion (caused due to excessive build-up of ama), unaccustomed foods and parasitic infections

(worms). This is called agantuja chardi. Even in this type of vomiting, the symptoms of doshas (described earlier) shall be considered.

Krimija Chardi - In krimija chardi (vomiting caused by parasitic infection) pain in the abdomen and nausea are prominent. Apart from this, the symptoms of krimija hrdroga (heart disease produced by worms) will also be found. (12-13)

Symptoms of incurability of chardi

kṣīṇasya yā chardiratiprasaktā sopadravā śoṇitapūyayuktā |
sacandrikāṃ tāṃ pravadedasādhyāṃ sādhyāṃ cikitsennirupadravāṃ ca ||14||
(ca| ci| a| 23) |
Vomiting is incurable when it occurs in emaciated persons, when the vomiting is continuous with too many bouts, is associated with complications and when the vomited material consists of blood, pus and white shining particles. The vomiting devoid of complications shall be considered as curable and should be treated promptly. (14)

Chardi Upadrava – complications of vomiting

kāsaḥ śvāso jvaro hikkā tṛṣṇā vaicittyameva ca |
hṛdrogastamakaścaiva jñeyāścharderupadravāḥ ||15||
(The complications of vomiting are – cough, dyspnoea (increased / difficult respiration), fever, hiccough, thirst, mental torpidity, heartache (heart disease) and feeling of being in darkness (darkness in front of the eyes or feeling as if enveloped by darkness).

iti śrīmādhavakaraviracite mādhavanidāne chardinidānaṃ samāptam ||15||
Thus ends the chapter on Chardi.

CHAPTER SIXTEEN

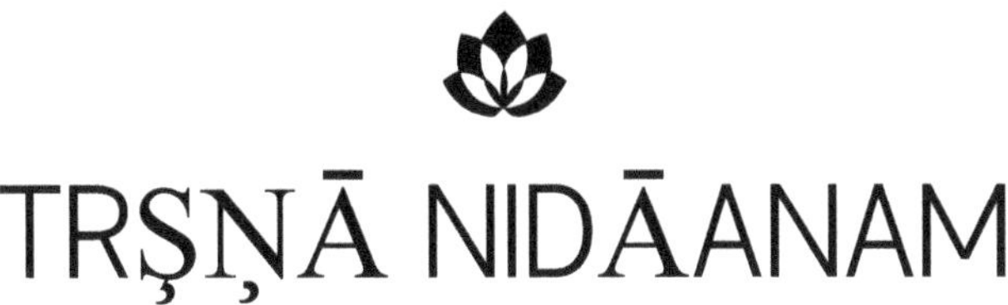

TRṢṆĀ NIDĀANAM

Trsna Samprapti - Pathogenesis of Trsna

bhayaśramābhyāṃ balasaṅkṣayādvā hyūrdhvaṃ citaṃ pittavivardhanaiśca |
pittaṃ savātaṃ kupitaṃ narāṇāṃ tāluprapannaṃ janayet pipāsām |
srotassvapāṃvāhiṣu dūṣiteṣu doṣaiśca tṛṭ sambhavatīha jantoḥ ||1||
Pitta which has undergone increase due to its etiological factors (pitta aggravating factors like excessive consumption of pungent, hot, corrosive foods, anger, consumption of alcohol etc) gets association of vata which has undergone increase due to fear, physical exhaustion (fatigue) and loss of strength. Now, this pitta along with vata reaches the palate, gets lodged therein and produces severe thirst. This condition is called Trsna.
Also, trsna – thirst may be manifested when the vitiated doshas contaminate the channels transporting water (organs controlling the water balance and supply in the body). (1)

Pathway of pathogenesis of Trsna

Pitta aggravated by its own etiological factors

↓

Finds association of vata which has undergone aggravation due to fear, physical exertion and loss of physical strength

↓

Both doshas reach and get lodged in the palate (or contaminate the water transporting channels) and

↓

Cause severe thirst – this condition is called as trsna

Trsna Purvarupa, Rupa – Premonitory symptoms and symptoms of Trsna

tālvoṣṭha kaṇṭhāsya viśeṣa dāha santāpa moha bhrama pravilāpā: |
pūrvāṇi rūpāṇi bhavanti tāsāmuptatti kāle tu viśeṣato hi ||
Purvarupa – The premonitory symptoms of trsna are – dryness and also burning sensation of the palate, lips, throat and mouth, increased temperature in the entire body, dizziness, and delirium.
Rupa / Lakshanas – When the same symptoms mentioned in the premonitory symptoms clearly manifest in a stronger way they become the lakshanas or symptoms of trsna disease.

Types of Trsna

tisraḥ smṛtāstāḥ kṣatajā caturthī kṣayāttathā hyāmasamudbhavā ca |
bhaktodbhavā saptamiketi tāsāṃ nibodha liṅgānyanupūrvaśastu ||2||
(su| u| taṃ| a| 48) |
Trsna is of seven kinds, one from each dosa, the fourth from injury (ulcerations), the fifth one due to the depletion (loss) of body tissues, the sixth one from ama (excessive accumulation of undigested materials formed due to sluggish digestion in the stomach) and the seventh one is caused by food (consumption of bad foods). The symptoms of all these types of trsna will be described further. (2)

Note – The 7 types of Trsna are –

1. Vataja Trsna
2. Pittaja Trsna
3. Kaphaja Trsna
4. Kshataja Trsna
5. Kshayaja Trsna
6. Amaja Trsna
7. Bhaktodbhava Trsna

Symptoms of Vataja Trsna

kṣāmāsyatā mārutasambhavāyāṃ todastathā śaṅkhaśiraḥsu cāpi |
srotonirodho virasaṃ ca vaktraṃ śītābhiradbhiśca vivṛddhimeti ||3||
(su| u| taṃ| a| 48) |
The symptoms of Vataja Trsna are - pinched or dry face, pricking pain in the temples and head, obstruction of the channels of transportation of nutrition and water, manifestation of bad tastes in the mouth and increase of thirst on drinking cold water. (3)

Symptoms of Pittaja Trsna

mūrchānnavidveṣavilāpadāhā raktekṣaṇatvaṃ pratataśca śoṣaḥ |
śītābhinandā mukhatiktatā ca pittātmikāyāṃ paridūyanaṃ ca ||4||
(su| u| taṃ| a| 48) |
The symptoms of pittaja trsna are – fainting (loss of consciousness), aversion to food, delirium, burning sensation, reddish eyes, constant dryness (due to immense thirst all the tissues of the body dry up continuously), liking towards cold things / cold comforts, manifestation of bitter taste in the mouth, feel of discomfort in the entire body or smoke (hot fumes) being eliminated from the entire body, and yellowish discoloration of faeces, urine, eyes skin etc. (4)

Symptoms of Kaphaja Trsna

bāṣpāvarodhāt kaphasaṃvṛte'gnau tṛṣṇā balāsena bhavettathā tu |
nidrā gurutvaṃ madhurāsyatā ca tṛṣṇārditaḥ śuṣyati cātimātram ||5||
(su| u| taṃ| a| 48) |
Pathogenesis of kaphaja trsna – The kapha which has been aggravated due to its own causes (etiological factors causing aggravation of kapha) envelopes (destroys, puts off) the digestive fire. This leads to obstruction of heat in the channels of transportation of water. This will further lead to manifestation of trsna. Such a thirst caused by kapha is called kaphaja trsna. The symptoms of kaphaja trsna are – excessive sleep, heaviness of the body, manifestation of sweet taste in the mouth and excessive emaciation (quick emaciation) of the body of the patient. (5)

Symptoms of Ksataja and Ksayaja Trsna

kṣatasya rukśoṇitanirgamābhyāṃ tṛṣṇā caturthī kṣatajā matā tu |6| (su| u| taṃ| a| 48) |
rasakṣayādyā kṣayasambhavā sā tayā'bhibhūtaśca niśādineṣu ||6||
pepīyate'mbhaḥ sa sukhaṃ na yāti tāṃ sannipātāditi kecidāhuḥ |
rasakṣayoktāni ca lakṣaṇāni tasyāmaśeṣeṇa bhiṣagvyavasyet ||7|| (su| u| taṃ| a| 48) |
Ksataja Trsna – This type of thirst manifests as a result of excessive bleeding and pain caused due to injury.
Ksayaja Trsna – This type of thirst manifests due to loss of rasa tissue (the first and predominantly watery tissue of the body). The person suffering from this type of thirst repeatedly drinks water during day time and also at night but the thirst is not relieved by any amount of water intake. Along with this, the symptoms of rasa ksaya (symptoms of decrease of rasa tissue including pain, tremors, feeling of dryness and emptiness in the region of heart, dryness of the mouth, skin etc) are also manifested.

Some authorities consider this type of trsna (ksayaja trsṇā)as sannipātaja (caused by all three doses together). (6-7)

Amaja and Bhaktodbhava Trsna
tridoṣaliṅgā''masamudbhavā ca hṛcchūlaniṣṭhīvanasādakartrī |8| (su| u| taṃ| a| 48) |
snigdhaṃ tathā'mlaṃ lavaṇaṃ ca bhuktaṃ gurvannamevāśu tṛṣāṃ karoti ||8|| (su| u| taṃ| a| 48) |
Amaja Trsna – In this type of thirst, the combined symptoms of all the three doshas are seen. Apart from this – pain in the region of the heart, excessive expectoration / spitting of sputum and weakness (always lying down) are found as specific symptoms.
Bhaktodbhava / Annaja Trsna – This kind of thirst is produced by excessive consumption of unctuous (fatty), sour, salty and heavy foods. (8)

Upasargaja Trsna – signs of thirst manifested as a complication of other diseases

dīnasvaraḥ pratāmyan dīnaḥ saṃśuṣkavaktragalatāluḥ |
bhavati khalu yopasargāttṛṣṇā sā śoṣiṇī kaṣṭā ||9||

It is very difficult to treat patients of thirst in whom there is manifestation of –

- Suppression of voice / feeble voice
- Repeated fainting (goes into state of unconsciousness repeatedly)
- Tiredness / restless (feel of helplessness)
- Dryness of mouth, throat and palate
- Excessive emaciation

This type of thirst caused as a complication of other diseases is called as upasargaja trsna. (9)

Complications of Trsna

jvaramohakṣayakāsaśvāsādyupasṛṣṭadehānām |10| (ca| ci| a| 22) |
sarvāstvatiprasaktā rogakṛśānāṃ vamiprayuktānām |
ghoropadravayuktāstṛṣṇā maraṇāya vijñeyāḥ ||10|| (ca| ci| a| 22) |
Fever, delusion, emaciation, cough, dyspnoea (increased / difficult respiration) are the complications of trsnā. (According to others these are the causes of upasargaja trsna mentioned above i.e., people suffering from these diseases can develop upasargaja trsna).
Any type of trsnā, which is very severe and persists for long (continuously present) is incurable. Thirst manifesting in persons who have been debilitated or emaciated by other diseases, in those who have continuous bouts of vomiting and those associated with complications will definitely cause death. (10-11)

iti śrīmādhavakaraviracite mādhavanidāne tṛṣṇānidānaṃ samāptam ||16||
Thus ends the chapter on Trsnā.

CHAPTER SEVENTEEN

MŪRCHĀ, BHRAMA, NIDRĀ, TANDRĀ, SANNYASA NIDĀNAM

Nidana and Samprapti of Murcha – Etiological factors and pathogenesis of fainting

kṣīṇasya bahudoṣasya viruddhāhārasevinaḥ |
vegāghātādabhighātāddhīnasattvasya vā punaḥ ||1||
karaṇāyataneṣūgrā bāhyeṣvābhyantareṣu ca |
niviśante yadā doṣāstadā mūrchanti mānavāḥ ||2||
Etiological factors (persons prone to suffer from murcha) of murcha – The aggravated doshas cause murcha – fainting in - persons who are emaciated (debilitated), in whom the doshas have undergone profound increase, those who indulge in incompatible (foods which are mutually opposite in nature) foods and suppression of urges, those who are injured and those who are mentally weak.
Pathogenesis – Due to the above said factors the doshas undergo severe aggravation. These doshas get entry into and lodged in the external and internal organs related to the mind and cause the disease murcha – fainting. (1-2)

How does murcha develop? – extended pathogenesis & types of murcha

sañjñāvahāsu nāḍīṣu pihitāsvanilādibhiḥ |
tamo'bhyupaiti sahasā sukhaduḥkhavyapohakṛt ||3||

sukhaduḥkhavyapohācca naraḥ patati kāṣṭhavat |
moho mūrcheti tāmāhuḥ ṣaḍvidhā sā prakīrtitā ||4||
vātādibhiḥ śoṇitena madyena ca viṣeṇa ca |
ṣaṭsvapyetāsu pittaṃ tu prabhutvenāvatiṣṭhate ||5||
(su| u| taṃ| a| 46) |
When the sajñāvaha srotas (channels that carry sensations) are blocked by the increased vata and other doshas, the person experiences darkness in front of his eyes (goes into utter darkness). Due to this, the person will not be able to differentiate between pleasure and pain. He falls on the ground like a dry log of wood and undergoes unconsciousness.
This condition is known as moha or mūrchā.
Types of Murcha – Murcha is of 6 kinds, one from each dosha, one from rakta (blood), one from madya (alcoholic beverages), and another from visa (poisons). Pitta will be the predominant dosha in all these types of murcha. (3-5)

Murcha Purvarupa – Premonitory symptoms of fainting

hṛtpīḍā jṛmbhaṇaṃ glāniḥ sañjñādaurbalyameva ca |
sarvāsāṃ pūrvarūpāṇi, yathāsvaṃ tā vibhāvayet ||6||
(su| u| taṃ| a| 46) |
The premonitory symptoms of all types of murcha are – pain in the heart, excessive yawning, and weakness, improper or inadequate knowledge (inability of sense organs to perceive their respective sense objects leading to inadequate knowledge of things around us). These are the general premonitory symptoms of all types of murcha. Along with this the premonitory symptoms of the other types of murcha shall be understood by seeing the presence of their symptoms along with these general symptoms. Example – if along with these premonitory symptoms, the symptoms of vataja type of murcha are present, they shall be considered as the premonitory symptoms of vataja murcha. (6)

Vataja Murcha Symptoms

nīlaṃ vā yadi vā kṛṣṇamākāśamathavā'ruṇam |
paśyaṃstamaḥ praviśati śīghraṃ ca pratibudhyate ||7||
vepathuścāṅgamardaśca prapīḍā hṛdayasya ca |

kārśyaṃ śyāvā'ruṇā chāyā mūrchāye vātasambhave ||8||
(ca| sū| a| 24) |
In vātaja mūrchā – while fainting (going into unconsciousness) the person sees the sky (or his surroundings) in blue, black or crimson colours, goes into darkness (experiences darkness in front of his eyes), falls down unconscious but regains consciousness quickly. He would also have tremors, pain all over the body, and severe pain in the heart, emaciation, blackish red discolouration of the body. (7-8)

Pittaja Murcha Symptoms

raktaṃ haritavarṇaṃ vā viyat pītamathāpi vā |
paśyaṃstamaḥ praviśati sasvedaśca prabudhyate ||9||
(sapipāsaḥ sasantāpo raktapītākulekṣaṇaḥ) |
jātamātre patati ca śīghraṃ ca pratibudhyate |
sambhinnavarcāḥ pītābho mūrchāye pittasambhave ||10||
(ca| sū| a| 24) |
In pittaja murcha – while fainting (going into unconsciousness), the person sees the sky and surroundings in red, green or yellow colours. The person faints and goes into unconsciousness and would sweat a lot when he regains consciousness (gains consciousness along with sweating). (In this stage the person would experience thirst, increase in temperature of the body, red or yellow colour of the eyes, would go into a state of unconsciousness along with these symptoms and quickly regain consciousness). Diarrhoea and yellowish discolouration of the body are the other symptoms of pittaja type of murcha. (9-10)

meghasaṅkāśamākāśamāvṛtaṃ vā tamoghanaiḥ |
paśyaṃstamaḥ praviśati cirācca pratibudhyate ||11||
gurubhiḥ prāvṛtairaṅgairyathaivārdreṇa carmaṇā |
saprasekaḥ sahṛllāso mūrchāye kaphasambhave ||12||
(ca| sū| a| 24) |
In kaphaja mūrchā - while fainting (going into unconsciousness), the person sees the sky covered with thick clouds, falls unconscious. In this condition, the person regains consciousness after a long time. He feels as though his body is covered with heavy moist leather. Excessive salivation and nausea are the other symptoms of kaphaja type of murcha. (11-12)

Symptoms of Sannipataja Murcha

sarvākṛtiḥ sannipātādapasmāra ivāgataḥ |
sa jantuṃ pātayatyāśu vinā bībhatsaceṣṭitaiḥ ||13||
(ca| sū| a| 24) |
In sannipātaja type (caused by all the doşhas together) there will be manifestation of all the symptoms (of all the doshas) together. Leaving out 'bibhatsa chesta – disgusting or loathsome activities' the person would have all the other symptoms of apasmara disease (epilepsy, memory disorders). The bouts of fainting will be similar to those seen or experienced in apasmara. In this condition the person will faint (go into a state of unconsciousness) very quickly. (13)
Bibhatsa Cesta - Froth coming out of the mouth, grinding of teeth, rolling of eyes, hallucinations and convulsions are known as bibhatsa cestā and are invariably seen in apasmāra (epilepsy).

Symptoms of Raktaja Murcha

pṛthivyāpastamorūpaṃ raktagandhastadanvayaḥ |
tasmādraktasya gandhena mūrchanti bhuvimānavāḥ ||14||
dravyasvabhāva ityeke dṛṣṭvā yadabhimuhyati |
(su| u| taṃ| a| 46) |
The prthvi and ap bhutas (earth and water elements) are predominant in tamo guna. The smell of blood is also predominant in prthvi and ap bhutas and hence predominant in tamo guna (the disease murcha is also predominant in tamo guna). This is the reason that some persons who are predominant in tamo guna (in their constitution) become unconscious and faint, falling to the ground when they smell (and also sight) the blood. Some consider this to be the specific property of the blood. (14)

Symptoms of Visha-Madhyaja Murcha

guṇāstīvrataratvena sthitāstu viṣamadyayoḥ ||15||
ta eva tasmāttābhyāṃ tu mohau syātāṃ yatheritau |
(su| u| taṃ| a| 46) |
The properties (qualities) of poison and alcoholic drinks are very intense

/ sharp and damaging in comparison to any other things having intense / sharp quality. Therefore, the vishaja and madhyaja murcha are produced due to the effect of these qualities. In mürcha caused by poisons and alcoholic drinks the symptoms are very profound.

Symptoms of Raktaja, Madhyaja and Vishaja Murcha

stabdhāṅgadṛṣṭistvasṛjā gūḍhocchvāsaśca mūrchitaḥ ||16||
madyena vilapaṃśchete naṣṭavibhrāntamānasaḥ |
gātrāṇi vikṣipan bhūmau jarāṃ yāvanna yāti tat ||17||
vepathusvapnatṛṣṇāḥ syustamaśca viṣamūrchite |
veditavyaṃ tīvrataraṃ yathāsvaṃ viṣalakṣaṇaiḥ ||18||
(su| u| taṃ| a| 46) |

Raktaja Murcha - In raktaja murcha stiffness of the body, fixed gaze and deep (difficult) breathing – severe dyspnoea is seen.

Madyaja (alcoholic) Murcha – In Madyaja Murcha inconsistent (irrelevant) speech (delirium), falling on the ground with loss of consciousness and mental activities are seen. The person makes in-coordinated movements of the body parts (throwing of hands and feets), falls unconscious and stays in that state until the alcohol is digested in the body. (This means to tell that the symptoms of this type of murcha disappear once the alcohol gets digested).

Visaja (due to poison) Murcha – In Visaja Murcha there are tremors (rigors), sleep, thirst and feeling of darkness (in front of the eyes). Apart from this, the other symptoms specific to the particular (specific) poisons too will be present. The symptoms will be specific to the poison and can be mild, severe or harmful depending on the sharpness and intensity of the poison involved. (15-18)

Dosha predominance in murcha, bhrama, tandra and nidra
mūrchā pittatamaḥprāyā rajaḥpittānilādbhramaḥ |
tamovātakaphāttandrā nidrā śleṣmatamobhavā ||19||
(su| śā| a| 4) |
Mürcha (fainting, unconsciousness) is caused by predominance of pitta and

tamas.
Bhrama (dizziness, giddiness) is caused by predominance of rajas, pitta and vata.
Tandra (stupor) is caused by predominance of tamas, vata and kapha.
Nidra (sleep) is caused by predominance of kapha and tamas. (19)

Bhrama

(cakravadbhramato gātraṃ bhūmau patati sarvadā |
bhramaroga iti jñeyo rajaḥpittānilātmakaḥ) |

The body reeling like a turning (spinning) wheel and the person falling on the ground (repeatedly) always is known as bhrama roga (giddiness). It is caused due to predominance of rajas, pitta and vata.

Tandra

indriyārtheṣvasaṃvittirgauravaṃ jṛmbhaṇaṃ klamaḥ |
nidrārtasyeva yasyehā tasya tandrāṃ vinirdiśet ||20||
(su| śā| a| 24) |
The symptoms of tandra (stupor) include - non-perception of the sense objects by their related sense organs, feeling of heaviness (of the body), excessive yawning, weakness / fatigue (even without physical work) and the person appearing as though sleeping. (20)

Difference between mada, murcha and sannyasa

doṣeṣu madamūrchāyāḥ kṛtavegeṣu dehinām |
svayamevopaśāmyanti sannyāso nauṣadhairvinā ||21||
(ca| sū| a| 24) |
In cases of mada and all types of mürcha, etc. the person recovers soon after the bouts produced by doshas are over and even without medicines. On the other hand, sannyasa (another similar disease – compared to coma) does not subside without appropriate treatment. (21)

Sannyasa

vāgdehamanasāṃ ceṣṭāmākṣipyātibalā malāḥ |

sannyasyantyabalaṃ jantuṃ prāṇāyatanamāśritāḥ ||22||
sa nā sannyāsasannyastaḥ kāṣṭhībhūto mṛtopamaḥ |
prāṇairvimucyate śīghraṃ muktvā sadyaḥphalāṃ kriyām ||23||
(ca| sū| a| 24) |

The doshas which have become very powerful invade the chief seat of prana and obstruct the functions of speech, body and mind and makes a debilitated person unconscious and fall on the ground. This condition is known as sannyasa (coma). In this condition the person falls down on the ground like a dry log of wood or like a dead person. If this condition is not addressed immediately and if proper and quick restorative treatment is not given the person will surely die. (22-23)

iti śrīmādhavakaraviracite mādhavanidāne mūrchābhramanidrātandrāsannyāsanidānaṃ samāptam ||17||
Thus ends the chapter on Murchā etc.

CHAPTER EIGHTEEN

PĀNĀTYAYA, PARAMADA, PĀNĀJIRNA-PĀNAVIBHRAMA NIDANAM

Relationship between madya and visha (alcohol and poison)

ye viṣasya guṇāḥ proktāste'pi madye pratiṣṭhitāḥ |
tena mithyopayuktena bhavatyugro madātyayaḥ ||1||
All the qualities and properties present in poisons are also found in madya (alcoholic beverages). Hence, indiscriminate use of madya – alcohol causes madatyaya (alcoholic intoxication). (1)

Properties of Alcoholic drinks

kintu madyaṃ svabhāvena yathaivānnaṃ tathā smṛtam |
ayuktiyuktaṃ rogāya yuktiyuktaṃ yathā'mṛtam ||2||
prāṇāḥ prāṇabhṛtāmannaṃ tadayuktyā hinastyasūn |
viṣaṃ prāṇaharaṃ tacca yuktiyuktaṃ rasāyanam ||3||
(ca| ci| a| 24) |
By nature, alcoholic drinks are considered to be similar to food. When it is used improperly it causes many diseases. On the other hand, when it is used properly it acts like nectar. Food sustains life. But if the same food is taken improperly (violating the basic rules and regulations of food consumption, in terms of quality, quantity and time of eating) it takes away life. Similarly, the basic nature of the poison is to take away the life but when used judiciously it acts like a rejuvenator. (2-3)

vidhinā mātrayā kāle hitairannairyathābalam |
prahṛṣṭo yaḥ pibenmadyaṃ tasya syādamṛtopamam ||4||
(ca| ci| a| 24) |
snigdhaistadannairmāṃsaiśca bhakṣyaiśca saha sevitam |
bhavedāyuḥprakarṣāya balāyopacayāya ca ||5||
kāmyatā manasastuṣṭistejo vikrama eva ca |
vidhivatsevyamāne tu madye sannihitā guṇāḥ ||6||
(su| u| taṃ| a| 47) |
Alcohol is considered to be similar to (acts like) nectar when it is taken in accordance with proper procedure (of consumption), dose & time (of intake), with right combinations of food and in accordance to one's physical strength. This type of consumption of alcohol gives happiness (joy) to the person.
Alcohol taken with unctuous foods (fatty foods), meats or other nurturing foods brings about an increase of lifespan, strength and development of the body.
The alcohol taken judiciously bestows beauty (good looking body), happiness of (pleasantness) of mind, physical strength and valour. (4-6)

Symptoms of prathama mada – effects of first stage of alcoholism

buddhismṛtiprītikaraḥ sukhaśca pānānnanidrārativardhanaśca |
sampāṭhagītasvaravardhanaśca prokto'tiramyaḥ prathamo mado hi ||7||
In the first stage of the alcoholic effect, there is an increase of intelligence, memory, pleasantness / desire and happiness (pleasure). It enhances desire towards drinks, foods and sleep. It enhances the capacity and interest in reading, singing and the quality of voice (speech). Thus, the first stage is said to provide a very pleasant experience. (7)

Symptoms of Madhya / dvitiya mada – effects of second (intermediary) stage of alcoholism

avyaktabuddhismṛtivāgviceṣṭaḥ sonmattalīlākṛtirapraśāntaḥ |
ālasyanidrābhihato muhuśca madhyena mattaḥ puruṣo madena ||8||
In the intermediary stage of alcoholic effect – the intellect, memory and speech of the person becomes heavily disturbed (opposite, abnormal). His

activities and appearance appear like those of an insane person. He becomes uncontrollable, becomes lazy and sleeps frequently. (8)

Symptoms of Trtiya Mada – effects of third stage of alcoholism

gacchedagamyānna gurūṃśca manyet khādedabhakṣyāṇi ca naṣṭasañjñaḥ |
brūyācca guhyāni hṛdi sthitāni made tṛtīye puruṣo'svatantraḥ ||9||
In the third stage of alcoholic effect - the person indulges in forbidden acts and things, does not care for (disrespect) elders, eats things which are not to be eaten, having lost control speaks out secrets hidden in his mind.(9)

Symptoms of Chaturtha Mada – effects of fourth stage of alcoholism

caturthe tu made mūḍho bhagnadārviva niṣkriyaḥ |
kāryākāryavibhāgajño mṛtādapyaparo mṛtaḥ ||10||
ko madaṃ tādṛśaṃ gacchedunmādamiva cāparam |
bahudoṣamivāmūḍhaḥ kāntāraṃ svavaśaḥ kṛtī ||11||
In the fourth stage of alcoholic effect - the person falls to the ground and stays inactive (unconsciousness) just like a cut tree or dry log of wood. The person will not know the difference between activity and inactivity (confused so as to what to do and what not to, becomes incapable of doing any activity) and his condition becomes worse than a dead body. Which intelligent person would wish to be in such a worst intoxicated condition which almost makes the man insane? Which person would develop a strange desire to enter and stroll in a dense forest which is inhabited (by the fear of) by many cruel animals like lion etc.

Note – Here the fearful forest inhabited animals are compared to the 4th stage of alcoholic intoxication. Just like a person entering into the jungle becomes a prey for these animals and would not come back, the person entering into the 4th stage of alcoholic intoxication too becomes a victim of this condition and would not return back. (10-11)

Effects of taking alcohol in an unmethodical way

nirbhaktamekāntata eva madyaṃ niṣevyamāṇaṃ manujena nityam |
āpādayetkaṣṭatamānvikārānāpādayeccāpi śarīrabhedam ||12||

(sa| u| a| 47) |
Only such a person who drinks (alcoholic beverages) on empty stomach and in solitude daily becomes a victim of very difficult diseases. This can also cause loss of life (death). (12)

Other causative factors which are responsible for Madhya vikaras (diseases caused due to alcoholic intoxication)

kruddhena bhītena pipāsitena śokābhitaptena bubhukṣitena |
vyāyāmabhārādhvaparikṣatena vegāvarodhābhihatena cāpi ||13||
atyambubhakṣāvatatodareṇa sājīrṇabhuktena tathā'balena |
uṣṇābhitaptena ca sevyamānaṃ karoti madyaṃ vividhānvikārān ||14||
(su| u| taṃ| a| 47) |
Alcoholic drinks produce many diseases in persons afflicted with anger, fear, thirst, grief and hunger. Similarly, it produces many diseases in those debilitated by physical exercises, lifting heavy weights, too much of walking (travelling), and those who suppress natural urges of the body, those drinking large quantities of water, eating too much quantity of food or eating foods while having indigestion (before the previously taken food is digested), those who are very weak and those who are very much exposed to the heat. (13-14)

Diseases caused due to unmethodical consumption of alcohol

pānātyayaṃ paramadaṃ pānājīrṇamathāpi vā |
pānavibhramamugraṃ ca teṣāṃ vakṣyāmi lakṣaṇam ||15||
(su| u| taṃ| a| 47) |
Pānātyaya, paramada, pānājīrna and pānavibhrama are diseases caused due to excessive consumption of alcohol in an unmethodical way. The symptoms of these conditions will be described further. (15)

Symptoms of dosha predominant 'alcoholic excess' / alcoholic intoxication

hikkāśvāsaśiraḥkampapārśvaśūlaprajāgaraiḥ |
vidyādbahupralāpasya vātaprāyaṃ madātyayam ||16||
tṛṣṇādāhajvarasvedamohātīsāravibhramaiḥ |

vidyāddharitavarṇasya pittaprāyaṃ madātyayam ||17||
chardyarocakahṛllāsatandrāstaimityagauravaiḥ |
vidyācchītaparītasya kaphaprāyaṃ madātyayam |
jñeyastridoṣajaścāpi sarvaliṅgairmadātyayaḥ ||18||
(ca| ci| a| 24) |
Vataja Madatyaya - Hiccough, dyspnoea (increased respiration), shaking of the head, pain in the flanks, excessive awakening (loss of sleep) and excessive talking (delirium) are symptoms of pānātyaya in which vāta is the predominant dosha.
Pittaja Madatyaya - Thirst, burning sensation, fever, perspiration (excessive sweating), delusion, diarrhoea, giddiness and greenish discolouration of the body are symptoms of pānātyaya in which pitta is dominant.
Kaphaja Madatyaya - Vomiting, anorexia, nausea, stupor, feeling as if the body has been wrapped with wet cloth (laziness), feeling of heaviness and cold are symptoms of pānātyaya in which kapha is predominant.
Tridoshaja Madatyaya - Presence of all the symptoms together (symptoms of all the three doshas) is found in tridoshaja pānātyaya. (16-18)

Symptoms of Paramada

śleṣmocchrayo'ṅgagurutā virasāsyatā ca viṇmūtrasaktiratha tandriraroсakaśca |
liṅgaṃ parasya ca madasya vadanti tajjñāstṛṣṇā rujā śirasi sandhiṣu cāpi bhedaḥ ||19||
(su| u| taṃ| a| 47) |
According to expersts paramada is a type of madatyaya in which the below mentioned symptoms are seen –

- increase of kapha (seen as excess salivation, running in the nose, etc.)
- feeling of heaviness of the body,
- bad taste in the mouth (manifestation of abnormal tastes in the mouth),
- non-elimination of faeces and urine;
- stupor,
- anorexia,
- thirst,
- pain in the head and joints. (19)

Symptoms of Panajirna and Pana-vibhrama

ādhmānamugramatha codgiraṇaṃ vidāhaḥ pāne'jarāṃ samupagacchati lakṣaṇāni |20|
(su| u| taṃ| a| 47) |
hṛdgātratodakaphasaṃsravakaṇṭhadhūmā
mūrchāvamijvaraśirorujanapradāhāḥ ||20||
dveṣaḥ surānnavikṛteṣvapi teṣu teṣu taṃ pānavibhramamuśantyakhilena dhīrāḥ |
(su| u| taṃ| a| 47) |
Panajirna – Panajirna means indigestion of alcoholic drink. In this condition the symptoms including profound distension of the abdomen, vomiting, burning sensation and the drink not undergoing digestion at all – are seen.
Pana Vibhrama – Pricking (throbbing) pain in the region of the heart and of the whole body, excess salivation and running in the nose, feeling as though hot fumes are coming out of the throat, fainting, vomiting, fever, headache, severe burning sensation in the body, hatred even towards different kinds of alcoholic drinks and food are the symptoms of pānavibhrama as described by experts. (20)

Symptoms of incurability of madatyaya

hīnottarauṣṭhamatiśītamamandadāhaṃ tailaprabhāsyamapi pānahataṃ tyajettu ||21||
jihvauṣṭhadantamasitaṃ tvathavā'pi nīlaṃ pīte ca yasya nayane rudhiraprabhe vā |
(su| u| taṃ| a| 47) |
Hanging down of upper lip, feeling of excessive cold externally (outside of the body) and excessive heat or burning sensation internally (inside the body) i.e., the body is cold to touch but is very hot inside (burns from within), face of the person appears as if smeared with oil, blackish or bluish discolouration of the tongue, lips and teeth, and eyes very red, seen in a patient intoxicated by alcohol should be refused treatment. (21)

Upadrava – complications of madatyaya

hikkājvarau vamathuvepathupārśvaśūlāḥ kāsabhramāvapi ca pānahataṃ bhajante ||22||
(su| u| taṃ| a| 47)
The complications of alcoholic intoxication are – hiccough, fever, vomiting, rigors, pain in the flanks, cough and giddiness. (22)

iti śrīmādhavakaraviracite mādhavanidāne pānātyayaparamadapānājīrṇapānavibhramanidānaṃ samāptam ||18||
Thus ends the chapter on Madātyaya.

CHAPTER NINETEEN

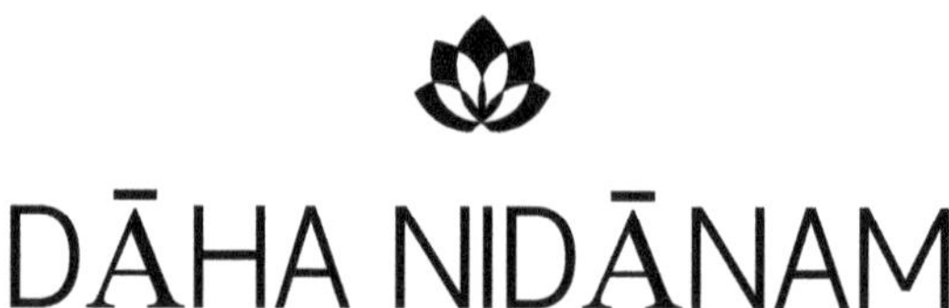

DĀHA NIDĀNAM

Daha Nidanam – etiological factors of burning sensation

tvacaṃ prāptaḥ sa pānoṣmā pittaraktābhimūrchitaḥ |
dāhaṃ prakurute ghoraṃ pittavattatra bheṣajam ||1||
The heat produced by indiscriminate (violating the ideal procedure of alcoholic consumption as mentioned in the texts) consumption of alcoholic drinks gets associated with pitta and rakta (blood), reaches the skin and gets localized therein and produces a severe burning sensation. The treatment for burning sensation is similar to that of pitta (pitta mitigating treatments). (1)

Raktaja Daha – Burning sensation caused by blood
kṛtsnadehānugaṃ raktamudriktaṃ dahati dhruvam |
sa uṣyate tṛṣyate ca tāmrābhastāmralocanaḥ ||2||
lohagandhāṅgavadano vahninevāvakīryate |
(su| u| taṃ| a| 47) |
The rakta which has aggravated to severe proportions would spread all over the body and cause burning sensation. In this condition the person feels as if his body is being burnt by fire. Apart from this there would be severe thirst, coppery red coloration of the skin and eyes, smell of iron from the body and face (mouth). These are the symptoms of raktaja daha. (2)

Pittaja Daha – Burning sensation caused by pitta
pittajvarasamaḥ pittātsa cāpyasya vidhiḥ smṛtaḥ ||3||
(su| u| taṃ| a| 47) |
In dāha caused due to pitta aggravation, the symptoms and treatment are similar to those of pitta jwara (fever caused by aggravated pitta). (3)

Trshna Nirodhaja Daha – Burning Sensation caused by suppressing the thirst

tṛṣṇānirodhādabdhātau kṣīṇe tejaḥ samuddhatam |
sabāhyābhyantaraṃ dehaṃ pradahenmandacetasaḥ ||4||
saṃśuṣkagalatālvoṣṭho jihvāṃ niṣkṛṣya vepate |
(su| u| taṃ| a| 47) |
By suppressing thirst (not drinking water even when thirsty) the water component (body fluids) of the body gets depleted. This increases teja (pitta, heat of the body). This heat produces burning sensation internally as well as externally (inside the body and on the surface of the body). The activity of the mind of the person gets reduced (causes unconsciousness or semi-conscious state) and he suffers from dryness of the throat, palate and lips. The person puts his tongue out of his mouth and experiences shaking of body parts (tremors, convulsions). These are the symptoms of trsna nirodhaja daha. (4-5)

Raktapurna Koshtaja Daha – Burning Sensation caused due to 'blood filled visceral organs'

asṛjaḥ pūrṇakoṣṭhasya dāho'nyaḥ syāt suduḥsahaḥ ||5||
(su| u| taṃ| a| 47) |
Another kind of dāha occurs due to accumulation of blood in the various visceral organs caused by injury. This type of burning sensation is called as raktapurna koshtaja daha. This condition is dreadful. (5)

Dhatu Kshayaja and Kshataja Daha – Burning sensation caused due to depletion of tissues and injury

dhātukṣayottho yo dāhastena mūrchātṛḍarditaḥ |
kṣāmasvaraḥ kriyāhīnaḥ sa sīdedbhṛśapīḍitaḥ ||6||
(su| u| taṃ| a| 47) |
Dhatu Kshayaja Daha is the burning sensation which is caused as an effect of depletion of the body tissues. This produces fainting (unconsciousness), thirst and feeble (tired) voice (loss of voice). The person becomes inactive (or unfit to undergo any kind of treatment – no treatment would give

him relief) and might also face death. This type of daha is called as dhatu kshayaja daha. (6)

Kshataja Daha –

kṣatajo'naśnataścānnaṃ śocato vā'pyanekadhā |
tenāntardahyate'tyarthaṃ tṛṣṇāmūrchāpralāpavān ||7||

Kshataja Daha –

This type of burning sensation is caused in a person who becomes incapable of eating food due to injury and also gets afflicted with many types of grief / worries. The symptoms of Kshataja Daha include burning sensation experienced in the interior of the body, excessive thirst, unconsciousness and delirium.

Marmabhighataja Daha – Burning Sensation caused by injury to vital organs

marmābhighātajo'pyasti so'sādhyaḥ saptamo mataḥ |
sarva eva ca varjyāḥ syuḥ śītagātrasya dehinaḥ ||8||
(su| u| taṃ| a| 47) |

Marmabhighataja Daha is the seventh type of burning sensation. This is caused due to the injury to the vital organs including heart, urinary bladder and head. This type of burning sensation is incurable. All types of daha – burning sensation should be refused treatment (should not be treated and rejected because they are incurable) if the body of the patient has become cold (in spite of severe burning sensation inside the body). (7)

iti śrīmādhavakaraviracite mādhavanidāne dāhanidānaṃ samāptam ||19||
Thus ends the chapter on daha.

CHAPTER TWENTY

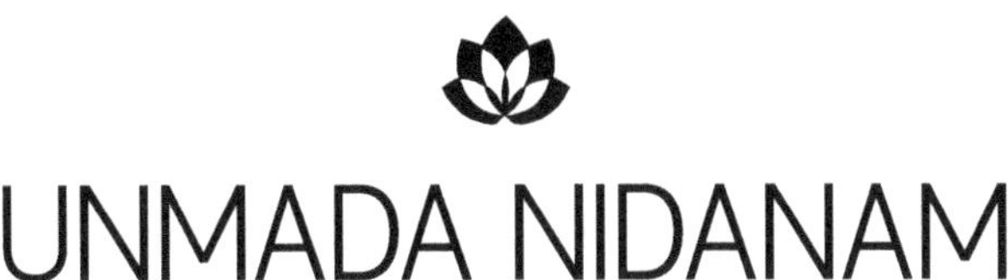

UNMADA NIDANAM

Unmada Nirukti – meaning and definition of unmada

madayantyudgatā doṣā yasmādunmārgamāgatāḥ |
mānaso'yamato vyādhirunmāda iti kīrtitaḥ ||1||
(su| u| taṃ| a| 62) |
Unmada is a disease in which the doshas which have undergone abnormal increase and traversing upwards (through the channels of the mind) get localized in the mind and cause its abnormality. (1)

Types of Unmada

ekaikaśaḥ sarvaśaśca doṣairatyarthamūrchitaiḥ |
mānasena ca duḥkhena sa ca pañcavidho mataḥ ||2||
viṣādbhavati ṣaṣṭhaśca yathāsvaṃ tatra bheṣajam |
sa cāpravṛddhastaruṇo madasañjñāṃ bibharti ca ||3||
(su| u| taṃ| a| 62) |
Unmada is basically of 6 types. They are, one from each dosa, the fourth type is from the combination of all the three doshas, fifth from grief etc mind factors and the sixth type is caused by poisons.
The treatment of these shall be done in accordance and as appropriate to the cause. When unmada is not completely developed and is of recent onset it will be called as mada. (2-3)

Unmada Nidana (samanya hetu) – common etiological factors of unmada

viruddhaduṣṭāśucibhojanani pradharṣaṇaṃ devagurudvijānām |
unmādaheturbhayaharṣapūrvo mano'bhighāto viṣamāśca ceṣṭāḥ ||4||

(ca| ci| a| 9) |

Below mentioned are the etiological factors of unmada –

- excessive indulgence in foods which are incompatible, spoilt (contaminated) and unclean;
- showing disrespect to gods, preceptors (elders) and the twice born (Brahmans)
- affection of the mind due to sudden emotions like fear, joy, etc. and
- violent physical activities (4)

Unmada Samprapti – Pathogenesis of Unmada

tairalpasattvasya malāḥ praduṣṭā buddhernivāsaṃ hṛdayaṃ pradūṣya |
srotāṃsyadhiṣṭhāya manovahāni pramohayantyāśu narasya cetaḥ ||5||
(ca| ci| a| 1) |
In persons who are mentally weak (the sattvika quality of the mind has been immensely decreased), the doṣhas having undergone abnormal increase invade and contaminate the hrdaya which is the seat of mind, get spread (lodged) in all the channels of the mind and bring about the derangement of the mind in quick time. This state of derangement of the mind is called as Unmada. (5)
Note – Hrdaya generally means heart. This word has also been mentioned to explain the brain. So, it has to be understood contextually. Therefore, it is good to consider hrdaya as the brain in this context of Unmada.

Unmada Samanya Lakshana – general symptoms of Unmada

dhīvibhramaḥsattvapariplavaścaparyākulādṛṣṭiradhīratāca|
abaddhavāktvaṃhṛdayaṃcaśūnyaṃsāmānyamunmādagadasyaliṅgam||6||
(ca|ci|a|9)
The generalized symptoms of Unmada are - improper understanding and unsteadiness of the mind, in-coordination of sight (seeing here and there or not making eye to eye coordination without any reason), lack of courage (feeling of fear), irrelevant talk, and feeling of emptiness of heart (mind). (6)

Causes, pathogenesis and symptoms of Vataja Unmad

rūkṣālpaśītānnavirekadhātukṣayopavāsairanilo'tivṛddhaḥ |
cintādiduṣṭaṃ hṛdayaṃ pradūṣya buddhiṃ smṛtiṃ cāpyupahanti śīghram ||7||
asthānahāsasmitanṛtyagītavāgaṅgavikṣepaṇarodanāni |
pāruṣyakārśyāruṇavarṇatāśca jīrṇe balaṃ cānilajasya rūpam ||8||
(ca| ci| a| 9) |
Causes - Vata gets abnormally increased in the body due to indulgence in foods which are dry, scanty (foods less in quantity) or cold, (frequent) purgation (inclusive of vomiting), depletion of tissues, fasting (starvation) and other factors.
Pathogenesis - This Vāta, in turn invades and further contaminates the hrdaya (brain) which has already been weakened (contaminated) by emotions like worry etc and further brings about derangement of intellect and memory, leading to manifestation of vataja unmada.

Symptoms – The signs and symptoms of unmada caused by abnormal increase of vata are –

- laughing, smiling, dancing, singing, speaking, making movement of body parts and weeping at improper time and place (unnecessarily and without any reason);
- hardness / roughness, emaciation, blackish red discolouration of the body and
- exacerbation of symptoms after digestion of food (7-8)

Causes, pathogenesis and symptoms of Pittaja Unmada

ajīrṇakaṭvamlavidāhyaśītairbhojyaiścitaṃ pittamudīrṇavegam |
unmādamatyugramanātmakasya hṛdi sthitaṃ pūrvavadāśu kuryāt ||9||
amarṣasaṃrambhavinagnabhāvāḥ santarjanātidravaṇauṣṇyaroṣāḥ |
pracchāyaśītānnajalābhilāṣaḥ pītā ca bhāḥ pittakṛtasya liṅgam ||10||
(ca| ci| a| 9) |
Causes – Pitta gets abnormally increased in the body due to indulgence in foods which are not properly cooked, very pungent or sour, corrosive

(cause heartburn), or those which are hot etc.
Pathogenesis – This aggravated pitta reaches the hrdaya – brain (which has already been weakened / contaminated by emotions like worry, anger etc) and affects the mind quickly as described earlier, in people who are not self controlled and further brings about derangement of intellect and memory, leading to the manifestation of pittaja unmada.

Symptoms - The signs and symptoms of unmada caused by abnormal increase of pitta are –

- intolerance,
- uncontrollability,
- casting away the clothes and remaining naked,
- threatening others,
- running away (to beat / harm others)
- feeling of excessive heat in the body (burning sensation),
- desiring shade, cold water and cold foods,
- yellowish discolouration of the body (9-10)

Causes, pathogenesis and symptoms of Kaphaja Unmada

sampūraṇairmandaviceṣṭitasya soṣmā kapho marmaṇi sampraduṣṭaḥ |
buddhiṃ smṛtiṃ cāpyupahatya cittaṃ pramohayan sañjanayedvikāram ||11||
vākceṣṭitaṃ mandamarocakaśca nārīviviktapriyatā'tinidrā |
chardiśca lālā ca balaṃ ca bhukte nakhādiśauklyaṃ ca kaphātmake syāt |
(ca| ci| a| 9) ||12||
Causes – Kapha along with pitta gets abnormally increased in the body due to excessive indulgence in over-eating, lack of physical exercise etc.
Pathogenesis - This Kapha (with pitta), in turn invades and further contaminates the hrdaya (brain) which has already been weakened (contaminated) by emotions like worry etc and further brings about derangement of intellect and memory, leading to manifestation of kaphaja unmada. This occurs on the backdrop of derangement of mind caused by kapha and pitta.

Symptoms - The signs and symptoms of unmada caused by abnormal increase of kapha are –

- slow / weak / sluggish voice (or talk) and body movements,
- anorexia,
- desire for women (or sex) and
- solitude,
- excessive sleep,
- vomiting,
- saliva dribbling out,
- symptoms pronounced immediately after taking food,
- whitish discoloration of nails, etc. (11-12)

Causes, pathogenesis and symptoms of Sannipataja Unmada

yaḥ sannipātaprabhavo'tighoraḥ sarvaiḥ samastaiḥ sa ca hetubhiḥ syāt |
sarvāṇi rūpāṇi bibharti tādṛgviruddhabhaiṣajyavidhirvivarjyaḥ ||13||
(ca| ci| a| 9) |
Causes and pathogenesis - Sannipataja unmäda is produced by increase of all the three došhas together by their respective causes.
Symptoms – This condition is said to be very dreadful. The symptoms of all the doṣas are seen in the patient. Since the treatment of this condition is mutually antagonistic (treatment to balance one dosha aggravates the other) it is regarded as incurable and hence treatment of this type of unmada shall be denied (refused). (13)

Causes and symptoms of Shokadi Janya Unmada

corairnarendrapuruṣairaribhistathā'nyairvitrāsitasya
dhanabāndhavasaṅkṣayādvā |
gāḍhaṃ kṣate manasi ca priyayā riraṃsorjāyeta cotkaṭatamo manaso vikāraḥ ||14||
citraṃ bravīti ca mano'nugataṃ visañjño gāyatyatho hasati roditi cāpi mūḍhaḥ |
(su| u| taṃ| a| 62) |
Causes and pathogenesis - Getting frightened by (sudden appearance or presence) of robbers, government officials (like police, etc.) enemies and others (wild animals, weapons and anything causing fear), loss of money (or wealth), death of relatives (next of kin such as wife, lover, sons,

daughters, parents etc.) excessive desire for sex with beloved partner and not being able to obtain that and such other factors cause great injury to the mind and produce dreadful mental disorder - unmada.
Symptoms - Person so affected talks indifferently, which he likes most and sometimes reveals even the secrets hidden in his mind, sings, laughs or weeps on his own accord and behaves senselessly. (14-15)

Symptoms of Visha janya unmada

raktekṣaṇo hatabalendriyabhāḥ sudīnaḥ śyāvānano viṣakṛte'tha bhavedvisañjñaḥ ||15||
(su| u| taṃ| a| 62) |
In unmada produced by poisons, the person will have red shot eyes, loss of strength of body, senses and complexion. He will have a sense of helplessness, black / bluish-black discolouration of the mouth or face and loss of consciousness. (15)

Symptoms of incurability of Unmada

avāñcī vā'pyudañcī vā kṣīṇamāṃsabalo naraḥ |
jāgarūko hyasandehamunmādena vinaśyati ||16||
(su| u| taṃ| a| 62) |
Patient of unmāda who is found always keeping his head bent down or bent up, whose muscles have decreased (is emaciated), whose strength has been decreased (weak) and always awake (without sleep) is sure to die. (16)

General symptoms of Bhutonmada

amartyavāgvikramavīryaceṣṭo jñānādivijñānabalādibhiryaḥ |
unmādakālo'niyataśca tasya bhūtotthamunmādamudāharettam ||17||
(ca| ci| a| 9) |
Bhütonmāda (unmāda caused due to possession by "spirits") is described as the disease in which the speech, valour, strength, activities, intellect and knowledge of the affected person are super-human and the time of onset of the symptoms is unspecific (not in accordance with that of the doshas). (17)

Symptoms of Devajushta Unmada (possession by Gods)

santuṣṭaḥ śuciratidivyamālyagandho nistandrīravitathasaṃskṛtaprabhāṣī |
tejasvī sthiranayano varapradātā brahmaṇyo bhavati naraḥ sa devajuṣṭaḥ ||18||
(su| u| taṃ| a| 60) |

The symptoms of a person possessed by Deva Graha (Gods, Goddesses) are - contentment (not expressing any desires), cleanliness (engaged in keeping his body, dress, surroundings, etc. very clean), desire for very pleasant garlands and scents etc. (excessive smell of divine perfumed flowers or flower garlands emitted from his body without the person applying any such perfumes), not getting stupor or sleep (always alert and / or awake), always speaking refined (cultured) language and truth, possessing bright complexion (on the face), unruffled (un-winking) eyes, bestowing favours and blessings and such other acts as seen (done by) in brāhmaṇas or respecting and worshipping Brahmanas. (18)

Symptoms of Devashatru (Danava / Asura) jushta Unmada (possessed by demons)

saṃsvedī dvijagurudevadoṣavaktā jihmākṣo vigatabhayo vimārgadṛṣṭiḥ |
santuṣṭo na bhavati cānnapānajātairduṣṭātmā bhavati sa devaśatrujuṣṭaḥ ||19||
(su| u| taṃ| a| 60) |

The symptoms of a person possessed by Devashatru / Danava / Asura Graha (Demons) are – heavy perspiration (heavily sweating), always abusing brahmanas, teachers, gods, etc. having distorted look (crooked eyes / squint), absence of any fear, always taking wrong paths to achieve anything (critical of everything), never getting satisfied with foods and drinks and indulging in sinful acts. (19)

Symptoms of Gandharvajushta Unmada (possessed by Gandharva)

hṛṣṭātmā pulinavanāntaropasevī svācāraḥ priyaparigītagandhamālyaḥ |
nṛtyan vai prahasati cāru cālpaśabdaṃ gandharvagrahaparipīḍito manuṣyaḥ ||20||
(su| u| taṃ| a| 60) |

The symptoms of a person possessed by Gandharva are – always in contentment, loves to roam around river banks, gardens etc, indulging in good deeds (pure character), fond of good company, songs (music), scents, garlands, dancing with passion, laughing and speaking less (man of less words). (20)

Symptoms of Yaksha jushta Unmada (possessed by Yaksha)

tāmrākṣaḥ priyatanuraktavastradhārī gambhīro drutagatiralpavāksahiṣṇuḥ |
tejasvī vadati ca kiṃ dadāmi kasmai yo yakṣagrahaparipīḍito manuṣyaḥ ||21||
(su| u| taṃ| a| 60) |
The symptoms of a person possessed by Yaksha are – red shot eyes, desire for good (beautiful, likable), thin and red coloured dress, steadiness in all activities and quick pace (walking fast), very less speech, enduring any trouble (has good tolerance), bright complexion of the face (attractive), and enquiring others what they want from him (ready to help and give away anything, helping nature). (21)

Symptoms of Pitr jushta Unmada (possessed by Pitr - ancestor)

pretānāṃ sa diśati saṃstareṣu piṇḍān śāntātmā jalamapi cāpasavyavastraḥ
|
māṃsepsustilaguḍapāyasābhikāmastadbhakto bhavati pitṛgrahābhijuṣṭaḥ
||22||
(su| u| taṃ| a| 60) |
The symptoms of a person possessed by Pitr are – The person is engaged in the act of offering pinda (balls of cooked rice offered to the departed souls of ancestors / forefathers during ceremonial procedures) and water, on the seat prepared with kusha grass etc, by being calm and composed, and putting clothes etc on his right shoulder. He has developed desires towards foods prepared with mutton (meat), sesame, jaggery and milk puddings (sweets prepared in milk base) and is also a devotee of pitr (respects them immensely). (22)

Symptoms of Sarpa / Bhujanga Graha Jushta Unmada (possessed by snakes)

yastūrvyāṃ prasarati sarpavat kadācit sṛkkaṇyau vilihati jihvayā tathaiva

|
krodhālurguḍamadhudugdhapāyasepsurjñātavyo bhavati bhujaṅgamena juṣṭaḥ ||23||
(su| u| taṃ| a| 60) |
The symptoms of a person possessed by Sarpa / Bhujanga Graha are – The person afflicted by this graha is seen moving on the ground (crawling) lying on his chest, just like a snake does, keeps licking his lips with his tongue, is extremely angry (quickly gets angry), and develops desire for jaggery, honey, milk and milk puddings (sweet dish prepared on milk base). (23)

Symptoms of Rakshasa Graha Jushta Unmada

māṃsāsṛgvividhasurāvikāralipsurnirlajjo bhṛśamatiniṣṭhuro'tiśūraḥ |
krodhālurvipulabalo niśāvihārī śaucadviḍ bhavati sa rākṣasairgṛhītaḥ ||24||
(su| u| taṃ| a| 60) |
The symptoms of a person possessed by Rakshasa Graha are – This person possessed with Rakshasa Graha will show immense desire for foods prepared with meat (mutton) and blood, and various types of alcohols / intoxicating drinks. He is devoid of shyness; very cruel and very courageous (brave).He gets very angry and also has great strength. He roams around at night time and hates cleanliness. (24)

Symptoms of Pishaca Graha Jushta Unmada

uddhastaḥ kṛśaparuṣo acirapralāpī durgandho bhṛśamaśucistathā'tilolaḥ |
bahvāśī vijanavanāntaropasevī vyāceṣṭan bhramati rudan piśācajuṣṭaḥ ||25||
(su| u| taṃ| a| 60) |
The symptoms of a person possessed by Pishaca Graha are – the person is always seen keeping his shoulders elevated or keeping himself naked, is emaciated, speaks irrelevantly with intermittent gaps, emits bad smell from his body, is unclean (very dirty), is greedy, eats large quantities of food, roams around in deserted forests and uninhabited places, who does untoward (weird, opposite) activities, and roams around weeping loudly all alone. (25)

Symptoms of incurability in unmada

sthūlākṣo drutamaṭanaḥ sa phenalehī nidrāluḥ patati ca kampate ca yo hi |
yaścādridviradanagādivicyutaḥ syāt so'sādhyo bhavati tathā trayodaśābde ||26||
(su| u| taṃ| a| 60) ||
Below mentioned are the symptoms of incurability of Unmada –

- bulging out of the eyes,
- running / walking fast,
- licking the froth (saliva) coming out of his mouth,
- sleeping in excess,
- falling off suddenly,
- has tremors,
- unmada caused due to fall from a mountain, back of an elephant or tree,
- unmada persisting for 13 long years (any type of unmada which is 13 years old) (26)

Periodicity of attack of different grahas

devagrahāḥ paurṇamāsyāmasurāḥ sandhyayorapi |
gandharvāḥ prāyaśo'ṣṭamyāṃ, yakṣāśca pratipadyatha ||27||
pitryāḥ kṛṣṇakṣaye hiṃsyuḥ, pañcamyāmapi coragāḥ |
rakṣāṃsi rātrau, paiśācāścaturdaśyāṃ viśanti hi ||28||
(su| u| taṃ| a| 60) |
Deva grahas seize the person on full-moon days,
Asura grahas seize the person in the mornings (junction of night and early morning) or evening (junction of noon and evening)
Gandharva grahas seize the person on the eighth day,
Yaksa grahas seize the person on the first day,
Pitr grahas seize the person during the dark half of the month,
Naga grahas seize the person on the fifth day,
Raksasa grahas seize the person during nights and
Pisaca grahas seize the person on the fourteenth day. (27-28)

Analogy to describe the attack and presence of grahas

darpaṇādīn yathā chāyā śītoṣṇaṃ prāṇino yathā |
svamaṇiṃ bhāskarārciśca yathā dehaṃ ca dehadhṛk |
viśanti ca na dṛśyante grahāstadvaccharīriṇaḥ ||29||
(su| u| taṃ| a| 60) |
Just as an image enters into the mirror, the heat and cold which are invisible enter our body, the sunrays enter the suryakanti gem (or the heat enters the fire), the soul which cannot be seen enters the physical body and all these cannot be perceived by our physical eyes. We cannot see these happening. Similarly, the grahas also enter the human body but cannot be seen or perceived by our physical eyes. Though the grahas are present in the body they cannot be felt or seen. (29)

Entry and existence of (attack, seize) grahas as explained by other texts

praviśyāśu śarīraṃ hi pīḍāṃ kurvanti duḥsahām ||30||
Having entered the body (being invisible), the grahas (spirits) create intolerable sufferings. (30)

tapāṃsi tīvrāṇi tathaiva dānaṃ vratāni dharmo niyamaśca satyam |
guṇāstathā'ṣṭāvapi teṣu nityā vyastāḥ samastāśca yathāprabhāvam ||31||
na te manuṣyaiḥ saha saṃviśanti na vā manuṣyān kvacidāviśanti |
ye tvāviśantīti vadanti mohātte bhūtavidyāviṣayādapohyāḥ ||32||
teṣāṃ grahāṇāṃ paricārakā ye koṭīsahasrāyutapadmasaṅkhyāḥ |
asṛgvasāmāṃsabhujaḥ subhīmā niśāvihārāśca tathā''viśanti ||33||
Observance of austerities, charity, vows, right conduct, rigid discipline, truth, the eight extraordinary capabilities — are the qualities always found in the grahas, more in deva graha and less in others. Depending on the graha and their impact, the above said qualities are present either partially or in entirety. This means to tell that these qualities are found partially (few) in asura etc grahas and in entirety (full, almost) in deva graha. Being endowed with these good qualities the deva graha etc do not sit along with human beings nor do enter the unclean bodies of the human beings all by themselves. But those who still, due to ignorance, say that these grahas enter the human body, should be considered as having absolutely no knowledge of bhuta vidhya i.e., demonology.
It is in fact the thousands and millions of servants or retinue of the grahas,

who are fond of blood and flesh, who are very terrific and who roam about at nights, which enter into the human body and take possession of the person. (31-33)

iti śrīmādhavakaraviracite mādhavanidāna unmādanidānaṃ samāptam||20||
Thus ends the chapter on Unmāda.

The eight extraordinary capabilities are

(1) Anima - capacity to assume minute size
(2) Mahima - capacity to assume very huge size
(3) Garima - capacity to become very heavy
(4) Laghima - to become very light
(5) Prapti - obtaining any desired thing
(6) Prakamya - fulfilling all desires
(7) Isatwa – over-lordship on anything and
(8) Vasitva - subjugating or controlling anything

According to another version, the extraordinary powers are –

1. Capacity to enter into the body of another person
2. Extraordinary sense perception
3. To understand all sounds or meanings of all words / language
4. Capacity to see
5. Hear and
6. Remember things which are impossible by others
7. Unusual bright complexion and
8. Capacity to vanish out of sight-are the extraordinary powers.

CHAPTER TWENTY-ONE

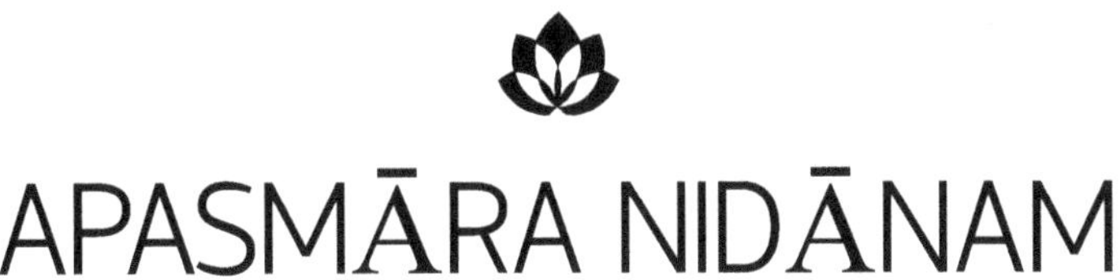

APASMĀRA NIDĀNAM

Apasmara Samprapti, Swarupa – Pathogenesis and nature of epilepsy

(cintāśokādibhirdoṣāḥ kruddhā hṛtsrotasi sthitāḥ |
kṛtvā smṛterapadhvaṃsamapasmāraṃ prakurvate) |
tamaḥpraveśaḥ saṃrambho doṣodrekahatasmṛteḥ |
apasmāra iti jñeyo gado ghoraścaturvidhaḥ ||1||
(The doshas having become increased (aggravated) by worry, grief, etc. get lodged in the channels of the hrdaya (mind, brain), make for loss of memory (knowledge, consciousness) and produce the disease apasmāra).
In Apasmāra the person experiences a feeling as if entering into a zone of utter darkness (the person experiences darkness in front of his eyes and he experiences entering into a zone of ignorance which is in the form of darkness, loss of consciousness), and does many types of activities including violent movements of the eyes, limbs (convulsions) etc. All these happen due to the destruction (loss) of memory caused by severely aggravated doshas. This dreaded disease is called Apasmara and is of four kinds. (1)
The four types of apasmara are – vataja, pittaja, kaphaja and tridoshaja.

Apasmara Purvarupa – Premonitory symptoms of apasmara

hṛtkampaḥ śūnyatā svedo dhyānaṃ mūrchā pramūḍhatā |
nidrānāśaśca tasmiṃśca bhaviṣyati bhavatyatha ||2||
(su| u| taṃ| a| 61) |
The premonitory symptoms of apasmara are – palpitation of the heart, feeling of emptiness (of the mind), perspiration, worry, fainting, destruction of activities of mind and senses (delusion), and loss of sleep. (2)

Symptoms of Vataja Apasmara

kampate pradaśeddantān phenodvāmī śvasityapi |
paruṣāruṇakṛṣṇāni paśyedrūpāṇi cānilāt ||3||
(ca| ci| a| 10) |
The symptoms of vataja apasmara are – tremors (convulsions), grinding of teeth, frothy vomiting, dyspnoea (increased respiration), and roughness of the body. All things around him appear to be of reddish black colour before the attack (before he falls and goes into unconsciousness). (3)

Symptoms of Pittaja Apasmara

pītaphenāṅgavaktrākṣaḥ pītāsṛgrūpadarśakaḥ |
satṛṣṇoṣṇānalavyāptalokadarśī ca paittikaḥ ||4||
(ca| ci| a| 10) |
The symptoms of pittaja apasmara are - yellow coloured froth around the mouth, yellowish skin, face and eyes. He sees all things around him being yellow or red coloured (before the attack, before going into unconsciousness). He also will have severe thirst, feeling of excessive heat in the body and would see the surroundings as if covered (burning) with fire (that everything around him is being burnt by the fire). (4)

Symptoms of Kaphaja Apasmara

śuklaphenāṅgavaktrākṣaḥ śītahṛṣṭāṅgajo guruḥ |
paśyechuklāni rūpāṇi ślaiṣmiko mucyate cirāt ||5||
(ca| ci| a| 10) |
The symptoms of kaphaja apasmara are - whitish froth at the mouth, white colour of the skin, face and eyes, (feeling of) coldness and heaviness of the body, horripilation, and seeing white coloured things (he sees all things around him being white in colour, before the attack). The attacks of this type of apasmara ends very late i.e. the person regains consciousness long time after the attack. (5)

Symptoms of Tridoshaja / Sannipataja Apasmara and symptoms of incurability of apasmara

sarvairetaiḥ samastaiśca liṅgairjñeyastridoṣajaḥ |
apasmāraḥ sa cāsādhyo yaḥ kṣīṇasyānavaśca yaḥ ||6||
(ca| ci| a| 10) |
In tridoshaja / sannipataja apasmara is caused by the aggravation of all the three doshas and the symptoms of all three doshas are seen in this condition.
This type of apasmara (tridoshaja), the apasmara manifested in persons who are emaciated and apasmara which is not of recent onset (chronic apasmara) - are all said to be incurable. (6)

Other symptoms of incurability of apasmara

pratisphurantaṃ bahuśaḥ kṣīṇaṃ pracalitabhruvam |
netrābhyāṃ ca vikurvāṇamapasmāro vināśayet ||7||
(ca| ci| a| 10) |
When apasmara occurs with too much of (severe and continuous) tremors (convulsions), emaciation, fierce movement of eyebrows (eyebrows deviated in upward direction) and eyes (deformities in the eyes), it would kill the person (it becomes incurable). (7)

Period of aggravation of apasmara

pakṣādvā dvādaśāhādvā māsādvā kupitā malāḥ |
apasmārāya kurvanti vegaṃ kiñcidathāntaram ||8||
(ca| ci| a| 10) |
deve varṣatyapi yathā bhūmau bījāni kānicit |
śaradi pratirohanti tathā vyādhisamucchrayāḥ ||9||
(su| u| taṃ| a| 61) |
The dosas get aggravated (regularly) on 5, 12 or 30-days intervals and produce episodes of apasmāra (epileptic seizures). Sometimes the episodes (attacks) can take place at any other interval of time, even apart from these intervals (whenever there is aggravation of accumulated and latent doshas).
Just as the seeds which lay in the earth even during rainy season sprout only during sarat ritu (autumn season) i.e., when the favourable season for their sprouting appears, the diseases also, (in spite of being latent in the body) develop only after a certain period of time. (8-9)

iti śrīmādhavakaraviracite mādhavanidāne'pasmāranidānaṃ samāptam ||21||
Thus ends the chapter on Apasmāra.

CHAPTER TWENTY-TWO

VĀTA VYĀDHI NIDĀNAM

Vata Vyadhi Nidana, Samprapti – Etiological Factors and Pathogenesis of Vata Vyadhi

rūkṣaśītālpalaghvannavyavāyātiprajāgaraiḥ |
viṣamādupacārācca doṣāsṛksravaṇādapi ||1||
laṅghanaplavanātyadhvavyāyāmādiviceṣṭitaiḥ |
dhātūnāṃ saṅkṣayāccintāśokarogātikarṣaṇāt ||2||
vegasandhāraṇādāmādabhighātādabhojanat |
marmābādhādgajoṣṭrāśvaśīghrayānāpataṃsanāt ||3||
dehe srotāṃsi riktāni pūrayitvā'nilo balī |
karoti vividhān vyādhīn sarvāṅgaikāṅgasaṃśrayān ||4||
(ca| ci| a| 28) |

Causes – The etiological factors of Vata Vyadhi include - excessive indulgence in foods which are dry, cold, scanty, light (quickly digestible); sexual intercourse, keeping awake at nights, improper treatments (administering Panchakarma treatments at wrong times, in wrong conditions or consuming foods and activities which are incompatible as well as opposite to the nature of land and season), excessive discharge (elimination) of doṣhas and blood from the body (during the course of treatments like emesis, purgation, bloodletting, etc.), jumping, swimming, long distance walking and such other exercises and untoward activities (opposite to one's nature); loss or depletion of body tissues, worry, grief, extreme debility due to protracted diseases, habit of suppression of natural urges of the body, production of āma (undigested intermediary metabolites), trauma, fasting or diseases of vital organs (pain or damage to vital organs), riding fast on elephants, camels and horses (other similar animals or vehicles), or falling during such rides.

Pathogenesis – Due to the above said etiological factors aggravation of vata takes place and the channels (of vāta) in the body become empty or dry. This aggravated vata later occupies (fills) these channels and produces different diseases affecting one or more parts of the body. (1-4)

Vata Vyadhi Purvarupa – Premonitory Symptoms of Vata Vyadhi

avyaktaṃ lakṣaṇaṃ teṣāṃ pūrvarūpamiti smṛtam |
ātmarūpaṃ tu yadvyaktamapāyo laghutā punaḥ ||5||
(ca| ci| a| 28) |
Premonitory stage of Vata Vyadhi is characterised by appearance of the symptoms of the disease which are in milder form. When the same symptoms (found in milder form in the premonitory stage) become well marked and severe, they denote the stage of manifestation of the disease (vata vyadhi).
On the other hand, absence of characteristic symptoms and lightness of the body (during the course of specific diseases to be described further on) are the signs of cure of such diseases.(5)

Vata Vyadhi Lakshanas – Symptoms of Vata Vyadhi

saṅkocaḥ parvaṇāṃ stambho bhaṅgo'sthnāṃ parvaṇāmapi |
romaharṣaḥ pralāpaśca pāṇipṛṣṭhaśirograhaḥ ||6||
khāñjyapāṅgulyakubjatvaṃ śotho'ṅgānāmanidratā |
garbhaśukrarajonāśaḥ spandanaṃ gātrasuptatā ||7||
śironāsākṣijatrūṇāṃ grīvāyāścāpi huṇḍanam |
bhedastodo'rtirākṣepo muhuścāyāsa eva ca ||8||
evaṃvidhāni rūpāṇi karoti kupito'nilaḥ |
hetusthānaviśeṣācca bhavedrogaviśeṣakṛt ||9||
(ca| ci| a| 28) |
The general symptoms of vata vyadhi are - contractures of small joints of hands and feet (body parts), rigidity of joints, fracture & dislocation of joints including small joints of hands and feet, horripilation, delirium, stiffness (gripping pain, rigidity) of hands, back and head, limping and lameness of one or both legs, curvature of the back (hunchback), wasting of the body parts, loss of sleep, loss or destruction of foetus, semen and ovum

(menstrual blood); tremors, and loss of sensation pain in the body parts. This also occurs crookedness (drawing in of) head, nose, eyes, shoulders and neck; cutting or throbbing type of pain in the body parts, frequent convulsions and tiredness. These and other (similar) symptoms are produced by increased väta. The aggravated vata also produces special and newer diseases corresponding to the specific causes and sites of affection. (6-9)

Symptoms of Koshtashrita Vata

tatra koṣṭhāśrite duṣṭe nigraho mūtravarcasoḥ |
bradhnahṛdrogagulmārśaḥpārśvaśūlaṃ ca mārute ||10||
If the increased (aggravated) vāta is localised in the kostha (alimentary tract) there will be obstruction to passage of urine and faeces, enlargement of the scrotum (swelling in the groin), heart diseases, tumours of the abdomen, haemorrhoids and pain in the flanks. (10)

Symptoms of Sarvanga Vata

sarvāṅgakupite vāte gātrasphuraṇabhañjanam |
vedanābhiḥ parītāśca sphuṭantīvāsya sandhayaḥ ||11||
(ca| ci| a| 28) |
If vāta gets increased all over the body, there will be tremors (throbbing, twitching, pulsations, etc.) cutting, crushing and other types of pain, feeling of pain in the joints and the person feels as if there is a blast (bursting) in the joints. (11)

Symptoms of Guda Sthita (Gudagata) Vata

graho viṇmūtravātānāṃ śūlādhmānāśmaśarkarāḥ |
jaṅghorutrikapātpṛṣṭharogaśoṣau gude sthite ||12||
When the aggravated vāta gets localized and occupies in the gudā (rectum), it causes stoppage of movement of urine, faeces and flatus; pain (colic) and distension of the abdomen, formation of urinary gravel (calculus), pain in the calves, thighs, pelvis, legs (feet) and back and emaciation. (12)

Symptoms of Amashaya Sthita (Amashaya gata) Vata

ruk pārśvodarahṛnnābhestṛṣṇodgāravisūcikāḥ |
kāsaḥ kaṇṭhāsyaśoṣaśca śvāsaścāmāśayasthite ||13||
(ca| ci| a| 28) |
If increased vāta resides in the āmāśaya (stomach) it causes pain in the flanks, abdomen, region of the heart and umbilicus, thirst, belching / eructation, vomiting and diarrhoea (occurring together), cough, dryness of throat and mouth and dyspnoea are found. (13)

Symptoms of Pakwasaya Sthita (Pakwasaya Gata) Vata

pakvāśayastho'ntrakūjaṃ śūlāṭopau karoti ca |
kṛcchramūtrapurīṣatvamānāhaṃ trikavedanām ||14||
If the aggravated vata gets lodged in the pakwāśaya (large intestine and rectum) it will cause intestinal gurgling and pain, gurgling sounds in the abdomen, difficulty for defecation and urination, flatulence (distension) of abdomen and pain in the sacral region. (14)

Symptoms of Srotradi Gata Vata

śrotrādiṣvindriyavadhaṃ kuryādduṣṭasamīraṇaḥ | (su| ni| a| 1) |
If vāta gets increased and localised in the Indriyas (sense organs) it will produce loss of function (loss of perception) of those organs.

Symptoms of Twak-Gata Vata

tvagrūkṣā sphuṭitā suptā kṛśā kṛṣṇā ca tudyate |
ātanyate sarāgā ca parvaruk tvaggate'nile ||15||
(ca| ci| a| 28) |
If the increased vata is located in the twak (skin), it produces dryness, cracks, loss of sensation, thinning, blackish discolouration, pricking pain, stretching, redness and pain in the small joints of the hands and feet (and other joints of the body). (15)

Symptoms of Raktagata Vata

rujastīvrāḥ sasantāpā vaivarṇyaṃ kṛśatā'ruciḥ |
gātre cārūṃṣi bhuktasya stambhaścāsṛggate'nile ||16||

(ca| ci| a| 28) |
If vata gets located in asrk (blood), it will cause severe pain, increased feeling of heat, discolouration, emaciation, loss of taste, appearance of ulcers or boils on the skin and stiffness of the body after meals. (16)

Symptoms of Mamsa-Medogata Vata

gurvaṅgaṃ tudyate'tyarthaṃ daṇḍamuṣṭihataṃ yathā |
saruk śramitamatyarthaṃ māṃsamedogate'nile ||17||
If vāta gets lodged in māmsa and medas (muscles and fat) it produces a feeling of heaviness of the body parts (body parts would become heavy and inactive) associated with severe throbbing (pricking) pain and pain as though beaten by a stick or fist. The person would also experience severe pain in the entire body and extreme exhaustion. (17)

Symptoms of Majja-Asthigata Vata

bhedo'sthiparvaṇāṃ sandhiśūlaṃ māṃsabalakṣayaḥ |
asvapnaḥ santatā ruk ca majjāsthikupite'nile ||18||
(ca| ci| a| 28) |
When the aggravated vata is located in the majjā (bone marrow) and asthi (bone) it causes splitting pain in the bones and joints of the body including the small joints of the hands and feet, loss of muscles and strength of the body, loss of sleep and constant pain of the body.(18)

Symptoms of Shukragata Vata

kṣipraṃ muñcati badhnāti śukraṃ garbhamathāpi vā |
vikṛtiṃ janayeccāpi śukrasthaḥ kupito'nilaḥ ||19||
(ca| ci| a| 28) |
If the aggravated vata gets localized in the shukra (semen, reproductive tissue) it would cause premature ejaculation or delayed expulsion (ejaculation) of semen. Similarly, the foetus created by such shukra (sperm) would either be delivered too soon (aborted / miscarriage) or would be delivered too late. This vata would also cause abnormalities of sperm (semen) and embryo. (19)

Symptoms of Siragata, Snayugata, Sandhigata Vata

kuryāt sirāgataḥ śūlaṃ sirākuñcanapūraṇam |
sa bāhyābhyantarāyāmaṃ khallīṃ kaubjyamathāpi vā ||20||
sarvāṅgaikāṅgarogāṃśca kuryāt snāyugato'nilaḥ | (ca| ci| a| 28) |
hanti sandhigataḥ sandhīn śūlāṭopau karoti ca ||21|| (su| ni| a| 17) |
Siragata Vata - Vata (aggravated) located in the siras (veins and arteries) would cause pain, contractures or shortening and engorgement (with accumulation of blood).
Snayugata Vata – When the aggravated vata gets located in the snayus (ligaments, tendons, nerves) it would cause bow-like bending of the body either inwards or outwards, contractures of the fingers, shortening of the body due to the abnormal curvature of the back, and other diseases of either the whole body or any particular part or parts of the body.
Sandhigata Vata - If the aggravated vata is localized in the joints, it causes destruction of joints (and their functions). Along with this, there also occurs pain and cracking sound (swelling) in the joints. (20-21)

Symptoms of Avarana of Vata subtypes by Pitta and Kapha
(prāṇodānau samānaśca vyānaścāpāna eva ca |
sthānasthā mārutāḥ pañca yāpayanti śarīriṇam) | (su| ni| a| 1) |
prāṇe pittāvṛte chardirdāhaścaivopajāyate |
daurbalyaṃ sadanaṃ tandrā vairasyaṃ ca kaphāvṛte ||22|| (su| ni| a| 1) |
udāne pittayukte tu dāho mūrchā bhramaḥ klamaḥ |
asvedaharṣau mando'gniḥ śītatā ca kaphāvṛte ||23||
svedadāhauṣṇyamūrchāḥ syuḥ samāne pittasaṃvṛte |
kaphena sakte viṇmūtre gātraharṣaśca jāyate ||24||
apāne pittayukte tu dāhauṣṇyaṃ raktamūtratā |
adhaḥkāye gurutvaṃ ca śītatā ca kaphāvṛte ||25||
vyāne pittāvṛte dāho gātravikṣepaṇaṃ klamaḥ |
stambhano daṇḍakaścāpi śūlaśothau kaphāvṛte ||26|| (su| ni| a| 1) |27|
Prana, Udana, Samana, Vyana and Apana are the five types of vata. In their normal state, these vata subtypes residing in their own seats would nourish and sustain the body and good health of the body.

Note – Avarana is a condition wherein vata and its normal functioning and movements are clouded (encompassed, masked, surrounded, blocked, obstructed or interfered) by pitta, kapha, tissues, food or excreta. One subtype of vata can cause avarana of another subtype of vata also.

Pittavrita Prana - If prana vata gets obstructed by pitta the person would have vomited and burning sensation.
Kaphavrta Prana – If prana vata is encompassed by kapha, the person would suffer from debility, tiredness (loss of strength), stupor and bad taste (manifestation of opposite tastes) in the mouth.
Pittavrita Udana – When udana vata is encompassed or enveloped by pitta it produces burning sensation, fainting (unconsciousness), dizziness and exhaustion.
Kaphavrita Udana – If Udana Vata is encompassed or enveloped by kapha it causes loss of perspiration, loss of enthusiasm, poor digestive ability and feeling of coldness.
Pittavrita Samana – When Samana Vata is encompassed by pitta it gives rise to perspiration, burning sensation, increased temperature and fainting (unconsciousness).
Kaphavrita Samana – When Samana Vata is enveloped by Kapha, it causes obstruction to the elimination of urine and faeces and horripilations in the body.
Pittavrita Apana – When Apana Vata is encompassed by pitta it causes burning sensation, increase of heat / temperature and elimination of blood mixed urine.
Kaphavrita Apana – When Apana Vata is obstructed by kapha, it causes heaviness of the lower portion of the body (limbs) and feeling of coldness.
Pittavrita Vyana – When Vyana Vata is encompassed by pitta it gives rise to burning sensation, abnormal movements of the parts of the body and exhaustion.
Kaphavrita Vyana – If Vyana Vata is clouded by Kapha the body becomes stiff like a log. Along with this there is pain and swelling.

Akshepaka

yadā tu dhamanīḥ sarvāḥ kupito'bhyeti mārutaḥ |
tadā''kṣipatyāśu muhurmuhurdehaṃ muhuścaraḥ ||27||
muhurmuhuścākṣepaṇādākṣepaka iti smṛtaḥ |
(su| ni| a| 1) |
When the increased vata gets localised in all the dhamanis (blood vessels)

of the body, it produces quick, frequent and jerky movements of the body. Since there are repeated convulsions, this condition is called Aksepaka (convulsions). (22-27)

Symptoms of Apatantraka and Apatanaka, Dandapatanaka

kruddhaḥ svaiḥ kopanairvāyuḥ sthānādūrdhvaṃ pravartate ||28||
pīḍayan hṛdayaṃ gatvā śiraḥśaṅkhau ca pīḍayan |
dhanurvannamayedgātrāṇyākṣipenmohayettadā ||29||
sa kṛcchrāducchvaseccāpi stabdhākṣo'tha nimīlakaḥ |
kapota iva kūjecca niḥsañjñaḥ so'patantrakaḥ ||30||
dṛṣṭiṃ saṃstabhya sañjñāṃ ca hatvā kaṇṭhena kūjati |
hṛdi mukte naraḥ svāsthyaṃ yāti mohaṃ vṛte punaḥ ||31||
vāyunā dāruṇaṃ prāhureke tadapatānakam |
(ca| si| a| 1) |
kaphānvito bhṛśaṃ vāyustāsveva yadi tiṣṭhati ||32||
daṇḍavat stambhayeddehaṃ sa tu daṇḍāpatānakaḥ |
(su| ni| a| 1) |

Note – Apatantraka and Apatanaka are the variants of Aksepaka.

Apatantraka - Vata undergoing increase by its own moves in an upward direction towards the head (leaving its seats of predominance like colon etc). While doing so, it causes pain in the heart, head and temples. It further makes the body bend like a bow and produces convulsions and loss of consciousness. The patient will find difficulty in breathing, the eyes are kept wide open at times (without the movement of lids) and at other times they remain half closed (or lids completely closed). The person remains in a state of unconsciousness and makes sounds from within the throat like a pigeon. This condition which is a variant of aksepaka is called apatantraka.

Apatanaka – Apatanaka is yet another variant of apatanaka (described by other scholars) in which the patient will have completely fixed gaze (incapable of perceiving any visual objects), complete loss of consciousness, produces cooing sounds in the throat, and will have intermittent relief of symptoms when the heart (brain) becomes free from the affliction of aggravated vata but once again enters into a state of unconsciousness when there is another attack. This dreadful disease caused by severely aggravated vata is called apatanaka.

Dandapatanaka – This is a variant of apatanaka. If in apatānaka, vāta gets associated with kapha, the body of the patient will become stiff like a log of wood. This condition is called as Dandāpatānaka. (28-32)

Symptoms of Dhanustambha, Abhyantarayama, Bahyayama

dhanustulyaṃ namedyastu sa dhanuḥstambhasañjñakaḥ ||33|| (su| ni| a| 1)
aṅgulīgulphajaṭharahṛdvakṣogalasaṃśritaḥ |
snāyupratānamanilo yadā''kṣipati vegavān ||34||
viṣṭabdhākṣaḥ stabdhahanurbhagnapārśvaḥ kaphaṃ vaman |
abhyantaraṃ dhanuriva yadā namati mānavam ||35||
tadā'syābhyantarāyāmaṃ kurute māruto balī |
bāhyasnāyupratānastho bāhyāyāmaṃ karoti ca ||36||
tamasādhyaṃ budhāḥ prāhurvakṣaḥkaṭyūrubhañjanam | (su| ni| a| 1) |

Dhanustambha – It is a condition wherein the aggravated vata makes the body bent like a bow.

Abhyantarayama (dhanustambha) – It is a variant of dhanustambha. Here the powerful (aggravated) vata affects the network of snayus (ligaments, tendons, nerves) located in the toes (and fingers), ankle joints, abdomen, and region of the heart, chest and throat. By doing so, it causes severe convulsive movements. The patient develops fixed gaze, stiffness of the jaw (lower) fracture (collapse or in-drawing) of the flanks, ribs), and vomiting of phlegm (mucus). Here the bending of the body will be inwards and is bent like a bow. This condition caused by severely aggravated vata is called as Abhyantharayama dhanustambha.

Bahyayama (dhanustambha) – It is also a variant of dhanustambha. When severely aggravated vata affects the tendons (nerves) of the external part of the body, the body of the person gets bent outwards like a bow. In this condition there is a threat of fracture (damage) to the chest, waist and thighs and hence is incurable. This condition is known as Bahyayama dhanustambha and in the opinion of scholars is an incurable condition.

(33-36)

Abhighataja Aksepaka - Dosha association in Aksepaka and symptoms of incurability of Apatanaka

kaphapittānvito vāyurvāyureva ca kevalaḥ ||37||
kuryādākṣepakaṃ tvanyaṃ caturthamabhighātajam |
garbhapātanimittaśca śoṇitātisravācca yaḥ ||38||
abhighātanimittaśca na sidhyatyapatānakaḥ | (su| ni| a| 1) |
Vata associated with kapha and pitta or even alone produces aksepaka. A fourth kind of aksepaka is caused due to trauma to the body parts and is called abhighataja aksepaka.
Apatanaka caused by abortions, excessive haemorrhage and trauma are incurable. (37-38)

Paksavadha – pathogenesis and symptoms

gṛhītvā'rdhaṃ tanorvāyuḥ sirāḥ snāyūrviśoṣya ca ||39||
pakṣamanyataraṃ hanti sandhibandhān vimokṣayan |
kṛtsno'rdhakāyastasya syādakarmaṇyo vicetanaḥ ||40||
ekāṅgarogaṃ taṃ kecidanye pakṣavadhaṃ viduḥ |
sarvāṅgarogastadvacca sarvakāyāśrite'nile ||41||
(vā| ni| a| 15) |
The aggravated vata gets lodged in and affects any half side of the body (right or left side of the body), causes dryness (destruction) of the siras and snayus (blood vessels and ligaments / tendons / nerves), causes looseness of the joints and destroys the functions and sensation of half side of the body. This condition is called as Ekanga Roga by some people and Paksavadha by some others. When the entire body i.e., both halves of the body are affected in a similar way by the aggravated vata, it is called Sarvanga Vata. (39-41)

Dosha association and symptoms of incurability in Paksavadha

dāhasantāpamūrchāḥ syurvāyau pittasamanvite |
śaityaśothagurutvāni tasminneva kaphānvite ||42||
śuddhavātahataṃ pakṣaṃ kṛcchrasādhyatamaṃ viduḥ |

sādhyamanyena saṃyuktamasādhyaṃ kṣayahetukam ||43||
(su| ni| a| 1) |
In the above disease (paksavadha), if vāta is associated with pitta, there will be burning sensation, increase of temperature of the affected parts and fainting (unconsciousness).
In paksavadha if vata is associated with kapha, there will be coldness, swelling and heaviness of the affected parts.
Pakşavadha caused by vāta alone is difficult to cure. Paksavadha caused by vata associated with other doshas (pitta and kapha) is easily curable. Pakdavadha caused by destruction of tissues (emaciation, wasting) is incurable. (42-43)

Other symptoms of incurability of Paksavadha

garbhiṇīsūtikābālavṛddhakṣīṇeṣvasṛksrute |
pakṣāghātaṃ pariharet vedanārahito yadi) |
(Paksāghāta seen in pregnant women, in women who has recently delivered, children, old people, emaciated persons and that caused by heavy bleeding and that in which the patient has no pain (sensation) at all in the affected limbs (and affected parts) should be refused treatment because this condition is incurable.)

Ardita – causes, pathogenesis, symptoms

uccairvyāharato'tyarthaṃ khādataḥ kaṭhināni vā |
hasato jṛmbhato vā'pi bhārādviṣamaśāyinaḥ ||44||
śironāsauṣṭhacibukalalāṭekṣaṇasandhigaḥ |
ardayatyanilo vaktramarditaṃ janayatyataḥ |
vakrībhavati vaktrārdhaṃ grīvā cāpyapavartate ||45||
śiraścalati vāksaṅgo netrādīnāṃ ca vaikṛtam |
grīvācibukadantānāṃ tasmin pārśve ca vedanā ||46||
Causes – Speaking in loud voice (high pitch) for long periods, eating (biting) hard food substances, excessive laughing (by opening the mouth), excessive yawning, carrying heavy loads on the head, and sleeping in uneven or irregular posture.

Pathogenesis - The vata getting aggravated by the above said etiological factors spreads to and occupies the head, nose, lips, chin, forehead and joints of the eye affects the face and causes a disease called as Ardita.

Symptoms – In this condition one half of the face gets crooked (deviated to the other side) and the neck also becomes crooked (turned outwards). There is also shaking of the head, obstruction of voice / speech (inability to speak), and deformities of eyes, nose, neck, jaw and teeth. The person also experiences pain (in the mentioned parts) on the afflicted side. (44-46)

Premonitory symptoms and symptoms of incurability of ardita

(yasyāgrajo romaharṣo vepathurnetramāvilam |
vāyurūrdhvaṃ tvaci svāpastodo manyāhanugrahaḥ) |
tamarditamiti prāhurvyādhiṃ vyādhivicakṣaṇāḥ |
kṣīṇasyānimiṣakṣasya prasaktāvyaktabhāṣiṇaḥ ||47||
na sidhyatyarditaṃ gāḍhaṃ trivarṣaṃ vepanasya ca |
(su| ni| a| 1) |
(The premonitory symptoms of ardita include horripilations, tremors, accumulation of dirt in the eyes (dirty looking eyes), belching (eructation), loss of sensation in the skin (of the face), pricking pain, stiffness of the neck and lower jaw.)
Expert clinicians call this disease Ardita.
Symptoms of incurability of ardita - Ardita is said to be incurable in emaciated persons, in those who do not wink their eyes, whose speech is slurred and incoherent and in whom ardita is persisting for more than three years. (47)

Attacks and episodes of Aksepaka and other disorders
gate vege bhavet svāsthyaṃ sarveṣvākṣepakādiṣu ||48|| (vā| ni| a| 15) |
In all types of aksepakas (convulsive disorders) the patient gets periods of health (normalcy) when the episodes of attack pass off. (48)

Causes and Symptoms of Hanugraha

jihvānirlekhanācchuṣkabhakṣaṇādabhighātataḥ |
kupito hanumūlasthaḥ sraṃsayitvā'nilo hanum ||49||
karoti vivṛtāsyatvamathavā saṃvṛtāsyatām |

hanugrahaḥ sa tena syāt kṛcchrāccarvaṇabhāṣaṇam ||50|| (vā| ni| a| 15) |
Causes – opening the mouth in excess and for long periods (and also putting out the tongue) for the purpose of cleaning the teeth (brushing) and tongue with the help of brushes and tongue cleaners, eating foods which are dry, and injury are the etiological factors of hanugraha.
Pathogenesis – Due to the above said causes, the vata located at the root of the jaw causes loosening and dislocation of the joints of the jaw.
Symptoms – The mouth of the person will either remain open or closed tight all the time. This would cause difficulty in chewing the food as well as speaking. This disease is known as Hanugraha. (49-50)

Causes and Symptoms of Manyastambha

divāsvapnāsanasthānavivṛtordhvanirīkṣaṇaiḥ |
manyāstambhaṃ prakurute sa eva śleṣmāṇa''vṛtaḥ ||51|| (su| ni| a| 1) |
Causes – Excessive sleeping during daytime, sleeping at irregular places and in irregular postures and looking in upward direction for long periods are the causes of manyastambha.
Pathogenesis and symptoms – Vata aggravated due to the above said etiological factors either singly or in association with kapha will afflict the sides of the neck and cause manyastambha.
Symptoms – Stiffness of the neck is the main symptom of this disease, which is also the name of the disease. (51)

Symptoms of Jihwastambha

vāgvāhinīsirāsaṃstho jihvāṃ stambhayate'nilaḥ |
jihvāstambhaḥ sa tenānnapānavākyeṣvanīśatā ||52||
(vā| ni| a| 15) |
Jihwa stambha (stiffness or loss of movement of the tongue) is caused when the aggravated vata affects the tendons / nerves near the voice box (responsible for the production of voice) and causes inability for chewing the food, drinking or talking. (52)

Symptoms of Siragraha

raktamāśritya pavanaḥ kuryānmūrdhadharāḥ sirāḥ |

rūkṣāḥ savedanāḥ kṛṣṇāḥ so'sādhyaḥ syāt sirāgrahaḥ ||53||
(vā| ni| a| 15) |
Vāta increases, getting localised in the blood makes the blood vessels of the neck dry, painful and black coloured.
This condition is known as Siragraha (or sirograha) and is incurable. (53)

Pathogenesis and Symptoms of Grdhrasi

sphikpūrvā kaṭipṛṣṭhorujānujaṅghāpadaṃ kramāt |
gṛdhrasī stambharuktodairgṛhṇāti spandate muhuḥ ||54||
vātādvātakaphāttandrāgauravārocakānvitā | (ca| ci| a| 28) |
vātajāyāṃ bhavettodo dehasyāpi pravakratā |
jānukaṭyūrusandhīnāṃ sphuraṇaṃ stabdhatā bhṛśam ||55||
vātaśleṣmodbhavāyāṃ tu nimittaṃ vahnimārdavam |
tandrā mukhaprasekaśca bhaktadveṣastathaiva ca ||56||
Pathogenesis of Grdhrasi - Vata either alone or associated with kapha produces (a disease called) Grdhrasi. This condition is characterised by a peculiar type of pain. The pain typically starts from the buttock and descends downwards encroaching (spreading in, radiating) the back portions of pelvis (lumbar region), thigh, knee joint, calf muscles (back of the leg – the portion of the lower limb between knee and ankle joints) and foot.
Vataja Grdhrasi - Due to this there is also (apart from pain) stiffness (inability to move), severe pain and throbbing (pricking pain) in the regions mentioned above along with repeated (and intermittent) pulsations. These symptoms are characteristic of Vataja (vata predominant) Grdhrasi.
Vata-Kaphaja Grdhrasi - In Grdhrasi if there is association of kapha with vata the person will experience stupor, heaviness and anorexia.
(Vataja Grdhrasi presents with pricking pain, crookedness of the body parts (irregular shape of the body parts), throbbing and severe stiffness in the joints of the knee, pelvis and thigh (hip). In Vata-Kaphaja Grdhrasi sluggishness of digestive fire / capacity (poor digestive capacity), stupor, excessive salivation and aversion towards food are predominantly seen as symptoms.) (54-60)

Symptoms of Visvaci

talaṃ pratyaṅgulīnāṃ yāḥ kaṇḍarā bāhupṛṣṭhataḥ ||57||
bāhvoḥ karmakṣayakarī viśvācī ceti socyate |
(su| ni| a| 1) |
Visvaci is an affection of the tendons / nerves of the fingers, the arms and the shoulders, leading to loss of function of the arm as caused by the aggravated vata.
The aggravated vata afflicts the tendons / nerves of the upper limb beginning from the back of the arm and reaching up to the back of the fingers and also involving the upper portions of the forearm and hands ultimately leading to the loss of functions in these regions. (57)

Symptoms of Krostuka Sirsa

vātaśoṇitajaḥ śotho jānumadhye mahārujaḥ ||58||
jñeyaḥ kroṣṭukaśīrṣastu sthūlaḥ kroṣṭukaśīrṣavat | (su| ni| a| 1) |
Vata and rakta getting affected together produces a very painful swelling of the knee joint (in the centre of the knee joint). The swelling is big and resembles the head of a fox and hence is known by the name Krostuka-Sirsa. (58)

Symptoms of Khanja and Pangu

vāyuḥ kaṭyāśritaḥ sakthnaḥ kaṇḍarāmākṣipedyadā ||59||
khañjastadā bhavejjantuḥ paṅguḥ sakthnordvayorvadhāt |
(su| ni| a| 1) |
Khanja – The aggravated vata gets lodged in the waist of the person, affects the tendons of one lower limb and causes loss of functions therein. This condition is called Khanja. Here the person cannot walk properly and experiences limping.
Pangu – When the aggravated vata, instead of one lower limb, affects the tendons and nerves of both the lower limbs and causes loss of functions therein the person would become lame. This condition is called as Pangu. (59)

Symptoms of Kalayakhanja

prakrāman vepate yastu khañjanniva ca gacchati ||60||

kalāyakhañjaṃ taṃ vidyānmuktasandhiprabandhanam |
(su| ni| a| 1) |
A condition in which there are tremors (in the legs, lower limbs) when the person begins to walk and later walks with a limp (limping gait, just like a person who has limp) is called Kalayakhanja. In this condition there is also looseness of the joints of the lower limb. This condition is caused due to excessive consumption of Kalaya (pea, lentil, masura dala) and hence the name Kalayakhanja. (60)

Symptoms of Vatakantaka

ruk pāde viṣamenyaste śramādvā jāyate yadā ||61||
vātena gulphamāśritya tamāhurvātakaṇṭakam |
(vā| ni| a| 15) |
Due to improper placing of the feet on the ground (walking on an irregular surface) while walking or exhaustion due to exertion of walking, the vata gets aggravated and gets localized in the ankle joints and causes severe pain therein. This condition is called as Vatakantaka. (61)

Symptoms of Padadaha

pādayoḥ kurute dāhaṃ pittāsṛksahito'nilaḥ ||62||
viśeṣataścaṅkramataḥ pādadāhaṃ tamādiśet |
(su| ni| a| 1) |
The vitiated Vata gets associated with pitta and rakta (blood) and causes burning sensation in the feet. The burning sensation is experienced more when the person walks. This condition is called as Padadaha. (72)

Symptoms of Padaharsa

hṛṣyete caraṇau yasya bhavetāṃ cāpi suptakau ||63||
pādaharṣaḥ sa vijñeyaḥ kaphavātaprakopataḥ |
(su| ni| a| 1) |
Vitiated vata along with kapha produces a feeling of pins and needles or feeling of loss of sensation in the feet. This condition is called as padaharsa. (63)

Symptoms of Amsa Shosha and Apabahuka

aṃsadeśasthito vāyuḥ śoṣayedaṃsabandhanam ||64|| (su| ni| a| 1) |
sirāścākuñcya tatrastho janayedavabāhukam |65| (su| ni| a| 1) |
Amsa Sosa - Vāta located in the region of the shoulder (shoulder blade) causes emaciation (of muscles) of
the shoulder joint. (This is known as Amsa sosa.)
Avabahuka / Apabahuka – The aggravated vata located in the region of the shoulder (blades) causes constriction / dryness of the tendons / nerves located therein and causes another condition called as Apabahuka. (64)

Symptoms of Mukadi

āvṛtya vāyuḥ sakapho dhamanīḥ śabdavāhinīḥ ||65||
narān karotyakriyakānmūkaminminagadgadān |
(su| ni| a| 1) |
The aggravated vata along with kapha invades and obstructs the shabda vahini dhamanis (vessels / nerves which are responsible for the production of voice, vessels and nerves around the voice box) and cause inability to speak in the person. The person would become mute or would develop nasal speech or stammer. (65)

Symptoms of Tuni and Pratituni

adho yā vedanā yāti varcomūtrāśayotthitā ||66||
bhindatīva gudopasthaṃ sā tūnī nāma nāmataḥ | (su| ni| a| 1) |
gudopasthotthitā yā tu pratilomaṃ pradhāvitā ||67||
vegaiḥ pakvāśayaṃ yāti pratitūnīti socyate |(su| ni| a| 1) |
Tuni - The disease in which severe cutting pain begins in the colon (rectum?) and urinary bladder and moves downwards towards anus and penis is called Tuni.
Pratituni – In this condition the movement of the pain is in reverse direction as compared to that of tuni. Here the cutting type of pain first starts in the anus and penis and moves upwards towards the colon (large intestine). Here the pain quickly moves up in bouts, as if thrown in an upward direction (colic). (66-67)

Symptoms of Adhmana and Pratyadhmana

sāṭopamatyugrarujamādhmātamudaraṃ bhṛśam ||68||
ādhmānamiti taṃ vidyād ghoraṃ vātanirodhajam |
vimuktapārśvahṛdayaṃ tadevāmāśayotthitam ||69||
pratyādhmānaṃ vijānīyāt kaphavyākulitānilam |
(su| ni| a| 1) |

Adhmana - Adhmana is a condition caused due to the obstruction to the movements of vata. It is characterised by gurgling noise in the abdomen (intestines), severe pain and distension of the abdomen. This is considered to be a dreadful condition (life threatening).

Pratyadhmana – When the same symptoms of adhmana manifest in the stomach excluding (not manifesting) the regions of flanks and heart and is caused by vata associated with kapha, it is known as Pratyadhmana. (68-69)

Symptoms of Vatasthila and Pratyasthila

nābheradhastāt sañjātaḥ sañcārī yadi vā'calaḥ ||70||
aṣṭhīlāvadghano granthirūrdhvamāyata unnataḥ |
vātāṣṭhīlāṃ vijānīyādbahirmārgāvarodhinīm ||71||
etāmeva rujopetāṃ vātaviṇmūtrarodhinīm |
pratyaṣṭhīlāmiti vadejjaṭhare tiryagutthitām ||72||
(su| ni| a| 1) |

Ashthila / Vatashthila – A tumour / cyst (like outgrowth / protuberance) occurring below the umbilicus, which is either mobile or immobile, hard like a stone, which projects upwards and causes obstruction to the passage of faeces and urine is called as Vatashthila or Ashthila.

Pratyashthila – If the same stony projection (as that found in ashthila) is found lying obliquely in the abdomen, produces pain and obstruction to flatus, faeces and urine it is called as pratyashthila. (70-72)

Mutravarodha

mārute'nuguṇe bastau mūtraṃ samyak pravartate |
vikārā vividhāścātra pratilome bhavanti ca ||73||
(su| ni| a| 3) |

When the vata (present in the urinary bladder) has its normal downward movement (anuloma), it causes proper elimination of urine from teh urinary bladder. But when the same vata moves in an upward direction (pratiloma), it causes many disorders (like mutrakrchchra, mutraghata, ashmari etc). (73)

Symptoms of Kampavata / Vepathu and Khalli

sarvāṅgakampaḥ śiraso vāyurvepathusañjñakaḥ |74|
khallī tu pādajaṅghorukaramūlāvamoṭanī ||74||
(ca| ci| a| 28) |
Vepathu - Vepathu is that condition caused by vata in which there will be tremors in the entire body or all the parts of the body including the head. (Vepathu may occur with or without shaking or tremors in the head).
Khalli - Khalli is that condition in which there will be cramps (distortions) of the foot (legs), calves, thighs, chest and wrist joints (arms). (74)

Symptoms of Urdhvavata

adhaḥ pratihato vāyuḥ śleṣmaṇā mārutena vā |
karotyudgārabāhulyamūrdhvavātaḥ sa ucyate ||75||
Vata, getting obstructed in its downward movement either by kapha or by itself (another subtype of vata), begins to move upwards and produces too many belchings (eructation). This condition is known as Urdhvavata. (75)

Anukta Vataroga – other vatavyadhi which are not explained

sthānanāmānurūpaiśca liṅgaiḥ śeṣān vinirdiśet |
sarveṣveteṣu saṃsargaṃ pittādyairupalakṣayet ||76||
(ca| ci| a| 28) |
Symptoms of the remaining kinds of vata vyadhis are to be diagnosed with respect to their site of affection and names. Similarly, the association of pitta, kapha and ama with vata shall be inferred based on the existing symptoms (of the associated dosha in the disease). (76)

Incurability of Vata Vyadhi

hanustambhārditākṣepapakṣāghātāpatānakāḥ |

kālena mahatā vātā yatnāt sidhyanti vā na vā ||77||
narān balavatastvetān sādhayennirupadravān |
(ca| ci| a| 28) |
Hanustambha, ardita, aksepa, paksaghata, apatanaka, become severe and difficult to cure or even incurable with lapse of time. These diseases, in the availability of all equipments and facilities of treatment and with proper treatment being administered will sometimes get cured and sometimes not. Treatment of these conditions shall be attempted in patients who are physically strong and when they are not associated with complications. (77-78)

Upadravas – complications of Vata

visarpadāharuksaṅgamūrchārucyagnimārdavaiḥ ||78||
kṣīṇamāṃsabalaṃ vātā ghnanti pakṣavadhādayaḥ |
Visarpa (erysipelas), burning sensation, severe pain, stiffness of body parts (ankylosis) or non-elimination of flatus, faeces, urine, etc. fainting (unconsciousness), anorexia, poor digestive capacity, wasting of muscles, and loss of strength are the complications of vata vyadhi. In the presence of these diseases / conditions, the vata disorders such as paksawadha become fatal. (78)

śūnaṃ suptatvacaṃ bhagnaṃ kampādhmānanipīḍitam |
|rujārtimantaṃ ca naraṃ vātavyādhirvināśayet ||79||
(su| sū| a| 33) |
Swelling of the body (or its parts), loss of tactile sensation, fractures of bones, tremors, distension of the abdomen (flatulence) or severe pain found in vata vyadhis are also to be considered as fatal signs. (79)

Symptoms of Prakrutastha Vata

avyāhatagatiryasya sthānasthaḥ prakṛtisthitaḥ |
vāyuḥ syāt so'dhikaṃ jīvedvītarogaḥ samāḥ śatam ||80||
(ca| ci| a| 28) |
The person in whom the movements (functions) of vata are not obstructed anywhere in the body, the subtypes of vata (Prana, Udana, Vyana, Samana and Apana Vata) remaining in their normal locations render normal

functions, will live for hundred years without suffering from any disease. (80)

iti śrīmādhavakaraviracite mādhavanidāne vātavyādhinidānaṃ samāptam ||22||
Thus ends the chapter on Vātavyādhi.

CHAPTER TWENTY-THREE

VĀTA RAKTA NIDĀNAM

Vatarakta Nidana - Samprapti – Etiological Factors and Pathogenesis of Vatarakta

lavaṇāmlakaṭukṣārasnigdhoṣṇājīrṇabhojanaḥ |
klinnaśuṣkāmbujānūpamāṃsapiṇyākamūlakaiḥ ||1||
kulatthamāṣaniṣpāvaśākādipalalekṣubhiḥ |
dadhyāranālasauvīraśuktatakrasurāsavaiḥ ||2||
viruddhādhyaśanakrodhadivāsvapnaprajāgaraiḥ |
prāyaśaḥ sukumārāṇāṃ mithyāhāravihāriṇām |(ca| ci| a| 29) |
sthūlānāṃ sukhināṃ cāpi kupyate vātaśoṇitam ||3|| (su| ci| a| 1) |
hastyaśvoṣṭrairgacchataścāśnataśca vidāhyannaṃ savidāho'śanasya |
kṛtsnaṃ raktaṃ vidahatyāśu tacca srastaṃ duṣṭaṃ pādayoścīyate tu |
tat sampṛktaṃ vāyunā dūṣitena tatprābalyāducyate vātaraktam ||4|| (su| ni| a| 1) |
Etiological Factors of Vatarakta –

Excessive indulgence in foods which are salty, sour, pungent, alkaline, unctuous (fatty), hot or uncooked (unprocessed),

- Excessive consumption of flesh of animals or birds belonging to marshy or desert like regions – which are either wet (soaked in water for long time) or dry (devoid of moisture)
- Excessive consumption of eatables having sesame paste, radish, horse gram, black gram, cow pea, green leafy vegetables, meat (mutton), sugarcane (juice),
- Excessive consumption of curds, fermented drinks like aranala, sauviraka, sukta, takra (fermented buttermilk), sura, asava etc

- Excessive consumption of incompatible (foods having opposite qualities),
- Eating food in excess
- Anger
- Habit of sleeping during day time and keeping awake at night (and many such other unhealthy foods and activities)

The above-mentioned etiological factors produce a disease called Vatarakta especially in those who are very tender (those people who are not accustomed to hardships of life, those having soft and tender organs or body parts), who are obese and people who are always happy and content (have not experienced hardships or misery of any kind.
Pathogenesis of Vatarakta – Excessive riding on elephants, horses, camels etc (animal back) for long durations of time or regularly (as a habit or part of profession) and excessive indulgence (consumption of) in foods which cause burning sensation (inside the body) during or after digestion etc will burn the food which in turn would quickly burn (vitiate or contaminate) the blood. This burnt and improperly processed blood will flow downwards and accumulate in the foot. Here this blood gets associated with vata which has been aggravated due to its etiological factors (like riding on the elephants etc mentioned above) and causes the disease therein. Since vata is predominant in this disease it is called as Vatarakta. (1-4)

Vatarakta Purvarupa – Premonitory Symptoms of Vatarakta

svedo'tyarthaṃ na vā kārṣṇyaṃ sparśājñatvaṃ kṣate'tiruk |
sandhiśaithilyamālasyaṃ sadanaṃ piḍakodgamaḥ ||5||
jānujaṅghorukaṭyaṃsahastapādāṅgasandhiṣu |
nistodaḥ sphuraṇaṃ bhedo gurutvaṃ suptireva ca ||6||
kaṇḍūḥ sandhiṣu rugbhūtvā bhūtvā naśyati cāsakṛt |
vaivarṇyaṃ maṇḍalotpattirvātāsṛkpūrvalakṣaṇam ||7||
(ca| ci| a| 29) |
The premonitory symptoms of vatarakta include - excessive or absence of perspiration, black discolouration, loss of tactile sensation, severe pain even on slight injury (pain in the seat of injury), looseness of joints, laziness (lethargy), debility, appearance of boils (eruptions, blisters) in joints of

knee, leg, thigh (hip), pelvis (waist), shoulder (blade, axillary region), hands (fingers), feet (toes) and the entire body. There will also be severe pain which present in different ways, like throbbing (gnawing), pulsating and cutting (in the above-mentioned joints and body) along with heaviness and loss of sensation. Apart from these, there is itching, the pain keeps coming and going in the joints (intermittent pain), discolouration and appearance of circular rashes. (5-7)

Vatadhika Vatarakta

vāte'dhike'dhikaṃ tatra śūlasphuraṇabhañjanam |
śothasyaraukṣyaṃ kṛṣṇatvaṃ śyāvatā vṛddhihānayaḥ ||8||
dhamanyaṅgulisandhīnāṃ saṅkoco'ṅgagraho'tiruk |
śītadveṣānupaśayau stambhavepathusuptayaḥ ||9||
If vāta is very predominant in vatarakta, there will be excessive (severe) pain, like pulsating or tearing (cutting) pain. The swelling over the joints will appear dry, black or blue (bluish black). The symptoms increase or decrease often. There will be contractures of arteries (blood vessels) and joints of the fingers, stiffness of the body parts and severe pain. The person will have dislike (aversion) towards cold things and the symptoms would increase by consumption of or exposure to cold things, stiffness, tremors and loss of sensation etc (in other parts of the body). (8-9)

Raktadhika Vatarakta

rakte śotho'tiruktodastāmraścimicimāyate |
snigdharūkṣaiḥ śamaṃ naiti kaṇḍūkledasamanvitaḥ ||10||
If in vatarakta, rakta is affected profoundly; the swelling will be having severe pain, pricking or a feeling of pins and needles, coppery red in colour, and tingling sensation. There will be no relief with unctuous (oily) or dry comforts (like massage etc). The person will also have itching and exudation from the joints. (10)

Pittadhika Vatarakta

pitte vidāhaḥ sammohaḥ svedo mūrchā madastṛṣā |
sparśāsahatvaṃ rugrāgaḥ śothaḥ pāko bhṛśoṣmatā ||11||

If pitta is predominant (in vatarakta) the person would experience burning sensation in the body, delusion, perspiration, unconsciousness (fainting), intoxication and thirst. There will also be tenderness, pain, redness, swelling, suppuration (formation of pus) and increased heat (temperature). (11)

Kaphadhika Vatarakta, Dwandwa & Sannipataja Vatarakta

kaphe staimityagurutāsuptisnigdhatvaśītatāḥ |
kaṇḍūrmandā ca rugdvandvaṃ sarvaliṅgaṃ ca saṅkarāt ||12||
(vā| ni| a| 16) |
If kapha is predominant (in vatarakta), the person would feel as if his body has been wrapped with wet cloth and would experience heaviness of the body, loss of sensation, unctuousness (greasy feel), coldness, itching and mild pain (in the joints).
When there is predominance of two doshas in vatarakta, the symptoms of both doshas will be present mixed together.
When there is predominance of three doshas in vatarakta, the symptoms of all the three doshas will be present mixed together. (12)

Mode of spread of vatarakta

pādayormūlamāsthāya kadāciddhastayorapi |
ākhorviṣamiva kruddhaṃ taddehamupasarpati ||13|| (su| ni| a| 1) |
The (pain of) vatarakta usually starts from the root of the legs (toes or ankle joint) or from the root of the hands (fingers or wrist joint) and spreads to the other parts of the body, slowly, just like a rat poison. (13)

Symptoms of incurability of Vatarakta

ājānu sphuṭitaṃ yacca prabhinnaṃ prasrutaṃ ca yat |
upadravaiśca yajjuṣṭaṃ prāṇamāṃsakṣayādibhiḥ ||14||
vātaraktamasādhyaṃ syādyāpyaṃ saṃvatsarotthitam | (su| ni| a| 1) |
asvapnārocakaśvāsamāṃsakothaśirograhāḥ ||15||
sammūrchāmadaruktṛṣṇājvaramohapravepakāḥ |
hikkāpāṅgulyavīsarpapākatodabhramaklamāḥ ||16||
aṅgulīvakratāsphoṭadāhamarmagrahārbudāḥ |

etairupadravairvarjyaṃ mohenaikena vā'pi yat ||17||
akṛtsnopadravaṃ yāpyaṃ, sādhyaṃ syānnirupadravam |
ekadoṣānugaṃ sādhyaṃ navaṃ, yāpyaṃ dvidoṣajam |
tridoṣajamasādhyaṃ syādyasya ca syurupadravāḥ ||18|| (ca| ci| a| 29) |
Vatarakta is said to be incurable if –

- It has started in the toe and has spread to the knee joint (all the joints from foot to knee are affected)
- The skin over the joints has peeled off or has cracked and if there is exudation from the cracked skin
- It is associated with many complications (like loss of sleep etc enumerated below) which bring about
- Destruction of muscles (muscular wasting) and loss of vital functions of the body (prana)

Vatarakta is said to be manageable (persists for the rest of the life but would require regular treatment to keep it under control – yapya) if it has not existed for more than one year.

Vatarakta associated with complications is also incurable. The complications of vatarakta are – loss of sleep, anorexia, dyspnoea (increased / difficult respiration), putrefaction of muscles, headache, unconsciousness (fainting), intoxication, pain (colic), thirst, fever, delusion, rigors (tremors), hiccough, lameness (inability to walk), herpes / erysipelas (or other skin diseases), suppuration, pricking sensation (pain), giddiness, exhaustion (tiredness), crookedness / contractures of fingers (or toes), blisters, burning sensation, diseases / pain in the vital organs and appearance of tumours (nodules). The patient of vatarakta having these complications shall be refused treatment. Vatarakta is incurable even if unconsciousness is the only complication associated with it.

When vatarakta is not associated with all the above-mentioned complications (only few complications exist), the condition is said to be manageable (disease would persist for life but would require regular treatment).

When vatarakta is devoid of any of the above-mentioned complications it is

said to be curable.
Vatarakta is caused by only one dosha and that which is of recent onset is curable.
Vatarakta caused by two doshas is manageable (persists for life but needs regular treatment).
Vatarakta caused by all three aggravated doshas is incurable. Similarly, vatarakta associated with complications is also incurable. (14-18)

iti śrīmādhavakaraviracite mādhavanidāne vātaraktanidānaṃ samāptam ||23||
Thus ends the chapter on Vātarakta.

CHAPTER TWENTY-FOUR

URUSTAMBHA NIDĀNAM

Nidana, Samprapti & Lakshanas of Urustambha – etiological factors, pathogenesis & symptoms of urustambha (stiffness of the thigh)

śītoṣṇadravasaṃśuṣkagurusnigdhairniṣevitaiḥ |
jīrṇājīrṇe tathā''yāsasaṅkṣobhasvapnajāgaraiḥ ||1||
saśleṣmamedaḥpavanaḥ sāmamatyarthasañcitam |
abhibhūyetaraṃ doṣamūrū cet pratipadyate ||2||
sakthyasthinī prapūryāntaḥ śleṣmaṇā stimitena ca |
tadā stabhnāti tenorū stabdhau śītāvacetanau ||3||
parakīyāviva gurū syātāmatibhṛśavyathau |
dhyānāṅgamardastaimityatandrācchardyarucijvaraiḥ ||4||
saṃyuktau pādasadanakṛcchroddharaṇasuptibhiḥ |
tamūrustambhamityāhurāḍhyavātamathāpare ||5||
(vā| ni| a| 15) |
Etiological factors –

- Excessive indulgence in foods and other activities which are mixture of opposites such as cold and hot, watery and dry, heavy and light, fatty (unctuous) and non-fatty (non-unctuous), cooked and uncooked (eating food when the previously taken food is not digested or partially digested), etc.
- Severe exertion, mental strain, over-sleeping or keeping awake and such other factors

Pathogenesis -
Due to the above said factors – the aggravated vata getting associated with

excessively accumulated ama (intermediate products of digestion or products formed due to sluggish digestion in the stomach), kapha and meda (adipose tissue) taking the pitta together with them, moves downwards and accumulate in the thigh. The thick consolidated kapha fills up the bones of the thighs and causes stiffness of the thighs.
Symptoms of Urustambha – This condition causes stiffness of lower limbs (thighs), coldness and loss of sensation (loss of control). The patient feels heaviness in his lower limbs, as if his legs are not his own and his legs have been replaced by someone else's legs (he feels as though his legs belong to somebody else and that is why they are heavy to him). He will also experience severe pain in the lower limbs. The patient also experiences grief or anxiety, pain in the body parts, immobility of lower limbs (as if his limbs are covered by wet clothes), stupor, vomiting, anorexia, fever, weakness in the legs (lower limbs), difficulty in lifting the legs and loss of sensation in the lower limbs. This disease is known as Urustambha. Others call the same condition as Adhyavata. (1-5)

Urustambha Purvarupa – Premonitory symptoms of urustambha

prāgrūpaṃ tasya nidrā'tidhyānaṃ stimitatā jvaraḥ |
romaharṣo'ruciśchardirjaṅghorvoḥ sadanaṃ tathā ||6||
The premonitory symptoms of urustambha are – excessive sleep, too much worry, loss of movements, (feeling as if the body or affected parts have been covered by a wet leather or cloth), fever, horripilation, anorexia, vomiting, and weakness in the legs and thighs. (6)

Anupashaya, Sadhyasadhyata – conditions in which the symptoms of urustambha get aggravated, symptoms of curability and incurability (prognosis)

vātaśaṅkibhirajñānāttasya syāt snehanāt punaḥ |
pādayoḥ sadanaṃ suptiḥ kṛcchrāduddharaṇaṃ tathā ||7||
jaṅghoruglāniratyarthaṃ śaśvaccādāhavedane |
pādaṃ ca vyathate nyastaṃ śītasparśaṃ na vetti ca ||8||
saṃsthāne pīḍane gatyāṃ cālane cāpyanīśvaraḥ |
anyasyeva hi sambhagnāvūrū pādau ca manyate ||9||
Without knowing the specific features of this disease (urustambha) and

suspecting it to be a disease of vata (on observing vata predominant symptoms like numbness, contracture, tremor etc), if unctuous remedies like oil massage etc. are done (considering that oil remedies are the best in treating vata disorders and vata symptoms), the symptoms will exacerbate (increase) quickly, causing severe debility in the legs, and loss of sensation, difficulty in lifting the lower limbs, severe exhaustion (tiredness) of the legs and thighs, constant mild burning sensation (heat) and pain. The patient gets pain on placing the foot on the ground, and he (his feet) will not be able to appreciate cold touch.

The patient suffering from urustambha will be unable to stand (keep the leg in any one posture), press something from his foot, move the foot, walk around or do any type of activity. The patient will feel that his thigh and feet has been replaced by someone else's thighs or that his thighs have been fractured. (7-9)

yadā dāhārtitodārto vepanaḥ puruṣo bhavet |
ūrustambhastadā hanyāt, sādhayedanyathā navam ||10||(ca| ci| a| 27) |
If urustambha is associated with complications like burning sensation, severe pain, pricking pain and tremors in the legs it is considered as incurable. At the same time if urustambha is not associated with these symptoms (complications) and if it has developed very recently, it is curable. (10)

iti śrīmādhavakaraviracite mādhavanidāne ūrustambhanidānaṃ samāptam ||24||
Thus ends the chapter on Ūrustambha

CHAPTER TWENTY-FIVE

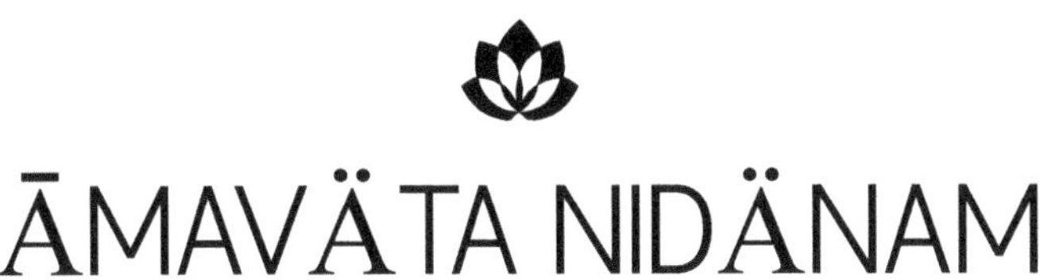

ĀMAVĀTA NIDĀNAM

Amavata Nidana, Samprapti – Etiological factors and Pathogenesis of amavata

viruddhāhāraceṣṭasya mandāgnerniścalasya ca |
snigdhaṃ bhuktavato hyannaṃ vyāyāmaṃ kurvatastathā ||1||
vāyunā prerito hyāmaḥ śleṣmasthānaṃ pradhāvati |
tenātyarthaṃ vidagdho'sau dhamanīḥ pratipadyate ||2||
vātapittakaphairbhūyo dūṣitaḥ so'nnajo rasaḥ |
srotāṃsyabhiṣyandayati nānāvarṇo'tipicchilaḥ ||3||
janayatyāśu daurbalyaṃ gauravaṃ hṛdayasya ca |
vyādhīnāmāśrayo hyeṣa āmasañjño'tidāruṇaḥ ||4||
yugapatkupitāvantastrikasandhipraveśakau |
stabdhaṃ ca kuruto gātramāmavātaḥ sa ucyate ||5||
Etiological factors –

- indulgence in incompatible (mutually opposite, incompatible and antagonistic) foods and habits,
- having low digestion fire (capacity),
- lack of physical activity, or
- doing exercise (indulgence in physical activities) immediately after taking unctuous (fatty) foods

Pathogenesis - The above said etiological factors produce plenty of ama (improperly digested food, intermediate products of digestion produced due to the action of weak digestive fire in the stomach on the food consequently leading to sluggish and incomplete digestion). The vata too is

aggravated.
This ama being stimulated and pushed by aggravated vata moves towards different seats of kapha and gets lodged therein.
Being excessively contaminated (further) and pushed further by the aggravated vata, this ama reaches the dhamanis (blood vessels).
This ama is further contaminated by all the three doshas i.e., vata, pitta and kapha located in the dhamanis.
Due to the contamination by all the three doshas, ama acquires different colours and becomes excessively sticky (slimy), produces excessive fluidity in all the channels of the body and causes obstruction therein.
All these events produce quick weakness (debility) and heaviness in the region of the heart (in the heart).This ama becomes the root source and causative factors of many diseases and hence is considered dreadful and dangerous.
These vata and ama aggravated simultaneously would enter and lodge in the trika sandhi – pelvis and other joints of the body.
This dreadful disease which produces stiffness of the entire body in due course of time is called as amavata. (1-5)

(Note - Trika Sandhi shall be considered as the joints in the pelvis or the meeting of three bones in the region of shoulder blade / shoulder girdle. This also includes sacro-iliac and sacro-coccygeal joints including lower lumbar vertebrae. Some have considered the words trika and sandhi separately. In this condition trika sandhi should be understood as the pelvis and other joints of the body.)

Amavata Lakshanas – General symptoms of amavata

aṅgamardo'rucistṛṣṇā ālasyaṃ gauravaṃ jvaraḥ |
apākaḥ śūnatā'ṅgānāmāmavātasya lakṣaṇam ||6||
The general symptoms of amavata include – pain all over the body (in all parts of the body and joints), tastelessness, thirst, laziness (loss of enthusiasm), heaviness of the body, fever, indigestion and swelling of the body parts (and joints). (6)

Pravruddha Amavata Lakshanas – Symptoms of advancing / advanced stage of amavata

sa kaṣṭaḥ sarvarogāṇāṃ yadā prakupito bhavet |
hastapādaśirogulphatrikajānūrusandhiṣu ||7||
karoti sarujaṃ śothaṃ yatra doṣaḥ prapadyate |
sa deśo rujyate'tyarthaṃ vyāviddha iva vṛścikaiḥ ||8||
janayet so'gnidaurbalyaṃ prasekārucigauravam |
utsāhahāniṃ vairasyaṃ dāhaṃ ca bahumūtratām ||9||
kukṣau kaṭhinatāṃ śūlaṃ tathā nidrāviparyayam |
tṛṭchardibhramamūrchāśca hṛdgrahaṃ viḍvibaddhatām |
jāḍyāntrakūjamānāhaṃ kaṣṭāṃścānyānupadravān ||10||

The severely aggravated and advanced stage of amavata (when it has become chronic due to long standing symptoms) is considered to be the most difficult one to treat in comparison to many other diseases i.e., it becomes incurable.

In this condition there is painful swelling of the joints of hands, feet, head, ankle, pelvis / waist, knee and thigh (hip), wherever the doshas tend to reach and get lodged. Apart from this, the person would experience severe pain resembling the pain of a scorpion sting in any place or joints of the body where the doshas reach (doshas here mean vata along with ama and other doshas as explained in the pathogenesis of amavata).

The other symptoms of amavata include – weakness of digestive fire (poor digestion), excessive salivation, anorexia, heaviness of the body, lack of enthusiasm and drive, manifestation of bad / odd tastes in the mouth, burning sensation, profuse (excessive) urination – polyuria, hardness of the abdomen, pain in the abdomen (colic), and erratic sleep patterns (excessive sleepiness in the morning and loss of sleep at night).

Along with these there is also excessive thirst, vomiting, giddiness, loss of consciousness, stiffness in the region of the heart, constipation, inability to do any work (loss of movements of the body parts – severe stiffness), gurgling sounds in the abdomen, flatulence (distension) and many other difficult complications. (7-10)

Symptoms of associated doshas in amavata

pittāt sadāharāgaṃ ca, saśūlaṃ pavanānugam |
stimitaṃ gurukaṇḍūṃ ca kaphaduṣṭaṃ tamādiśet ||11||

In amavata associated with pitta there will be burning sensation and redness of the affected joint (part).

If vata is predominant in amavata the patient would experience severe pain. In case of kapha predominance in amavata there will be feeling as if his joints (and other parts of the body) are covered by a wet leather or cloth, heaviness and itching. (11)

Prognosis / symptoms of incurability of amavata

ekadoṣānugaḥ sādhyo, dvidoṣo yāpya ucyate |
sarvadehacaraḥ śothaḥ sa kṛcchraḥ sānnipātikaḥ ||12||
Amavata caused by predominant involvement of any one dosha is curable. If amavata is caused by (involvement of) two doshas it will be manageable (persists for the rest of the life but needs regular and prompt treatment). Amavata, wherein all the three doshas are involved and presents with swelling which has spread all over the body (including all the joints) is said to be incurable. (12)

iti śrīmādhavakaraviracite mādhavanidāne āmavātanidānaṃ samāptam ||25||
Thus ends the chapter on Amavāta.

CHAPTER TWENTY-SIX

ŚŪLA PARIṆĀMAŚŪLA ANNADRAVAŚŪLA NIDĀNAM

Types of Sula

doṣaiḥ pṛthak samastāmadvandvaiḥ śūlo'ṣṭadhā bhavet |
sarveṣveteṣu śūleṣu prāyeṇa pavanaḥ prabhuḥ ||1||
Śūla (colic, pain in the abdomen) is of eight types; one from each doṣha, one from the combination of all three doshas, one each from the combination of two doṣhas and the eighth from āma. In all types, vāta is the predominant causative dosha. (1)

To sum up, sula is of 8 types and are named as mentioned below –

1. Vataja Sula
2. Pittaja Sula
3. Kaphaja Sula
4. Tridoshaja / Sannipataja Sula
5. Vata-Pittaja Sula
6. Kapha-Pittaja Sula
7. Kapha-Vataja Sula
8. Amaja Sula

Vataja Sula Nidana, Samprapti, Lakshanas – Etiological factors, pathogenesis and symptoms of Vataja Sula

vyāyāmayānādatimaithunācca prajāgarācchītajalātipānāt |

kalāyamudgāḍhakikoradūṣādatyartharūkṣādhyaśanābhighātāt ||2||
kaṣāyatiktātivirūḍhajānnaviruddhavallūrakaśuṣkaśākāt |
viṭśukramūtrānilavegarodhācchokopavāsādatihāsyabhāṣyāt ||3||
vāyuḥ pravṛddho janayeddhi śūlaṃ hṛtpārśvapṛṣṭhatrikabastideśe |
jīrṇe pradoṣe ca ghanāgame ca śīte ca kopaṃ samupaiti gāḍham ||4||
muhurmuhuścopaśamaprakopī viḍvātasaṃstambhanatodabhedaiḥ |
saṃsvedanābhyañjanamardanādyaiḥ snigdhoṣṇabhojyaiśca śamaṃ prayāti ||5||

Etiological factors –

- Excessive indulgence in physical exercises, riding, sexual intercourse, keeping awake at nights, and excessive drinking of very cold water
- Excessive ingestion of food articles like peas, green gram, tuvar dāl, kora dūsa and other foods which cause dryness inside the body,
- Excessive consumption of foods (over-eating)
- Injury / trauma,
- Consumption in excess of foods which are predominant in astringent and bitter taste; germinated grains and foods which have mutually opposite qualities (mutually incompatible foods), dried up flesh and dried leafy vegetables
- Suppression of urges of faeces, semen, urine and flatus;
- Excessive grief,
- Starvation or fasting,
- Excessive laughing and speaking

Pathogenesis – The vata gets abnormally increased due to the above said etiological factors and causes colic. This condition is called Vataja Sula.

Symptoms –

- pain is manifested in the region of the heart, flanks, back, waist and urinary bladder,
- pain gets exacerbated after the digestion of food, in the evenings, during cloudy (rainy season) and cold weather;
- pain frequently keeps increasing or decreasing on its own accord,
- there is obstruction to the movement (expulsion) of faeces and flatus,

- pain is of pricking or tearing nature
- the pain subsides on administration of sudation (hot fomentation), massage with oils, rubbing or tapping, and foods and drinks which are unctuous (fatty) and hot (2-5)

Pittaja Sula Nidana, Samprapti, Lakshanas – Etiological factors, pathogenesis and symptoms of Pittaja Sula

kṣārātitīkṣṇoṣṇavidāhitailaniṣpāvapiṇyākakulatthayūṣaiḥ |
kaṭvamlasauvīrasurāvikāraiḥ krodhānalāyāsaravipratāpaiḥ ||6||
grāmyātiyogādaśanairvidagdhaiḥ pittaṃ prakupyāśu karoti śūlam |
tṛṇmohadāhārtikaraṃ hi nābhyāṃ saṃsvedamūrchābhramacoṣayuktam ||7||
madhyandine kupyati cārdharātre vidāhakāle jaladātyaye ca |
śīte ca śītaiḥ samupaiti śāntiṃ susvāduśītairapi bhojanaśca ||8||
Etiological factors –

- Excessive consumption of foods which are alkaline, deep penetrating, excessive hot, which produces burning sensation (or heat),
- Excessive consumption of oils, cow-pea, and cake made from paste of sesame, horse gram soup
- Excessive consumption of foods which are predominant in pungent and sour taste
- Excessive consumption of fermented beverages like sauvira, sura etc
- Excessive anger
- Exposure to fire
- Fatigue / tiredness
- Prolonged exposure to heat of the sun
- Excessive indulgence in sexual intercourse

Pathogenesis - The consumption of the above-mentioned etiological factors will cause improper digestion of food (burning of food). This in turn causes aggravation of pitta and this aggravated pitta causes colic. This colic is called Pittaja Sula.

Symptoms –

- Severe thirst
- Delusion
- Severe burning sensation around the umbilicus
- Perspiration (excessive sweating)
- Unconsciousness
- Giddiness
- Localised burning sensation
- The pain increases during afternoon, midnight, during the digestion of food and in Sharad Ritu (autumn season)
- The pain subsides in cold season, by cold comforts, and by consumption of sweet and cold foods (6-8)

Kaphaja Sula Nidana, Samprapti, Lakshanas – Etiological factors, pathogenesis and symptoms of Kaphaja Sula

ānūpavārijakilāṭapayovikārairmāṃsekṣupiṣṭakṛśarātilaśaṣkulībhiḥ |
anyairbalāsajanakairapi hetubhiśca śleṣmā prakopamupagamya karoti śūlam ||9||
hṛllāsakāsasadanārucisamprasekairāmāśaye stimitakoṣṭhaśirogurutvaiḥ |
bhukte sadaiva hi rujaṃ kurute'timātraṃ sūryodaye'tha śiśire kusumāgame ca ||10||
Etiological factors –

- Excessive consumption of foods prepared from the flesh of animals and birds living in the marshy lands and also that prepared from the flesh of aquatic animals (animals living in water)
- Excessive consumption of Kilata (a buttermilk preparation) and milk products
- Excessive consumption of meat (mutton), sugarcane (and sugarcane juice), flour (made of black gram), krshara (gruel prepared using sesame, rice and black gram) and large round cake prepared from sesame
- Excessive consumption of other etiological factors (foods and activities) which tend to cause aggravation of kapha

Pathogenesis – Kapha gets abnormally increased due to the consumption of the above-mentioned etiological factors and causes colic. This type of colic is called Kaphaja Sula.

Symptoms –

- Nausea (oppression of the chest)
- Cough,
- Debility,
- Tastelessness,
- Excessive salivation (excessive production of phlegm in the mouth),
- Pain in the stomach,
- Loss of movement (hardness) and fullness in the abdomen,
- Heaviness in the head
- The pain increases immediately after taking the food, early in the morning, late winter (shishira rtu) and spring season (kusumagame – vasanta rtu) (9-10)

Symptoms and nature of Sannipataja Sula

sarveṣu doṣeṣu ca sarvaliṅgaṃ vidyādbhiṣak sarvabhavaṃ hi śūlam |
sukaṣṭamenaṃ viṣavajrakalpaṃ vivarjanīyaṃ pravadanti tajjñāḥ ||11||
The colic produced by the combination of all the three dosas together is called sannipataja sula.
This condition is marked by the presence of the symptoms of all the three doshas. This colic will occur in severe form and is troublesome. According to experts this condition is difficult to treat (incurable) just like poison and diamond and hence should be refused treatment. (11)

Symptoms of Amaja Sula

āṭopahṛllāsavamīgurutvastaimityakānāhakaphaprasekaiḥ |
kaphasya liṅgena samānaliṅgamāmodbhavaṃ śūlamudāharanti ||12||
They symptoms of amaja sula (colic caused due to material produced due to indigestion) are - gurgling sounds in the abdomen (intestines), nausea (oppression in the chest), vomiting, feeling of heaviness, feeling as if the body has been wrapped with wet leather or cloth, flatulence (distension of the abdomen), excessive salivation, and manifestation of other symptoms similar to those found in kaphaja type of colic. (12)

Symptoms of Dwidoshaja Sula (colic caused by predominant aggravation of two doshas)

bastau hṛtpārśvapṛṣṭheṣu sa śūlaḥ kaphavātikaḥ |
kukṣau hṛnnābhimadhyeṣu sa śūlaḥ kaphapaittikaḥ ||13||
dāhajvarakaro ghoro vijñeyo vātapaittikaḥ |14|
Kapha-Vataja Sula - If the pain / colic is found in the region of the urinary bladder, heart, flanks and back it is probably due to combined vitiation of kapha and vata.
Kapha-Pittaja Sula – If the pain / colic is found in the centre of abdomen, heart and umbilicus, it is probably due to combined vitiation of kapha and pitta.
Vata-Pittaja Sula – If there is burning sensation and fever accompanied by severe pain in the region of urinary bladder and navel, it is probably caused due to combined vitiation of vata and pitta. (13)

Prognosis of Sula

ekadoṣotthitaḥ sādhyaḥ, kṛcchrasādhyo dvidoṣajaḥ ||14||
sarvadoṣotthito ghorastvasādhyo bhūryupadravaḥ |15|
Colic produced by the increase of any one dosha is easily curable. The colic caused by simultaneously vitiating 2 doshas is said to be difficult to cure.
The colic caused by simultaneous vitiation of all three doshas, is severe and dreadful in nature, and associated with many complications is incurable. (14)

Parinama Sula – pathogenesis and symptoms

svairnidānaiḥ prakupito vāyuḥ sannihitastadā ||15||
kaphapitte samāvṛtya śūlakārī bhavedbalī |
bhukte jīryati yacchūlaṃ tadeva pariṇāmajam ||16||
tasya lakṣaṇamapyetat samāsenābhidhīyate |17|
Pathogenesis – The vata gets aggravated due to its own etiological factors (etiological factors responsible for aggravation of vata) on getting lodged in specific seats (in the stomach and intestine) will get powerful (severely aggravated), gets enveloped (blocked, obstructed) by kapha and pitta and

produces severe colic during the process of digestion of food. This colic occurs during the digestion of food (transformation of food) and hence called as parinama sula. This itself (colic appearing during the process of digestion of food) is the characteristic symptom of parinama sula. (15-16)

Symptoms of Parinama Sula based on the predominance of dosha

Vataja Parinama Sula Symptoms

ādhmānāṭopaviṇmūtravibandhārativepanaiḥ ||17||
snigdhoṣṇopaśamaprāyaṃ vātikaṃ tadvadedbhiṣak |
The symptoms of parinama sula caused due to vata predominance are – distension of the abdomen, gurgling sounds in the abdomen (intestines), obstruction to the elimination of (excretion of) faeces and urine, restlessness (not able to focus in any work) and tremors. The symptoms pacify by using unctuous and hot comforts (fatty and warm foods). (16-17)

Pittaja Parinama Sula Symptoms

tṛṣṇādāhāratisvedaṃ kaṭvamlalavaṇottaram ||18||
śūlaṃ śītaśamaprāyaṃ paittikaṃ lakṣayedbudhaḥ |
The symptoms of parinama sula caused due to pitta predominance are – thirst, burning sensation, restlessness and perspiration. The pain increases by use of pungent, sour and salty foods. On the other hand, the pain gets reduced due to use of cold foods and comforts. (18)

Kaphaja Parinama Sula Symptoms

chardihṛllāsasammohaṃ svalparugdīrghasantati ||19||
kaṭutiktopaśāntaṃ ca tacca jñeyaṃ kaphātmakam |
The symptoms of parinama sula caused due to kapha predominance are – vomiting, nausea, and unconsciousness. The pain is mild in nature and persists for a long duration. The pain gets reduced by use of pungent and bitter foods. (19)

Dwidoshaja Parinama Sula and Tridoshaja Parinama Sula Symptoms

saṃsṛṣṭalakṣaṇaṃ buddhvā dvidoṣaṃ parikalpayet ||20||
tridoṣajamasādhyaṃ tu kṣīṇamāṃsabalānalam |21|
When in parainama sula there are combined symptoms of two doshas it should be considered as dwidoshaja parinama sula.
Similarly, when there are combined symptoms of three doshas in parinama sula it should be considered as tridoshaja parinama sula.
Tridoshaja Sula is considered to be incurable. Likewise, any sula associated with loss of muscles (emaciation), loss of strength and decrease of digestive fire (digestive capacity) is considered to be incurable. (20)

Annadrava Sula Symptoms

jīrṇe jīryatyajīrṇe vā yacchūlamupajāyate ||21||
pathyāpathyaprayogeṇa bhojanabhojanana ca |
na śamaṃ yāti niyamāt so'nnadrava udāhṛtaḥ ||22||
(annadravākhyaśūleṣu na tāvat svāsthyamaśnute |
vāntamātre jaratpittaṃ śūlamāśu vyapohati) ||1||
When the colic occurs after the digestion of food, during the process of digestion of food and also before the digestion of food (immediately after consumption of food) i.e., the colic can occur at any time (and doesn't subside at any time) – it is called as annadrava sula. Such type of pain doesn't pacify with use of compatible or incompatible foods, by eating food on not eating it.
(In annadrava sula the pain persists constantly and the patient never feels relieved with anything. The pain subsides when the aggravated pitta is expelled out through vomiting i.e., when the patient vomits or is induced). (21-22)

iti śrīmādhavakaraviracite mādhavanidāne śūlapariṇāmaśūlānnadravaśūlanidānaṃ samāptam ||26||
Thus ends the chapter on Śūla etc.

CHAPTER TWENTY-SEVEN

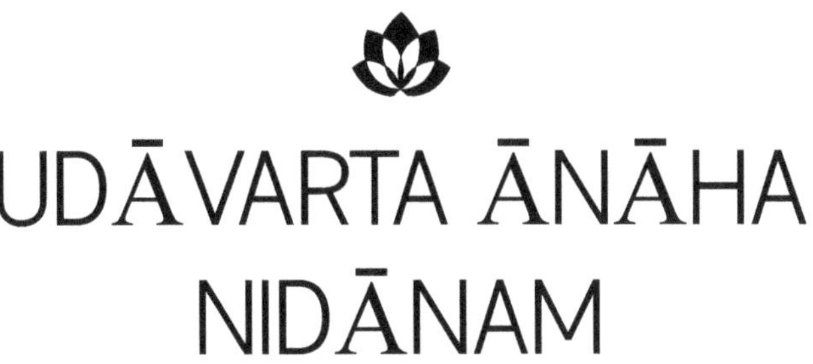

UDĀVARTA ĀNĀHA NIDĀNAM

Udavarta Nidana – Etiological Factors of Udavarta

vātaviṇmūtrajṛmbhāśrukṣavodgāravamīndriyaiḥ |
kṣuttṛṣṇocchvāsanidrāṇāṃ dhṛtyodāvartasambhavaḥ ||1||
Suppression of the urges of flatus, faeces, urine, yawning, tears, sneezing, belching, vomiting, semen, hunger, thirst, respiration and sleep, is the cause for the disease Udāvarta. (1)

Vata Nigrahaja Udavarta Symptoms

vātamūtrapurīṣāṇāṃ saṅgo dhmānaṃ klamo rujā |
jaṭhare vātajāścānye rogāḥ syurvātanigrahāt ||2||
(ca| sū| a| 7) |
The symptoms of 'suppression of urge (movement) of flatus' are –

- obstruction (difficulty in) to expulsion of flatus, faeces and urine
- distension of abdomen,
- weakness
- pain (in the abdomen or body parts)
- manifestation of other symptoms of abnormal increase of vata (in the abdomen) (2)

Purishaja Udavarta Symptoms

āṭopaśūlau parikartikā ca saṅgaḥ purīṣasya tathordhvavātaḥ |
purīṣamāsyādathavā nireti purīṣavege'bhihate narasya ||3||

(su| u| taṃ| a| 55) |
The symptoms of suppression of 'urge for defecation (expulsion or excretion of faeces)' are –

- gurgling sounds in the abdomen (intestines),
- pain in the abdomen (colic)
- cutting pain in the rectum (anus and also in the penis and urinary bladder)
- constipation (obstruction to excretion of faeces),
- excessive belching
- upward movement of flatus and faeces through the mouth (3)

Mutra Udavarta Symptoms

bastimehanayoḥ śūlaṃ mūtrakṛcchraṃ śirorujā |
vināmo vaṅkṣaṇānāhaḥ syālliṅgaṃ mūtranigrahe ||4||
(ca| sū| a| 7) |
The symptoms of suppression of 'urge for urination (expulsion or excretion of urine)' are –

- pain in the urinary bladder and penis,
- difficulty in urination (dysuria)
- headache
- bending of the body forwards
- distension / obstruction / tension / swelling in the groins (4)

Jrmbha Nirodhaja Udavarta Symptoms

manyāgalastambhaśirovikārā jṛmbhopaghātāt pavanātmakāḥ syuḥ |
tathā'kṣināsāvadanāmayāśca bhavanti tīvrāḥ saha karṇarogaiḥ ||5||
The symptoms of suppression of 'urge for yawning' are –

- stiffness of the nape of the neck and neck (throat)
- diseases of the head (headache)
- other symptoms / diseases of vata increase

- diseases of the eyes, nose, face (mouth)
- severe diseases of the ears (5)

Ashruja (ashru nirodhaja) Udavarta Symptoms

ānandajaṃ vā'pyatha śokajaṃ vā netrodakaṃ prāptamamuñcato hi |
śirogurutvaṃ nayanāmayāśca bhavanti tīvrāḥ saha pīnasena ||6||
(su| u| taṃ| a| 55) |
The symptoms of suppression of 'urge for tearing (weeping, shedding tears)' of pleasure or grief origin are –

- heaviness of the head
- disorders of the eyes
- severe nasal catarrh (6)

Kshavathu Nirodhaja Udavarta Symptoms

manyāstambhaḥ śiraḥśūlamarditārdhāvabhedakau |
indriyāṇāṃ ca daurbalyaṃ kṣavathoḥ syādvidhāraṇāt ||7||
(ca| sū| a| 7) |
The symptoms of suppression of 'urge for sneezing' are –

- stiffness of the neck (nape of the neck),
- headache
- facial paralysis
- headache on one side (hemicrania, migraine)
- weakness of the sense organs (inability or decreased ability of sense organs to perceive their respective objects) (7)

Udgara Nirodhaja Udavarta Symptoms

kaṇṭhāsyapūrṇatvamatīva todaḥ kūjaśca vāyorathavā'pravṛttiḥ |
udgāravege'bhihate bhavanti ghorā vikārāḥ pavanaprasūtāḥ ||8||
(su| u| taṃ| a| 55) |

The symptoms of suppression of 'urge for belching' are –

- feeling of fullness (obstruction) in the throat and mouth
- severe pricking pain in the throat
- gurgling sounds in the abdomen
- obstruction to breathing
- other diseases or symptoms of vata increase (8)

Chardi Nigrahajanya Udavarta Symptoms

kaṇḍūkoṭhārucivyaṅgaśothapāṇḍvāmayajvarāḥ |
kuṣṭhavīsarpahṛllāsāśchardinigrahajā gadāḥ ||9||
(ca| sū| a| 7) |
The symptoms of suppression of 'urge for vomiting' are –

- itching
- appearance of rashes
- tastelessness / anorexia
- black spots / patches on the face
- oedema
- anaemia
- fever
- leprosy / skin diseases
- erysipelas / herpes
- nausea (9)

Shukra Nirodhaja Udavarta Symptoms

mūtrāśaye vai gudamuṣkayośca śotho rujā mūtravinigrahaśca |
śukrāśmarī tatsravaṇaṃ bhavecca te te vikārā vihate ca śukre ||10||
The symptoms of suppression of 'urge for ejaculation of semen' are –

- oedema / swelling and pain in the urinary bladder, rectum (anus) and scrotum
- obstruction to the elimination of urine

- formation and discharge (expulsion) of stones / gravel in the seminal passages (seminal calculi) (10)

Kshuda Nirodhaja Udavarta Symptoms

tandrāṅgamardāvaruciḥ śramaśca kṣudhābhighātāt kṛśatā ca dṛṣṭeḥ |
The symptoms of suppression of 'urge for eating food (hunger)' are –

- stupor
- body aches,
- tastelessness (anorexia),
- exhaustion,
- darkness in front of the eyes / loss of vision

Trsna Nirodhaja Udavarta Symptoms

kaṇṭhāsyaśoṣaḥ śravaṇāvarodhastṛṣṇāvighātāddhṛdaye vyathā ca ||11||
The symptoms of suppression of 'urge for drinking water (thirst)' are –

- dryness of the throat and mouth,
- difficulty in hearing (deafness),
- pain in the region of heart (11)

Svasa Nigrahajanya Udavarta Symptoms

śrāntasya niḥśvāsavinigraheṇa hṛdrogamohāvathavā'pi gulmaḥ |
The symptoms of suppression of 'exertion induced dyspnoea' are –
Exertion causes difficulty in breathing for a short duration. If one suppresses this, it would cause –

- diseases of the heart,
- unconsciousness
- abdominal tumours

Nidra Nirodhaja Udavarta Symptoms

jṛmbhā'ṅgamardo'kṣiśiro'tijāḍyaṃ nidrābhighātādathavā'pi tandrā ||12||
(su| u| taṃ| a| 55) |
The symptoms of suppression of 'urge for ejaculation of sleep' are –

- yawning,
- body aches
- heaviness in the eyes and head
- stupor (12)

Vatajanya Udavarta

vāyuḥ koṣṭhānugo rūkṣaiḥ kaṣāyakaṭutiktakaiḥ |
bhojanaḥ kupitaḥ sadya udāvartaṃ karoti [1] hi ||13||
vātamūtrapurīṣāsṛkkaphamedovahāni vai |
srotāṃsyudāvartayati purīṣaṃ cātivartayet ||14||
tato hṛdbastiśūlārto hṛllāsāratipīḍitaḥ |
vātamūtrapurīṣāṇi kṛcchreṇa labhate naraḥ ||15||
śvāsakāsapratiśyāyadāhamohatṛṣājvarān |
vamihikkāśirorogamanaḥśravaṇavibhramān |
bahūnanyāṃśca labhate vikārān vātakopajān ||16||
(su| u| taṃ| a| 55) |
Vata located in the abdomen gets suddenly aggravated due to excessive consumption of foods which are dry and predominant in astringent, pungent and bitter tastes and produce a disease called udavarta instantly.

The normal direction of movement in the passages of flatus, urine, faeces, blood, kapha and medas (adipose tissue) gets reversed (or obstructed). The faeces would get dried up.
The person would experience severe pain in the region of the heart and urinary bladder, nausea & restlessness.

The flatus (fart), urine and faeces get eliminated with difficulty.
The other symptoms include – dyspnoea (increased respiration), cough,

running in the nose, burning sensation, unconsciousness / confusion, thirst, fever, vomiting, hiccough, headaches (diseases of the head), confusion (deviations in the mind), disorders of hearing (manifestation of abnormal sounds in the ears) and many other symptoms / diseases of vata increase. (13-16)

Anaha definition and types

āmaṃ śakṛdvā nicitaṃ krameṇa bhūyo vibaddhaṃ viguṇānilena |
pravartamānaṃ na yathāsvamenaṃ vikāramānāhamudāharanti ||17||
tasmin bhavantyāmasamudbhave tu tṛṣṇāpratiśyāyaśirovidāhāḥ |
āmāśaye śūlamatho gurutvaṃ hṛtstambha udgāravighātanaṃ ca ||18||
stambhaḥ kaṭīpṛṣṭhapurīṣamūtre śūlo'tha mūrchā śakṛtaśca chardiḥ |
śothaśca pakvāśayaje bhavanti tathā'lasoktāni ca lakṣaṇāni ||19||
(su| u| taṃ| a| 56) |
Anaha is a disease wherein gradually accumulated ama (undigested food, intermediated products of digestion caused by sluggishness of the digestive fire) in the stomach or faeces in the colon get obstructed in a more severe way as caused by aggravated vata and do not get eliminated through their normal routes.
Amaja Anaha – If anaha is caused by accumulation of ama in the stomach it produces – thirst, running in the nose, burning sensation in the head, pain and heaviness in the stomach, stiffness in the region of the heart, and absence of (obstruction of) belching.

Purishaja Anaha – If anaha is caused by accumulation of faeces in the large intestine (colon) it causes – stiffness of the waist and back, obstruction of faeces and urine, pain (colic), unconsciousness, vomiting of faecal material (vomited material appearing and smelling like faeces), dyspnoea, and other symptoms mentioned in the context of Alasaka disease. (17-19)

Symptoms of incurability of udavarta

tṛṣṇārditaṃ parikliṣṭaṃ kṣīṇaṃ śūlairabhidrutam |
śakṛdvamantaṃ matimānudāvartinamutsṛjet ||20||
(su| u| taṃ| a| 55) |
A patient of udavarta suffering from severe thirst, restlessness or severe

distress, emaciation, continuous obstinate abdominal pain and faecal vomiting should be refused treatment because this condition is incurable. (20)

iti śrīmādhavakaraviracite mādhavanidāne udāvartānāhanidānaṃ samāptam ||27||
Thus ends the chapter on Udāvarta.

CHAPTER TWENTY-EIGHT

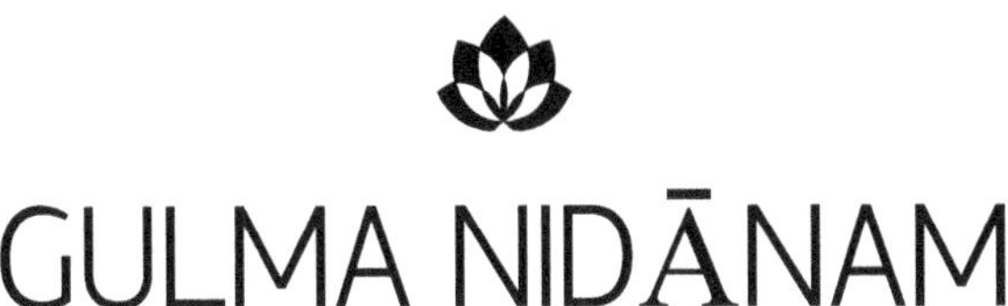

GULMA NIDĀNAM

Gulma Samprapti, Bheda – Pathogenesis and types of gulma

duṣṭā vātādayo'tyarthaṃ mithyāhāravihārataḥ |
kurvanti pañcadhā gulmaṃ koṣṭhāntargranthirūpiṇam |
tasya pañcavidhaṃ sthānaṃ pārśvahṛnnābhibastayaḥ ||1||
Pathogenesis of Gulma - Due to excessive indulgence in incompatible / erroneous foods and activities (habits and daily activities) Vata and other doshas undergo severe vitiation. These doshas cause five types of gulma which are of the form and shape of a cyst / tumour inside the abdomen (abdominal cavity).
Seats of Gulma – Gulma manifests in five seats. The five common sites of gulma are – two parsva (flanks, sides of the abdomen), hrdaya (heart, cardiac region, epigastrium), nabhi (umbilicus, umbilical region) and vasti (region of urinary bladder). (1)

Definition of Gulma

hṛnnābhyorantare granthiḥ sañcārī yadi vā'calaḥ |
vṛttaścayāpacayavān sa 'gulma' iti kīrtitaḥ ||2||
(su| u| taṃ| a| 42) |
Gulma is defined as a mass in between the region of the heart and the umbilicus, which is either moving (from one place to the other) or stationary, round in shape and undergoing increase or decrease in size. (2)

Gulma Bheda – types of gulma

sa vyastairjāyate doṣaiḥ samastairapi cocchritaiḥ |

puruṣāṇāṃ tathā strīṇāṃ jñeyo raktena cāparaḥ ||3||
(su| u| taṃ| a| 42) |
There are five types of gulma. Among these four types of gulma are caused in both men and women (common in men and women). These four types of gulma are caused due to vitiation of individual doshas i.e., vata, pitta, kapha, combined vitiation of all three doshas together. The fifth type of gulma is caused by an increase of rakta (blood) and is manifested only in women. (3)

In short, the five types of gulma are –

- Vataja Gulma
- Pittaja Gulma
- Kaphaja Gulma
- Sannipataja Gulma
- Raktaja Gulma (manifested only in women)

Gulma Purvarupa – Premonitory symptoms of Gulma

udgārabāhulyapurīṣabandhatṛptyakṣamatvāntravikūjanāni |
āṭopa ādhmānamapaktiśaktirāsannagulmasya vadanti cihnam ||4||
(vā| ni| a| 11) |
The premonitory symptoms of gulma are – excessive belching, constipation, disinterest towards food (a morbid feeling of contentment), lack of endurance, gurgling sounds in the abdomen (intestines), painful irritation in the abdomen, distension of abdomen and poor digestion capacity. (4)

Gulma Samanya Lakshana – general symptoms / presentation of gulma

aruciḥ kṛcchraviṇmūtravātatā'ntravikūjanam |
ānāhaścordhvavātatvaṃ sarvagulmeṣu lakṣayet ||5||
The symptoms commonly seen in all types of gulma are – loss of taste, difficulty in elimination of faeces, urine and flatus, gurgling sounds in the abdomen (intestines), flatulence, & upward movement of vata. (5)

Vataja Gulma – etiological factors and symptoms

rūkṣānnapānaṃ viṣamātimātraṃ viceṣṭanaṃ vegavinigrahaśca |
śoko'bhighāto'timalakṣayaśca nirannatā cānilagulmahetuḥ ||6||
yaḥ sthānasaṃsthānarujāṃ vikalpaṃ viḍvātasaṅgaṃ galavaktraśoṣam |
śyāvāruṇatvaṃ śiśirajvaraṃ ca hṛtkukṣipārśvāṃsaśirorujaṃ ca ||7||\
karoti jīrṇe tvadhikaṃ prakopaṃ bhukte mṛdutvaṃ samupaiti yaśca |
vātāt sa gulmo naca tatra rūkṣaṃ kaṣāyatiktaṃ kaṭu copaśete ||8||
(ca| ci| a| 5) |
Etiological factors – Excessive indulgence in dry foods and drinks (foods devoid of fats), imbalanced and incompatible foods, and excessive consumption of foods (in large quantities), unsuitable physical activities, suppression of natural urges, excessive grief, trauma, excessive depletion of faeces and starvation (not consuming food) are the etiological factors of vataja gulma.
Symptoms – In vataja gulma the seat, shape and nature of pain keeps changing constantly (they are not fixed or well defined, fluctuant in nature). The other symptoms include – obstruction to (non elimination) the elimination of faeces and flatus, dryness of throat and mouth, blackish or reddish discolouration, fever accompanied by cold, pain in the region of heart, abdomen, flanks, shoulder blades (shoulders) and head. The pain increases after the digestion of food and subsides immediately after consuming food. The pain and discomfort are not relieved (worsened, increased) by consumption of foods which are dry, astringent, bitter and pungent. (6-8)

Pittaja Gulma – etiological factors and symptoms

kaṭvamlatīkṣṇoṣṇavidāhirūkṣakrodhātimadyārkahutāśasevā |
āmābhighāto rudhiraṃ ca duṣṭaṃ paittasya gulmasya nimittamuktam ||9||
jvaraḥ pipāsā vadanāṅgarāgaḥ śūlaṃ mahajjīryati bhojana ca |
svedo vidāho vraṇavacca gulmaḥ sparśāsahaḥ paittikagulmarūpam ||10||
(ca| ci| a| 5) |
Etiological factors – Excessive indulgence in foods which are pungent, sour, penetrating, causing burning sensation (corrosive) and dry (devoid of fats and unctuous substances), anger, excessive use of alcohol, excessive exposure to sunlight and fire, excessive accumulation of ama in the body, injury, and vitiation (contamination) of blood are the causative factors for pittaja gulma.

Symptoms – The symptoms of pittaja gulma are – fever, thirst, redness of the face and body, severe pain (colic) in the abdomen experienced during the digestion of food, excessive sweating, burning sensation, and tenderness as found in (resembling) ulcers. (9-10)

Kaphaja Gulma – etiological factors and symptoms

śītaṃ guru snigdhamaceṣṭanaṃ ca sampūraṇaṃ prasvapanaṃ divā ca |
gulmasya hetuḥ kaphasambhavasya sarvastu duṣṭo nicayātmakasya ||11||
staimityaśītajvaragātrasādahṛllāsakāsārucigauravāṇi |
śaityaṃ rugalpā kaṭhinonnatatvaṃ gulmasya rūpāṇi kaphātmakasya ||12||
(ca| ci| a| 5) |
Etiological factors – Excessive indulgence in foods which are too cold, heavy to digest, and excessively unctuous (fatty), sedentary life devoid of any physical activities or exercise, eating foods till satiation (eating in excess) & excessive sleep during day time are the causative factors of kaphaja gulma.
Etiological factors of sannipataja Gulma – Sannipataja or Tridoshaja Gulma are caused by a combination of etiological factors mentioned for individual doshaja gulma.
Symptoms of kaphaja gulma – The symptoms of kaphaja gulma are – feeling as if the body (abdomen) has been covered by wet cloth, fever with cold, weakness, nausea, cough, tastelessness (anorexia), & heaviness of the body. The gulma is cold in touch (person feels cold), has mild pain, hard and elevated (bulged out). (11-12)

Dwandwaja Gulma – Tumours of abdomen caused by two doshas

nimittarūpāṇyupalabhya gulme dvidoṣaje doṣabalābalaṃ ca |
vyāmiśraliṅgānaparāṃśca gulmāṃstrīnādiśedauṣadhakalpanārtham ||13||
(ca| ci| a| 5) |
The combination of any two doshas will also cause three other types of gulma. This should be identified and diagnosed based on the availability of etiological factors, symptoms and strength of two doshas together. They are recognised for the purpose of providing suitable treatment. (13)

Sannipataja Gulma Symptoms

mahārujaṃ dāhaparītamaśmavadghanonnataṃ śīghravidāhi dāruṇam |
manaḥśarīrāgnibalāpahāriṇaṃ tridoṣajaṃ gulmamasādhyamādiśet ||14||
(ca| ci| a| 5) |
Sannipataja or Tridoshaja Gulma is marked by the presence of – severe pain and burning sensation, the mass is bulged out and has stone-like feel and consistency (on touch). The mass will undergo suppuration very quickly and is considered to be very dreadful. This condition would produce weakness of the mind, body, digestive fire and strength. This gulma is incurable in nature. (14)

Rakta Gulma – causes, symptoms

navaprasūtā'hitabhojana yā yā cāmagarbhaṃ visṛjedṛtau vā |
vāyurhi tasyāḥ parigṛhya raktaṃ karoti gulmaṃ sarujaṃ sadāham |
paittasya liṅgena samānaliṅgaṃ viśeṣaṇaṃ cāpyaparaṃ nibodha ||15||
(su| u| taṃ| a| 42) |
yaḥ spandate piṇḍita eva nāṅgaiścirāt saśūlaḥ samagarbhaliṅgaḥ |
sa raudhiraḥ strībhava eva gulmo māse vyatīte daśame cikitsyaḥ ||16||
(ca| ci| a| 5) |
Causes of Rakta Gulma – Consumption of unsuitable / incompatible foods and indulgence in incompatible activities by women who have recently delivered a child, have undergone miscarriage or abortion or during menstruation.
Pathogenesis – In women consuming the above-mentioned etiological factors, vata gets aggravated in the uterus (reproductive system of the women). This vata causes obstruction of rakta (menstrual blood) and causes gulma (tumour) along with pain and burning sensation. This condition is called rakta gulma.
Symptoms – Rakta Gulma is associated with pain and burning sensation. The symptoms are similar to those of pittaja gulma. In addition, this condition will also have some special symptoms. Due to the mass, the woman experiences all the signs of pregnancy but on palpation (by the doctor) the gulma pulsates in a single mass and not by organs i.e., the palpating hands of the physician can appreciate a pulsating mass (single) but will not be able to detect different parts of the fetus (since the foetus is not there in the womb). The pulsating pain occurs at long intervals along with signs of pregnancy. This condition occurs only in women. It shall

be treated only after the completion of ten months. (This is to rule out pregnancy in case of chance of wrong diagnosis. If it is pregnancy, the foetus will be naturally delivered at the end of 9 months. If it is rakta gulma it doesn't get delivered. This will confirm the diagnosis and hence shall be treated after 10 months.) (15-16)

Symptoms of incurability

sañcitaḥ kramaśo gulmo mahāvāstuparigrahaḥ |
kṛtamūlaḥ sirānaddho yadā kūrma ivotthitaḥ ||17||
daurbalyārucihṛllāsakāsacchardyaratijvaraiḥ |
tṛṣṇātandrāpratiśyāyairyujyate sa na sidhyati ||18||
gṛhītvā sajvaraṃ śvāsacchardyatīsārapīḍitam |
hṛnnābhihastapādeṣu śothaḥ karṣati gulminam ||19||
(ca| ci| a| 5) |
Gulma is incurable when the mass -

- grows steadily,
- has assumed very big size,
- occupies the entire abdomen
- is deeply rooted,
- has visible networks of veins on the abdomen (mass), i.e. accompanied with venous engorgement,
- is elevated like the shell of a tortoise,

It is also incurable when associated with the below mentioned symptoms –

- weakness / debility
- tastelessness
- nausea
- cough
- vomiting
- restlessness
- fever
- thirst
- drowsiness / stupor

- running in the nose,

  Other symptoms of incurability are –

- continuous fever
- dyspnoea
- vomiting
- diarrhoea
- swelling / oedema in the region of the heart, umbilicus, hands and feet (17-19)

Other symptoms of incurability of gulma

śvāsaḥ śūlaṃ pipāsā'nnavidveṣo granthimūḍhatā |
jāyate durbalatvaṃ ca gulmino maraṇāya vai ||20||
(su| sū| a| 33) |
Dyspnoea (difficulty in breathing), colic, thirst, aversion towards food, sudden disappearance of the mass (of gulma), and severe tiredness are the fatal signs of gulma. (20)

iti śrīmādhavakaraviracite mādhavanidāne gulmanidānaṃ samāptam ||28||
Thus ends the chapter on Gulma.

CHAPTER TWENTY-NINE

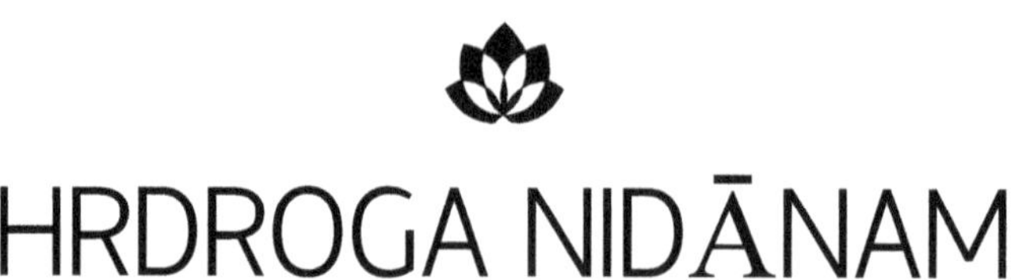

HRDROGA NIDĀNAM

Hrdroga Nidana – Etiological factors of heart diseases

atyuṣṇagurvannakaṣāyatiktaśramābhighātādhyaśanaprasaṅgaiḥ |
sañcintanairvegavidhāraṇaiśca hṛdāmayaḥ pañcavidhaḥ pradiṣṭaḥ ||1||
Regular and excessive consumption of foods which are very hot, heavy (hard to digest), predominantly astringent and bitter in taste, excess fatigue, injury, eating before the previous food has been digested, excessive worry, and suppression of the urges of the body are the causative factors of five kinds of heart diseases. (1)

Hrdroga Samprapti – pathogenesis of heart diseases

dūṣayitvā rasaṃ doṣā viguṇā hṛdayaṃ gatāḥ |
hṛdi bādhāṃ prakurvanti hṛdrogaṃ taṃ pracakṣate ||2||
(su| u| taṃ| a| 43) |
The doshas having undergone morbid increase by their etiological factors, vitiate the rasadhātu, and get localised in the heart which is the seat of rasa dhatu and causes disease (pain) in the heart. This condition is called as Hrdroga. (2)

Vataja Hrdroga Symptoms

āyamyate mārutaje hṛdayaṃ tudyate tathā |
nirmathyate dīryate ca sphoṭyate pāṭyate'pi ca ||3||
(su| u| taṃ| a| 43) |
In Vātaja hridroga – the pain in the heart is pulling (constricting), piercing / pricking, churning, bursting or tearing in nature. (3)

Pittaja Hrdroga Symptoms

tṛṣṇoṣmādāhacoṣāḥ syuḥ paittike hṛdayaklamaḥ |
dhūmāyanaṃ ca mūrchā ca svedaḥ śoṣo mukhasya ca ||4||
(su| u| taṃ| a| 43) |
In Pittaja Hrdroga – the person would have thirst, increased heat (temperature) in the body, burning sensation, localized heat, tiredness / weakness of the heart, feeling of movement of hot smoke (of hot air) inside the chest, unconsciousness (loss of consciousness), increased sweating and dryness of the mouth. (4)

Kaphaja Hrdroga Symptoms

gauravaṃ kaphasaṃsrāvo'ruciḥ stambho'gnimārdavam |
mādhuryamapi cāsyasya balāsāvatate hṛdi ||5||
(su| u| taṃ| a| 43) |
In Kaphaja Hrdroga – there will be feeling of heaviness of the body, excessive salivation (watery secretions from the mouth, nose, eyes), loss of taste (anorexia), stiffness of the body parts, weak digestive fire (poor digestion capacity), and manifestation of sweet taste in the mouth. (5)

Tridoshaja and Krimija Hrdroga Symptoms

vidyāttridoṣaṃ tvapi sarvaliṅgaṃ tīvrārtitodaṃ krimijaṃ sakaṇḍūm | (ca| ci| a| 26) |
utkledaḥ ṣṭhīvanaṃ todaḥ śūlaṃ hṛllāsakastamaḥ |
aruciḥ śyāvanetratvaṃ śothaśca krimije bhavet ||6|| (su| u| taṃ| a| 43) |
Tridoshaja Hrdroga – In this condition the symptoms of all the three doshas will be present in mixed proportions.
Krimija Hrdroga – There will be severe pain, pricking sensation and itching (in the chest or in the region of the heart). (Master Charaka)
According to Master Sushruta Krimija Hrdroga will manifest with nausea, severe and repeated spitting, pricking pain, severe pain, nausea (oppression in the chest), experiencing darkness in front of the eyes, tastelessness (loss of taste of food), blackish appearance of the eyes (around the eyes) and oedema (swelling). (6)

Hrdroga Upadrava - Complications of Heart diseases

klamaḥ sādo bhramaḥ śoṣo jñeyāsteṣāmupadravāḥ |
krimije krimijātīnāṃ ślaiṣmikāṇāṃ ca ye matāḥ ||8||
Debility, exhaustion, giddiness and emaciation are the complications of hrdroga. The complications explained in Kaphaja Krimi Roga (worm or parasitic infestation caused by excessive kapha) are found in Krimija Hrdroga also. (7)

iti śrīmādhavakaraviracite mādhavanidāne hṛdroganidānaṃ samāptam ||29||
Thus ends the chapter on Hrdroga.

CHAPTER THIRTY

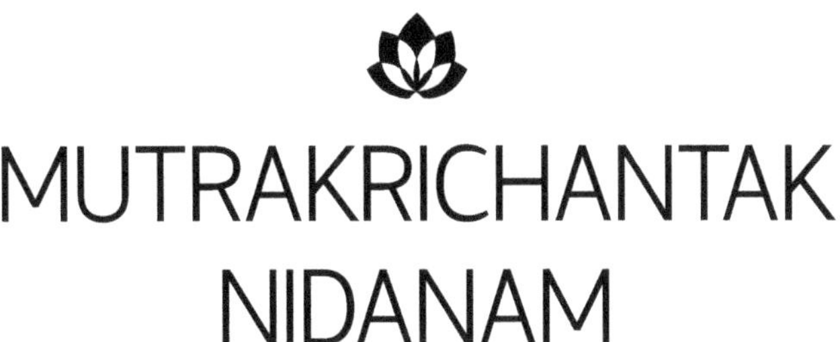

MUTRAKRICHANTAK NIDANAM

Mutrakrichra Nidana, Samprapti – Etiological factors and pathogenesis of Dysuria

vyāyāmatīkṣṇauṣadharūkṣamadyaprasaṅganityadrutapṛṣṭhayānāt |
ānūpamāṃsādhyaśanādajīrṇātsyurmūtrakṛcchrāṇi nṛṇāṃ tathā'ṣṭau ||1||
pṛthaṅmalāḥ svaiḥ kupitā nidānaiḥ sarve'thavā kopamupetya bastau |
mūtrasya mārgaṃ paripīḍayanti yadā tadā mūtrayatīha kṛcchrāt ||2|| (ca| ci| a| 26) |
Etiological Factors – Excessive indulgence in exercise, medicines which are penetrating in nature (heat producing), dry foods and alcoholic drinks, riding regularly on the backs of animals like horses which basically run fast (or riding any other vehicles with fast pace regularly), regular and excessive consumption of flesh of animals and birds living in the marshy places, eating food in excess and indigestion of foods are the etiological factors of mutra krchra.
Pathogenesis – The above-mentioned etiological factors aggravate one or all doshas and cause 8 kinds of mutrakrchra. The vata and other doshas aggravated by their respective etiological factors reach the urinary bladder (urinary tract) either singly or collectively and get lodged therein. These doshas cause constriction, pressure or irritation of the urinary passages. As an effect, the person will find difficulty in voiding the urine. This condition marked by 'difficulty in urination' is called Mutrakrchra. This is of 8 types. (1-2)

Note – The 8 types of Mutrakrchra are –

- Vataja Mutrakrchra
- Pittaja Mutrakrchra
- Kaphaja Mutrakrchra
- Sannipataja Mutrakrchra
- Shalyabhighataja Mutrakrchra (caused due to injury caused by foreign object)
- Purishaja / Shakrdvighataja Mutrakrchra (caused by forcibly holding the urge for defecation)
- Shukraja Mutrakrchra (dysuria caused by impaction of urinary passages by semen)
- Ashmarijanya Mutrakrchra (dysuria caused by urinary stones)

Symptoms of Vataja, Pittaja, Kaphaja, Sannipataja Mutrakrchra

tīvrārtirugvaṅkṣaṇabastimeḍhre svalpaṃ muhurmūtrayatīha vātāt |
pītaṃ saraktaṃ sarujaṃ sadāhaṃ kṛcchraṃ muhurmūtrayatīha pittāt ||3||
basteḥ saliṅgasya gurutvaśothau mūtraṃ sapicchaṃ kaphamūtrakṛcchre |
sarvāṇi rūpāṇi tu sannipātādbhavanti tatkṛcchratamaṃ hi kṛcchram ||4||
(ca| ci| a| 26) |
Vataja Mutrakrchra – In this type, severe pain in the groins, urinary bladder and penis, scanty and frequent urination are the symptoms.
Pittaja Mutrakrchra – In this type of dysuria the patient will pass urine which is yellow in colour and mixed with blood. The patient will experience pain and burning sensation along with difficulty in passing the urine.
Kaphaja Mutrakrchra – In this condition the patient will have heaviness and swelling in the region of the urinary bladder and penis. The urine will be thick and viscid (sticky, slimy).
Tridoshaja (Sannipataja) Mutrakrchra – In this condition all the above-mentioned symptoms in the individual doshaja types of mutrakrchra (vataja, pittaja, kaphaja) are found together and in severe form. (3-4)

Shalyabhighataja Mutrakrchra

mūtravāhiṣu śalyena kṣateṣvabhihateṣu vā |
mūtrakṛcchraṃ tadāghātājjāyate bhṛśadāruṇam ||5||

vātakṛcchreṇa tulyāni tasya liṅgāni nirdiśet |
This condition occurs due to the injury caused by the foreign bodies inside the urinary tract or due to external injury. The difficulty in urination is of a severe form and will have symptoms similar to those of vataja type of mutrakrchra. (5)

Shakrd Vighataja Mutrakrchra

śakṛtastu pratīghātādvāyurviguṇatāṃ gataḥ ||6||
ādhmānaṃ vātaśūlaṃ ca mūtrasaṅgaṃ karoti ca |
Due to the obstruction to the movement of the faeces as caused by habitual suppression of the urge for defecation will cause vata aggravation. This vata will move in an abnormal route (upward direction against its normal downward course) and produces distension of abdomen, colic of vataja type and difficulty in urination. (6)

Ashmarijanya & Shukraja Mutrakrchra

aśmarīhetu tatpūrvaṃ mūtrakṛcchramudāharet ||7||
(su| u| taṃ| a| 59) |
śukre doṣairupahate mūtramārge vidhāvite
saśukraṃ mūtrayet kṛcchrādbastimehanaśūlavān ||8||
Ashmarijanya Mutrakrchra - If mutrakrchra (dysuria) is caused due to asmari (urinary calculi) it is called Ashmarijanya Mutrakrchra. Here calculus is the cause and difficulty in urination is the effect.
Shukraja Mutrakrchra – When the semen which has been displaced from its place (and has not been ejaculated) gets vitiated and obstructed by the aggravated doshas in the urinary passages it leads to difficulty in micturation. Since this condition is caused by the obstruction of semen it is called shukraja (shukra = semen) mutrakrchra. In this condition the urine mixed with semen is eliminated with great difficulty. It is also associated with pain in the region of the urinary bladder and penis. (7-8)

Difference between Asmari and Sarkara

aśmarī śarkarā caiva tulyasambhavalakṣaṇe |
viśeṣaṇaṃ śarkarāyāḥ śṛṇu kīrtayato mama ||9||

pacyamānā'śmarī pittācchoṣyamāṇā ca vāyunā |
vimuktakaphasandhānā kṣarantī śarkarā matā ||10||
hṛtpīḍā vepathuḥ śūlaṃ kukṣāvagniśca durbalaḥ |
tayā bhavati mūrchā ca mūtrakṛcchraṃ ca dāruṇam ||11||
mūtraveganirastābhiḥ praśamaṃ yāti vedanā |
yāvadasyāḥ punarnaiti guḍikā srotaso mukham ||12||
(su| u| taṃ| a| 59) |

Asmarī (calculii) and sarkarā (gravel) are similar in their causes and symptoms. But there is a difference in both these conditions.

Sarkara – The asmari (calculus) undergoing processing by pitta, dried by vata (dehydration of asmari by vāta) and losing the property of cohesion (or sticking together) of kapha, broken into tiny particles and passed out is called as šarkarā (gravel).

Symptoms of dysuria (mutrakrchra) caused by ashmari or sarkara - pain in the region of the heart, shivering (tremors), pain in the abdomen (epigastrium), weakness of the digestive fire (poor digestive capacity), loss of consciousness (fainting) and great difficulty in urination are the symptoms caused by calculi or gravel.

Pain of the urinary tract subsides after the gravel gets eliminated along with the force of urination. The relief will be only until the urinary passage is impacted / obstructed by yet another gravel or stone. This means to tell that the symptoms recur (dysuria) when a new gravel or stone passes into the urinary tract and causes obstruction therein. (9-12)

iti śrīmādhavakaraviracite mādhavanidāne mūtrakṛcchranidānaṃ samāptam ||30||

Thus ends the chapter on Asmarī.

CHAPTER THIRTY-ONE

MŪTRĀGHĀTA NIDĀNAM

Mutraghata Nidana, Samkhya - Etiological factors and number of mutraghata

jāyante kupitairdoṣairmūtrāghātāstrayodaśa |
prāyo mūtravighātādyairvātakuṇḍalikādayaḥ ||1||
Causes – Suppression of natural urge for urination and other urges (like that of defecation, ejaculation etc) and consumption of dry foods (and other etiological factors which cause predominant vitiation of vata) are the chief causes of mutraghata – suppression of urine.
Pathogenesis and number of mutraghata – The doshas (one or more of the doshas), predominantly vata, aggravated by the above mentioned etiological factors cause thirteen types of mutraghata commencing with Vatakundalika. (1)

Vatakundalika

raukṣyādvegavighātādvā vāyurbastau savedanaḥ |
mūtramāviśya carati viguṇaḥ kuṇḍalīkṛtaḥ ||2||
mūtramalpālpamathavā sarujaṃ sampravartate |
vātakuṇḍalikāṃ tāṃ tu vyādhiṃ vidyāt sudāruṇam ||3||
(su| u| taṃ| a| 58) |
Excessive indulgence in dry foods, suppression of natural urges of the body etc are the etiological factors of Vatakundalika. These causes lead to aggravation of vata located in the urinary bladder. This vata moves all around in a circular way obstructing the urine and also causes pain in the urinary bladder.
There is either scanty urination (frequent passage of small quantities of

urine) or painful urination. This dreadful condition is known as Vatakundalika. (2-3)

Asthila

ādhmāpayan bastigudaṃ ruddhvā vāyuścalonnatām |
kuryāttīvrārtimaṣṭhīlāṃ mūtraviṇmārgarodhinīm ||4||
The vata which has abnormally increased in the urinary bladder causes distension of the urinary bladder and rectum and would cause an enlargement (cyst like structure) which resembles an asthila (round pebble or stone ball) and hence the name asthila. This is elevated and mobile. It will produce severe pain and obstruction in the passages of urine and faeces. (4)

Vatavasti / Vatabasti

vegaṃ vidhārayedyastu mūtrasyākuśalo naraḥ |
niruṇaddhi mukhaṃ tasya basterbastigato'nilaḥ ||5||
mūtrasaṅgo bhavettena bastikukṣinipīḍitaḥ |
vātabastiḥ sa vijñeyo vyādhiḥ kṛcchraprasādhanaḥ ||6||
(su| u| taṃ| a| 58) |
Vatavasti or Vatabasti is a condition caused in unwise persons who suppress their urge for urination and make the habit of the same (suppress urge for urination of long durations and long time). In these people the vata located in the urinary bladder gets aggravated and blocks the opening of the urinary bladder (urinary passages) and abdomen. This causes total retention of urine and also pain in the region of the urinary bladder. This disease is known as Vatavasti and is difficult to cure. (5-6)

Mutratita

ciraṃ dhārayato mūtraṃ tvarayā na pravartate |
mehamānasya mandaṃ vā mūtrātītaḥ sa ucyate ||7||
When a person is habituated to suppress the urge of urination for a long time (and also has suppressed it for a long time) he fails to void the urine with normal force (and speed). Even if he voids the urine, it will be in a very slow stream. This condition is called as Mūtrātīta. (7)

Mutrajathara

mūtrasya vege'bhihate tadudāvartahetukaḥ |
apānaḥ kupito vāyurudaraṃ pūrayedbhṛśam ||8||
nābheradhastādādhmānaṃ janayettīvravedanam |
tanmūtrajaṭharaṃ vidyādadhobastinirodhanam ||9||
(su| u| taṃ| a| 58) |
Suppression of the urge of urination is the cause for udāvarta (reverse / upward movement of vata). Apānavāta getting increased begins to move upwards and accumulates in the abdomen, causing distension of the abdomen below the umbilicus, along with severe pain and obstruction in the lower part (opening) of the urinary bladder. This condition is known as Mūtrajathara. (8-9)

Mutrotsanga

bastau vā'pyathavā nāle maṇau vā yasya dehinaḥ |
mūtraṃ pravṛttaṃ sajjeta saraktaṃ vā pravāhataḥ ||10||
sravecchanairalpamalpaṃ sarujaṃ vā'tha nīrujam |
viguṇānilajo vyādhiḥ sa mūtrotsaṅgasañjñitaḥ ||11||
(su| u| taṃ| a| 58) |
Mutrotsanga is a disease in which the urine which has left its seat (to get voided) gets obstructed in the urinary bladder, urethra or glans penis. If the person forcibly tries to void the urine in this condition (strains), the urine flows out mixed with blood or gets voided slowly and in small quantities, with or without pain. This condition is caused by aggravated vata. (10-11)

Mutraksaya

rūkṣasya klāntadehasya bastisthau pittamārutau |
mūtrakṣayaṃ sarugdāhaṃ janayetāṃ tadāhvayam ||12||
(su| u| taṃ| a| 58) |
In a person whose body is excessively dry and has fatigue, pitta and vata would undergo aggravation in the urinary bladder. They would cause reduction in the quantity of urine (mutraksaya) associated with pain and burning sensation. This condition is called as mutraksaya. (12)

Mutra Granthi

antarbastimukhe vṛttaḥ sthiro'lpaḥ sahasā bhavet |
aśmarītulyaruggranthirmūtragranthiḥ sa ucyate ||13||
(vā| ni| a| 9) |
A round, small and stationary cyst like mass developing quickly inside the urinary bladder, which resembles a stone and also presents pain (and other symptoms) similar to those of urinary calculi is called as Mutragranthi. (13)

Mutrasukra

mūtritasya striyaṃ yāto vāyunā śukramuddhatam |
sthānāccyutaṃ mūtrayataḥ prāk paścādvā pravartate ||14||
bhasmodakapratīkāśaṃ mūtraśukraṃ taducyate |
(vā| ni| a| 9) |
In a person who indulges in sexual intercourse suppressing the urge of urination, vata gets aggravated. By this, the semen which is dislodged from its seat gets obstructed and flows out of the body either before or after the urination. This disease in which the void urine resembles a solution of ash is called as Mutraksaya. (14)

Usnavata

vyāyāmādhvātapaiḥ pittaṃ bastiṃ prāpyānilānvitam ||15||
bastiṃ meḍhraṃ gudaṃ caiva pradahet srāvayedadhaḥ ||
mūtraṃ hāridramathavā saraktaṃ raktameva vā ||16||
kṛcchrāt punaḥ punarjantoruṣṇavātaṃ bruvanti tam |
(su| u| taṃ| a| 58) |
When a person is indulged in excessive physical exercises, long distance walking and exposure to the heat of the sun, the pitta gets aggravated and reaches the urinary bladder. Here it gets associated with vata and causes burning sensation in the urinary bladder, penis (urethra) and rectum (anus). The urine voided is deep yellow in colour (resembling the colour of turmeric) or mixed with blood or only the blood flows out. The urine frequently comes out in small quantities. This disease is known as Usnavata. (15-16)

Mutrasadam

pittaṃ kapho dvāvapi vā saṃhanyete'nilena cet ||17||
kṛcchrānmūtraṃ tadā pītaṃ śvetaṃ raktaṃ ghanaṃ sṛjet |
sadāhaṃ rocanāśaṅkhacūrṇavarṇaṃ bhavettu tat ||18||
śuṣkaṃ samastavarṇaṃ vā mūtrasādaṃ vadanti tam |
(vā| ni| a| 9) |
Pitta and kapha either alone or in combination will get condensed (solidified) by the aggravated vata. When this happens there is difficulty in urination. The urine is yellow, white or red in colour, is dense, associated with burning sensation, resembles the colour of the colour of ox bile or conch shell, is dry (the watery portion of the urine is less, non-viscid) and has different colours of all the doshas (due to the aggravation of tridoshas). This condition is called as Mutrasada. (17-18)

Vidvighata

rūkṣadurbalayorvātenodāvṛttaṃ śakṛdyadā ||19||
mūtrasroto'nupadyeta viṭsaṃsṛṣṭaṃ tadā naraḥ |
viḍgandhaṃ mūtrayet kṛcchrādviḍvighātaṃ vinirdiśet ||20||
(vā| ni| a| 9) |
In a person who has excessive dryness in the body and is also physically weak, the faeces are pushed in its opposite direction (upward direction) by the aggravated vata. The faeces enter the urinary bladder (urinary passages) and cause difficulty in urination. The urine which is void is either mixed with faeces or obtains the smell of faeces. This condition is called as Vidvighata. (19-20)

Vastikundala

drutādhvalaṅghanāyāsairabhighātāt prapīḍanāt |
svasthānādbastirudvṛttaḥ sthūlastiṣṭhati garbhavat ||21||
śūlaspandanadāhārto binduṃ binduṃ sravatyapi |
pīḍitastu sṛjeddhārāṃ saṃstambhodveṣṭanārtimān ||22||
bastikuṇḍalamāhustaṃ ghoraṃ śastraviṣopamam |
pavanaprabalaṃ prāyo durnivāramabuddhibhiḥ |24|
tasmin pittānvite dāhaḥ śūlaṃ mūtravivarṇatā ||23||
śleṣmaṇā gauravaṃ śothaḥ snigdhaṃ mūtraṃ ghanaṃ sitam |24|
śleṣmaruddhabilo bastiḥ pittodīrṇo na sidhyati ||24||
avibhrāntabilaḥ sādhyo, na tu yaḥ kuṇḍalīkṛtaḥ |25|
syādbastau kuṇḍalībhūte tṛṇmohaḥ śvāsa eva ca ||25||
By indulgence in fast walking, jumping and other exercises causing fatigue, injury (by blunt weapons) etc. or due to the pressure (on the urinary

bladder, the urinary bladder gets displaced upwards (due to the increased vata) towards the centre of the abdomen and also becomes upside down resembling a pregnant uterus.

In this condition there is pain in the urinary bladder, fluctuations in the region of bladder and burning sensation and the urine is voided with difficulty, drop by drop. The urine flows out in the stream when pressure is applied on the abdomen (the region of the urinary bladder is pressed with hands) but stops when the pressure is released. There is rigidity and cramps. Such a disease is called Vastikundala. It is very dreadful, just like a sharp weapon or poison or a sharp weapon (like an arrow) dipped in poison. Vata is predominantly aggravated in this condition, and should not be treated by a physician with less knowledge.

If pitta gets associated (involved) in Vastikundala it causes burning sensation, pain, and discolouration of urine.

If kapha is involved in Bastikundala it causes heaviness and swelling. The urine is oily, thick and white.

If the orifice of the urinary bladder is blocked by thick kapha or if the urinary bladder (inside) gets afflicted by pitta (inflamed or ulcerated) the disease becomes incurable. On the other hand, if the orifice of the bladder is not obstructed or if the bladder doesn't get rolled up into a ball like structure Vastikundala becomes curable.

If the urinary bladder becomes rolled up like a ball, it causes thirst, loss of consciousness (delusion) and dyspnoea. (21-26)

iti śrīmādhavakaraviracite mādhavanidāne mūtrāghātanidānaṃ samāptam ||31||

Thus ends the chapter on Mūtrāghāta.

CHAPTER THIRTY-TWO

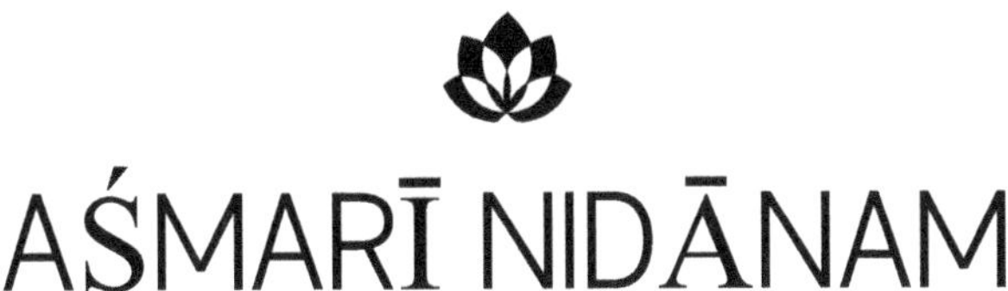

AŚMARĪ NIDĀNAM

Asmari Bheda – Types of calculus

vātapittakaphaistisraścaturthī śukrajā'parā |
prāyaḥ śleṣmāśrayāḥ sarvā aśmaryaḥ syuryamopamāḥ ||1||
Asmari is of four types, one from each dosha i.e., vataja, pittaja and kaphaja and the fourth one is that formed from sukra (semen). All types of asmari have predominance of kapha (kapha as the basic dosha involved in the formation of all kinds of asmari). This disease is considered to be dreadful, like the God of Death. (1)

Asmari Samprapti – Pathogenesis of Asmari

viśoṣayedbastigataṃ saśukraṃ mūtraṃ sapittaṃ pavanaḥ kaphaṃ vā |
yadā tadā'śmaryupajāyate tu krameṇa pitteṣviva rocanā goḥ ||2||
naikadoṣāśrayāḥ sarvāḥ||| |
(ca| ci| a| 26) |
Asmarī (stone, calculi) gets formed when vāta dries up the semen, urine, pitta or kapha located in the urinary bladder. These stones are formed in the same way as the bile gets dried up and solidified inside the gallbladder of the cow. All types of asmaris are caused by the combined vitiation of all the three doshas (no asmari is formed by predominance of only one dosha). Therefore, basically all types of asmaris are tridoshaja. (2)|
Note – Though all the asmaris (calculus) are caused by all three doshas, they are named as vataja, pittaja etc due to the predominance of that particular dosha in the combined vitiation. But for the formation of a stone or calculus kapha is the basic dosha which is required as a base substance or matrix. So, all kinds of asmaris are formed by tridoshas, any dosha may dominate the

picture (and hence different types of asmari based on dosha predominance) and kapha is the basic dosha required for the formation of structure of calculi of any type.

Asmari Purvarupa – Premonitory symptoms of asmari

... athāsāṃ pūrvalakṣaṇam |
bastyādhmānaṃ tadāsannadeśeṣu parito'tiruk ||3||
mūtre bastasagandhatvaṃ mūtrakṛcchraṃ jvaro'ruciḥ |
(vā| ni| a| 9) |
The premonitory symptoms of Aśmarīs are distension of the urinary bladder, severe pain in and around the urinary bladder, the smell of urine resembling that of a goat, difficulty in urination, fever and loss of taste in food. (3-4)

Asmari Samanya Lakshana – General Symptoms of Asmari

sāmānyaliṅgaṃ ruṅnābhisevanībastimūrdhasu ||4||
viśīrṇadhāraṃ mūtraṃ syāttayā mārge nirodhite |
tadvyapāyāt sukhaṃ mehedacchaṃ gomedakopamam ||5||
tatsaṅkṣobhāt kṣate sāsramāyāsāccātirugbhavet |
(vā| ni| a| 9) |
General signs and symptoms of asmari (calculi) include - pain in the region of the umbilicus, perineum and dome of the bladder. In this condition, since the urinary passage (flow) is interrupted or blocked by the stone, the flow of urine comes out in many streams. When the stone gets dislodged, the person easily voids urine which is clear, having the colour of gomedaka gem (yellowish red in colour), of blood coloured or mixed with blood (due to bleeding in the urinary tract). If the interior of the urinary bladder (and urinary passages) get injured due to the friction by stone, bleeding also occurs along with urine. When the person tries to void the urine forcibly in spite of the stone being present in the urinary passage, the pressure causes severe pain. (4-5)

Vataja Asmari

tatra vātādbhṛśaṃ cārto dantān khādati vepate ||6||

gṛhṇāti mehanaṃ nābhiṃ pīḍayatyaniśaṃ kvaṇan |
sānilaṃ muñcati śakṛnmuhurmehati binduśaḥ ||7||
śyāvāruṇā'śmarī cāsya syāccitā kaṇṭakairiva |
(vā| ni| a| 9) |
Symptoms of Vataja Asmari – The pain is so severe that the person bites his lips with his teeth and he will have tremors. He would constantly (repeatedly) squeeze his penis and would press his umbilicus constantly while crying. The faeces of the person are expelled along with flatus. Urine gets voided drop by drop frequently. The colour of the stone will be black or reddish black in colour and is surrounded by thorn like sprouts or projections. (6-7)

Paittika / Pittaja Asmari

pittena dahyate bastiḥ pacyamāna ivoṣmavān ||8||
bhallātakāsthisaṃsthānā raktapītā'sitā'śmarī |
(vā| ni| a| 9) |
Symptoms of Pittaja Asmari – The person would experience burning sensation inside the urinary bladder and heat similar to the ulcer which is in the process of being ripened (as though smeared by alkali). The region of the bladder is hot to touch. The stone resembles the seed of Bhallataka (Semecarpus anacardium). It is red, yellow or black in colour. (8)

Kaphaja Asmari

bastirnistudyata iva śleṣmaṇā śītalo guruḥ ||9||
aśmarī mahatī ślakṣṇā madhuvarṇā'thavā sitā |
(vā| ni| a| 9) |
Symptoms of Kaphaja Asmari - In this type there is pricking pain, coldness and heaviness in the urinary bladder. The stone will be big in size, smooth, resembles honey (slightly brownish) in colour or is white in colour. (9)

Asmari in children

etā bhavanti bālānāṃ teṣāmeva ca bhūyasā ||10||
āśrayopacayālpatvādgrahaṇāharaṇe sukhāḥ |
(vā| ni| a| 9) |

The above three types of asmari are common in young boys and girls. These stones can be easily removed through surgical process in children because of the small size of both the urinary bladder and the stone. (10)

Shukrasmari

śukrāśmarī tu mahatāṃ jāyate śukradhāraṇāt ||11||
sthānāccyutamamuktaṃ hi muṣkayorantare'nilaḥ |
śoṣayatyupasaṅgṛhya śukraṃ tacchukramaśmarī ||12||
bastiruṅmūtrakṛcchratvamuṣkaśvayathukāriṇī |
tasyāmutpannamātrāyāṃ śukrameti vilīyate ||13||
pīḍite tvavakāśe'smin||| |
(vā| ni| a| 9) |
Shukrasmari occurs in adults who withhold (suppress the urge) the ejaculation of the semen. Due to immense sexual excitation or during sex, the semen gets displaced from its seat (of production). In this condition if the person tries to withhold the urge for ejaculation the semen gets blocked (impacted) between the two testicles (in the urethra). The aggravated vata dries up this semen. Being dried by vata the semen becomes hard and assumes the shape and structure of a stone. This further leads to pain in the region of the urinary bladder, dysuria and swelling in the scrotum (testicles). On rubbing over the point of obstruction, the semen gets dissolved and released through the urethral passage. (11-13)

Sarkara – gravel

...aśmaryeva ca śarkarā |14|
aṇuśo vāyunā bhinnā sā tasminnanulomage ||14||
nireti saha mūtreṇa pratilome nirudhyate | (vā| ni| a| 9) |
mūtrasrotaḥpravṛttā sā saktā kuryādupadravān ||15||
daurbalyaṃ sadanaṃ kārśyaṃ kukṣiśūlamathārucim |
pāṇḍutvamuṣṇavātaṃ ca tṛṣṇāṃ hṛtpīḍanaṃ vamim ||16|| (su| ni| a| 3) |
Sarkarā (gravel) is the same as aśmari. The aggravated vata breaks the asmari into minute pieces. Due to the downward course (movement) of vata, the stone particles are expelled out mixed with urine. If the vata has an opposite course i.e., moves in the upward direction they remain inside (and are not expelled out).
The sarkara having got impacted inside the urinary passages due to the

reverse movement of vata causes many complications including debility, exhaustion, emaciation, pain in the lower part of the abdomen, loss of taste, anaemia, burning urination, thirst, pain in the region of the heart and vomiting. (14-16)

Symptoms of incurability of asmari

praśūnanābhivṛṣaṇaṃ baddhamūtraṃ rujāturam |
aśmarī kṣapayatyāśu sikatā śarkarānvitā ||17||
Asmari is going to kill the patient quickly if it is associated with severe swelling in the scrotum (testes) and umbilicus, total obstruction of urine, severe pain and presence of gravel in it (because such asmari is incurable). (17)

iti śrīmādhavakaraviracite mādhavanidāne'śmarīnidānaṃ samāptam ||32||
Thus ends the chapter on Aśmarī.

CHAPTER THIRTY-THREE

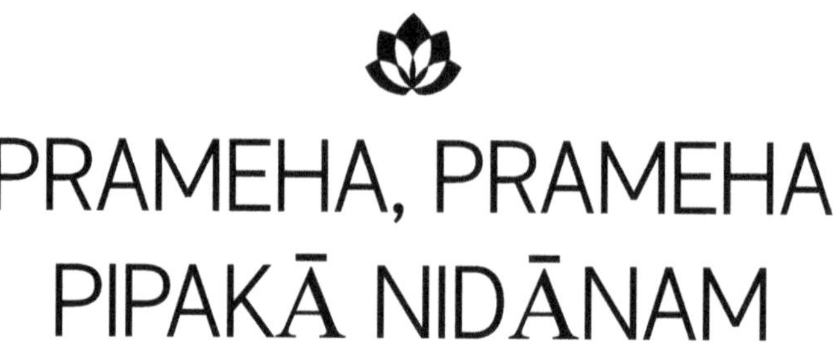

PRAMEHA, PRAMEHA PIPAKĀ NIDĀNAM

Prameha Nidana – Etiological Factors of Prameha

āsyāsukhaṃ svapnasukhaṃ dadhīni grāmyaudakānūparasāḥ payāṃsi |
navānnapānaṃ guḍavaikṛtaṃ ca pramehahetuḥ kaphakṛcca sarvam ||1||
(ca| ci| a| 7) |
Below mentioned are the etiological factors of prameha –

- sitting on soft cushions and comfortable beddings for long periods (thus avoiding physical activity),
- sleeping for long hours,
- excessive use of curds,
- excessive consumption of flesh of domestic animals (and birds) or of those living in aquatic or of marshy places,
- excessive consumption of milk and its products / preparations,
- excessive use of fresh grains and fresh water (rain water),
- excessive use of puddings made of jaggery / sugar (and other edibles made of jaggery or sugar) and
- all other similar factors which bring about increase of kapha in the body (kapha aggravating foods and activities) (1)

Prameha Samprapti – pathogenesis of prameha

medaśca māṃsaṃ ca śarīrajaṃ ca kledaṃ kapho bastigataḥ pradūṣya |
karoti mehān samudīrṇamuṣṇaistāneva pittaṃ paridūṣya cāpi ||2||

kṣīṇeṣu doṣeṣvavakṛṣya dhātūn sandūṣya mehān kurute'nilaśca |
Pathogenesis of Kaphaja Prameha - Kapha which has undergone increase due to its own etiological factors and located in the urinary bladder, vitiates the medas (fat), māṁsa (muscle) and kleda (body fluids), and causes kaphaja prameha.
Pathogenesis of Pittaja Prameha – Pitta which has been aggravated due to excessive consumption of foods which are hot in nature (and other pitta aggravating foods and activities) and located in the urinary bladder vitiates the fat, muscle and body fluids (as described in kaphaja prameha) and causes pittaja prameha.
Pathogenesis of Vataja Prameha – The vata aggravated due to decrease of kapha and pitta would vitiate muscle-fat, bone marrow, ojus (essence of all the tissues) and serum (plasma), pulls them into the urinary bladder and causes vataja prameha.

Prognosis of doshaja types of prameha

sādhyāḥ kaphotthā daśa, pittajāḥ ṣaḍ yāpyā, na sādhyaḥ pavanāccatuṣkaḥ ||3||
samakriyatvādviṣamakriyatvānmahātyayatvācca yathākramaṃ te |
(ca| ci| a| 6) |
The ten kinds produced by kapha are easily curable. This is due to the similarity in properties of the causative doshas and vitiated tissues. Due to this similarity the treatment for doshas and tissues will be similar and hence makes these conditions curable.
The six kinds of pittaja prameha are manageable (controllable). This is due to the dissimilarity in the properties of the causative doshas and vitiated tissues. Due to this dissimilarity the treatment for the involved doshas and tissues will be opposite in nature. Therefore, this condition becomes manageable (persists throughout the life but would be under control if timely and prompt treatment is given i.e., requires frequent treatment to manage the disease and have it under control).
The four kinds of vataja prameha are said to be incurable. This is due to the grave consequences and severe complications caused due to severe and quick destruction of tissues due to aggravation of vata and also due to the opposite nature of the treatment for the involved doshas and tissues. (2-3)

Doshas and Dushyas (tissues and other components of the body) involved in the pathogenesis of Prameha

kaphaḥ sapittaḥ pavanaśca doṣā medo'sraśukrāmbuvasālasīkāḥ |
majjā rasaujaḥ piśitaṃ ca dūṣyāḥ pramehiṇāṃ viṃśatireva mehāḥ ||4||
(ca| ci| a| 6) |
Involved doshas - In all the twenty varieties of prameha, vāta, pitta and kapha together form the causative doshas.
Involved dushyas – medas (fat), asrk (blood), sukra (semen), ambu (body fluids), vasa (muscle fat), lasika (tissue fluid), majja (marrow), rasa (lymph), oja (essence of all the dhātus) and pishita (muscle tissue) are the dushyas involved in the causation of prameha. (4)

Premonitory symptoms of Prameha

dantādīnāṃ malāḍhyatvaṃ prāgrūpaṃ pāṇipādayoḥ |
dāhaścikkaṇatā dehe tṛṭ svādvāsyaṃ ca jāyate ||5||
Premonitory symptoms of prameha are accumulation of dirt on the teeth (mouth, palate, throat, tongue, eyes, nose, and ears), feeling of burning sensation in the palms and soles, stickiness of the skin all over the body, thirst and manifestation of sweet taste in the mouth. (5)

Prameha Samanya Lakshana – General symptoms of Prameha

sāmānyaṃ lakṣaṇaṃ teṣāṃ prabhūtāvilamūtratā |
doṣadūṣyāviśeṣe'pi tatsaṃyogaviśeṣataḥ ||6||
mūtravarṇādibhedena bhedo meheṣu kalpyate |
(vā| ni| a| 10) |
Increased quantity and turbidity of urine are the characteristic features of prameha. Due to the specificity of doshas and tissues and combination of doṣhas and dūṣyas, different colours are seen in the urine and the prameha (diabetes) are classified depending upon the colour of the urine, etc. (6-7)

Kaphaja Prameha – their types and symptoms

acchaṃ bahu sitaṃ śītaṃ nirgandhamudakopamam ||7||
mehatyudakamehena kiñcidāvilapicchilam |
ikṣo rasamivātyarthaṃ madhuraṃ cekṣumehataḥ ||8||
sāndrībhavet paryuṣitaṃ sāndramehena mehati |

surāmehī surātulyamuparyacchamadho ghanam ||9||
saṃhṛṣṭaromā piṣṭena piṣṭavadbahalaṃ sitam |
śukrābhaṃ śukramiśraṃ vā śukramehī pramehati ||10||
mūrtāṇūn sikatāmehī sikatārūpiṇo malān |
śītamehī subahuśo madhuraṃ bhṛśaśītalam ||11||
śanaiḥ śanaiḥ śanairmehī mandaṃ mandaṃ pramehati |
lālātantuyutaṃ mūtraṃ lālāmehena picchilam ||12||
(vā| ni| a| 10) |
Udakameha Symptoms are – The urine is clear, more in quantity (copious), white, cold, odourless, resembles water, with little turbidity and stickiness.
Iksumeha Symptoms – The urine is sweet – like the juice of sugarcane.
Sandrameha Symptoms – In this condition, the urine kept undisturbed for a while in a vessel becomes thick and dense.
Surameha Symptoms – Here, the urine resembles sura i.e., alcoholic beverages prepared with flour, clear at the top and thick sediments at the bottom.
Pistameha Symptoms – In this condition the urine appears thick like flour (as if mixed with flour) & is white in colour. The patient will experience horripilations.
Sukrameha Symptoms – Here, the urine either resembles (appears like) semen or is mixed with semen.
Sikatameha Symptoms – In this condition the urine contains small particles which resemble sand.
Shitameha Symptoms – In this condition the urine is large in quantity (copious), sweet in taste and very cold.
Sanairmeha Symptoms – In this condition the urine is voided frequently and very slowly.
Lalameha Symptoms – Here the urine resembles saliva along with the appearance of thread like structures and is sticky in nature.
(These ten varieties are predominantly kaphaja.)(7-12)

Pittaja Prameha – their types and symptoms

gandhavarṇarasasparśaiḥ kṣāreṇa kṣāratoyavat |
nīlamehena nīlābhaṃ kālamehī masīnibham ||13||
hāridramehī kaṭukaṃ haridrāsannibhaṃ dahat |
visraṃ māñjiṣṭhamehena mañjiṣṭhāsalilopamam ||14||

visramuṣṇaṃ salavaṇaṃ raktābhaṃ raktamehataḥ |15|
(vā| ni| a| 10) |

Ksarameha Symptoms – In this condition the urine resembles the solution of alkali in smell, colour, taste and touch.

Nilameha Symptoms – The urine is blue in colour in nilameha.

Kalameha Symptoms – In this type the urine resembles the colour of ink.

Haridrameha Symptoms – In this condition the colour of the urine resembles that of turmeric (deep yellow). The urine is pungent in taste and the patient experiences a burning sensation during urination.

Manjisthameha Symptoms – The urine in this type of pittaja prameha resembles the decoction of Manjistha (Rubia cordifolia) and smells foul.

Raktameha Symptoms – The urine in this condition has a foul smell, hot, has salty taste and resembles blood in colour (is blood red in colour). (13-14)

(The above six varieties are predominantly pittaja.)

Vataja Prameha – their types and symptoms

vasāmehī vasāmiśraṃ vasābhaṃ mūtrayenmuhuḥ ||15||
majjābhaṃ majjamiśraṃ vā majjamehī muhurmuhuḥ |
kaṣāyaṃ madhuraṃ rūkṣaṃ kṣaudramehaṃ vadedbudhaḥ ||16||
hastī matta ivājasraṃ mūtraṃ vegavivarjitam |
salasīkaṃ vibaddhaṃ ca hastimehī pramehati ||17||
(vā| ni| a| 10) |

Vasameha Symptoms – In this condition the urine voided is either mixed with muscle fat and resembles muscle fat in colour, smell etc and is voided frequently.

Majjameha Symptoms – In this condition the person frequently voids urine mixed with marrow and also appears like marrow in colour, smell etc.

Ksaudrameha Symptoms – It is a condition in which the urine is astringent and sweet in taste and is dry (non-sticky, non-unctuous).

Hastimeha Symptoms – The person suffering from this condition continuously passes urine like an intoxicated elephant. The urine is mixed with laskia i.e., tissue fluid and is composed of matted (small nodular) material.

(The above four varieties are predominantly vātaja.) (15-17)

Prameha Upadrava – complications of prameha

avipāko‘ruciśchardirnidrā kāsaḥ sapīnasaḥ |
upadravāḥ prajāyante mehānāṃ kaphajanmanām ||18||
Complications of Kaphaja Prameha are - indigestion, loss of taste, vomiting, excessive sleep, cough, and running nose. (18)

bastimehanayostodo muṣkāvadaraṇaṃ jvaraḥ |
dāhastṛṣṇā'mlikā mūrchā viḍbhedaḥ pittajanmanām ||19||
Complications of Pittaja Prameha are – pricking pain in the urinary bladder and penis, cracking pain in the scrotum, fever, burning sensation, thirst, sour belching, loss of consciousness and diarrhoea. (19)

vātajānāmudāvartaḥ kampahṛdgrahalolatāḥ |
śūlamunnidratā śoṣaḥ kāsaḥ śvāsaśca jāyate ||20||
(vā| ni| a| 10) |
Complications of Vataja Prameha are – movement of vata in upward direction in the abdomen (retrograde peristalsis), tremors, stiffness or gripping pain in the heart (region of the heart), immense desire to eat foods having all tastes, pain in the abdomen (bladder and penis), loss of sleep, emaciation, cough and dyspnoea. (20)

Prameha Asadhyata – Symptoms of incurability

yathoktopadravāviṣṭamatiprasrutameva ca |
piḍakāpīḍitaṃ gāḍhaḥ prameho hanti mānavam ||21||
(su| sū| a| 33) |
Prameha of long duration (which has become chronic), associated with the above-mentioned complications, in which there is elimination of very large quantities of urine and appearance of carbuncles / tubercles (or ulcers) on the body is going to kill the patient (is incurable). (21)

jātaḥ pramehī madhumehino vā na sādhya uktaḥ sa hi bījadoṣāt |
ye cāpi kecit kulajā vikārā bhavanti tāṃstān pravadantyasādhyān ||22||
(ca| ci| a| 6) |
A person who is born with prameha (hereditary diabetes) or a person who is suffering from madhumeha are said to be incurable because of

defect in genes. Likewise, many other hereditary diseases also are said to be incurable. (22)

Transformation of all kinds of prameha into madhumeha

sarva eva pramehāstu kālenāpratikāriṇaḥ |
madhumehatvamāyānti tadā'sādhyā bhavanti hi ||23|| (su| ni| a| 6) |
madhumehe madhusamaṃ jāyate sa kila dvidhā |
kruddhe dhātukṣayādvāyau doṣāvṛtapathe'thavā ||24||
All varieties of prameha, if not treated at appropriate time, will ultimately get transformed into madhumeha. In this condition they will become incurable. Madhumeha - In Madhumeha, the urine is like honey (sweet in taste). Madhumeha is of two kinds. One type of madhumeha is caused by vata increase caused by dhatu ksaya – depletion of tissues. The other type of madhumeha is caused by obstruction of (the channels / passages of) vata by other doshas. (23-24)

āvṛto doṣaliṅgāni so'nimittaṃ pradarśayan |
kṣaṇāt kṣīṇaḥ kṣaṇāt pūrṇo bhajate kṛcchrasādhyatām ||25||
(vā| ni| a| 10) |
In case of madhumeha caused by avarana i.e., obstruction of vata by other doshas, the symptoms of doshas which appear are sometimes mild and sometimes severe in nature. Gradually the disease becomes difficult to cure.

Definition of Madhumeha

madhuraṃ yacca meheṣu prāyo madhviva mehati |
sarve'pi madhumehākhyā mādhuryācca tanorataḥ ||26||
(vā| ni| a| 10) |
Any variety of prameha in which the urine is sweet like honey and the whole body also becomes sweet is to be named as Madhumeha. (25-26)

Prameha Pidaka – Diabetic carbuncles

śarāvikā kacchapikā jālinī vinatā'lajī |
masūrikā sarṣapikā putriṇī savidārikā ||27||
vidradhiśceti piḍakāḥ pramehopekṣayā daśa |

sandhimarmasu jāyante māṃsaleṣu ca dhāmasu ||28||
(vā| ni| a| 10) |
The ten types of carbuncles caused by (related to) prameha are –

- saravika
- kacchapika,
- jalini,
- vinata
- alaji,
- masurika,
- sarsapika,
- putrini,
- vidarika,
- vidradhika

They appear on joints, vital parts and other fleshy parts of the body. (27-28)
(सु.नि.अ.६)

Symptoms of Prameha Pidakas

antonnatā tu tadrūpā nimnamadhyā śarāvikā |
gaurasarṣapasaṃsthānā tatpramāṇā ca sarṣapī ||29||
sadāhā kūrmasaṃsthānā jñeyā kacchapikā budhaiḥ |
jālinī tīvradāhā tu māṃsajālasamāvṛtā ||30||
avagāḍharujākledā pṛṣṭhe vā'pyudare'pi vā |
mahatī piḍakā nīlā vinatā nāma sā smṛtā ||31||
mahatyalpacitā jñeyā piḍakā cāpi putriṇī |
masūrākṛtisaṃsthānā vijñeyā tu masūrikā ||32||
raktā sitā sphoṭacitā dāruṇā tvalajī bhavet |
vidārīkandavadvṛttā kaṭhinā ca vidārikā ||33||
vidradherlakṣaṇairyuktā jñeyā vidradhikā tu sā |34| (su| ni| a| 6) |
ye yanmayāḥ smṛtā mehāsteṣāmetāstu tanmayāḥ ||34|| (su| ni| a| 6) |
Saravika – It resembles a saucer with elevated edges and a depressed centre.
Sarsapika – It is similar to white mustard seeds in colour and size.
Kacchapika – This resembles the shell of a tortoise and is associated with

burning sensation.
Jalini – This carbuncle appears like a sieve of muscle fibres and presents with severe burning sensation.
Vinata – It usually appears on the back or abdomen. The carbuncles are hard, blue, blue in colour, big in size and are associated with pain and exudation.
Putrini – It manifests in the form of a big eruption surrounded by smaller eruptions all around it.
Masurika – It resembles the shape and size of a masura (pea).
Alají – It is surrounded by red or white coloured blisters and is considered to be a dreadful condition.
Vidarika – It is round and hard just like the tuber of Vidari (Pueraria tuberosa).
Vidradhika – This is an eruption (carbuncle) which will present with all the features of an abscess.

These prameha pidakas are also caused by the same doshas which cause the pramehas which are responsible for the manifestation of these pidakas. (The same dosha which causes a particular prameha will also be responsible for the causation of a pidaka resulting from that particular prameha. To put it in simple words, the dosha causing a particular type of prameha and its pidaka is the same.) (29-34)

vinā pramehamapyetā jāyante duṣṭamedasaḥ |
tāvaccaitā na lakṣyante yāvadvāstuparigrahāḥ ||35||
(ca| sū| a| 17) |
The pidakas might also occur without the presence of prameha when the medas i.e. fat / adipose tissue gets severely contaminated (vitiated). (This means that pidakas need not be essentially caused by prameha. Severe vitiation of fat tissue may also cause these pidakas independently). But they cannot be recognized (their specific symptoms will not become evident) until they get localized in specific parts of the body. (35)

gude hṛdi śirasyaṃsye pṛṣṭhe marmasu cotthitāḥ |
sopadravā durbalāgneḥ piḍakāḥ parivarjayet ||36||
(su| ni| a| 6) |
The patients who have developed these pidakas in the anal region (rectum),

region of the heart, head, shoulders (scapular regions, shoulder blades), back and vital parts of the body, associated with complications and manifesting in those who have poor digestive fire (capacity) are to be refused treatment (because these conditions are incurable). (36)

iti śrīmādhavakaraviracite mādhavanidāne pramehapramehapiḍakānidānaṃ samāptam ||33||
Thus ends the chapter on Prameha.

CHAPTER THIRTY-FOUR

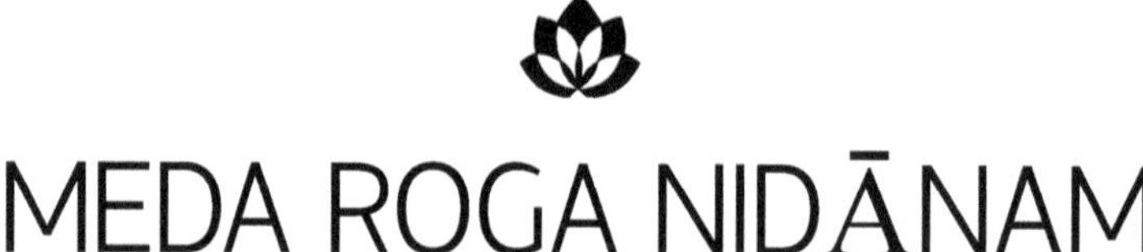

MEDA ROGA NIDĀNAM

Medo Roga Nidana, Samprapti – Etiological Factors and pathogenesis of Medo Roga

avyāyāmadivāsvapnaśleṣmalāhārasevinaḥ |
madhuro'nnarasaḥ prāyaḥ snehānmedaḥ pravardhayet ||1||
medasā''vṛtamārgatvāt puṣyantyanye na dhāvataḥ |
medastu cīyate tasmādaśaktaḥ sarvakarmasu ||2||
kṣudraśvāsatṛṣāmohasvapnakrathanasādanaiḥ |
yuktaḥ kṣutsvedadurgandhairalpaprāṇo'lpamaithunaḥ ||3||
medastu sarvabhūtānāmudareṣvasthiṣu sthitam |
ata evodare vṛddhiḥ prāyo medasvino bhavet ||4||
medasā''vṛtamārgatvādvāyuḥ koṣṭhe viśeṣataḥ |
caran sandhukṣayatyagnimāhāraṃ śoṣayatyapi ||5||
tasmāt sa śīghraṃ jarayatyāhāramabhikāṅkṣati |
vikārāṃścāpnute ghorān kāṃścit kālavyatikramāt ||6||
etāvupadravakarau viśeṣādagnimārutau |
etau tu dahataḥ sthūlaṃ vanadāvo vanaṃ yathā ||7||
medasyatīva saṃvṛddhe sahasaivānilādayaḥ |
vikārān dāruṇān kṛtvā nāśayantyāśu jīvitam ||8||
Etiological Factors – Below mentioned are the important causative factors of medo roga –

- not doing exercises (absence of physical activities, sedentary life)
- excessive sleeping during daytime
- excessive intake of foods which cause aggravation of kapha

Pathogenesis of Medoroga – Due to the above said etiological factors the end product of digestion becomes abnormally sweet and unctuous. This causes an increase of fat. This abnormally increased fat causes obstruction of the nutrient channels of the body. This would supply less or no nutrients to the other tissues of the body. The tissues are not nourished due to the deprivation of nutrition. This further leads to accumulation of only fat tissue in large quantities in the body. This makes the person incapable of doing all activities.

Symptoms of Medoroga – The symptoms of medoroga are – difficulty in breathing even after doing small activities or little exertion, thirst, delusion, excessive sleep, sudden obstruction of breathing, exhaustion (laxity of body parts), excessive hunger, excessive sweating, bad smell of the body, poor physical and sexual capacity.

The abdomen and the small bones are fat depots in the body. This is the reason there is enlargement of the abdomen in people who have excessive fat in their body (the excess fat accumulates around the abdomen).

The channels of vāta become obstructed by the increased fat mainly inside the abdomen. The vata thus obstructed quickly travels in the entire intestine and increases the digestive fire (activity). This causes very quick drying (parching, destruction) of food. The food will get quickly digested. This will cause voracious hunger and craving for large quantities of food frequently. In this condition if food is nor provided it will lead to many distressing symptoms and complications in due course of time. All complications are caused mainly by aggravated vata and severe digestive fire.

These two (vata and agni) would destroy the body of the person (kill the person) just like the forest fire destroys the entire forest.

When the fat increases to severe proportions vata and other doshas also undergo severe aggravation, produce many severe complications and even cause death in quick time. (1-8)

Definition of Atisthula

medomāṃsātivṛddhatvāccalasphigudarastanaḥ |
ayathopacayotsāho naro'tisthūla ucyate ||9|| (ca| sū| a| 21) |

A person is said to be very obese when his buttocks, abdomen and breasts begin to show movement (they sag and are pendulous during activity) due to abnormal increase and accumulation of fat and muscles, and when his muscle mass (body built) and enthusiasm are found to be disproportionate. (9)

iti śrīmādhavakaraviracite mādhavanidāne medonidānaṃ samāptam ||34||
Thus ends the chapter on Medaroga.

CHAPTER THIRTY-FIVE

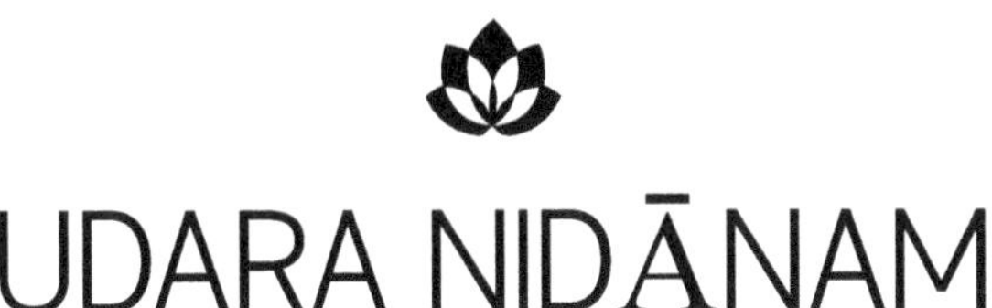

UDARA NIDĀNAM

Udara Roga Nidana – Etiological Factors for Udara Roga

rogāḥ sarve'pi mande'gnau sutarāmudarāṇi ca |
ajīrṇānmalinaiścānnairjāyante malasañcayāt ||1||
(vā| ni| a| 12) |
All diseases in the body, mainly the udara rogas (enlargement of abdomen) are caused by mandāgni (poor digestive fire or activity), indigestion of food, and excessive consumption of dirty or spoiled (contaminated) foods and accumulation of waste products in the body (excreta and other metabolic wastes). (1)

Udara Roga Samprapti – Pathogenesis of enlargement of abdomen

ruddhvā svedāmbuvāhīni doṣāḥ srotāṃsi sañcitāḥ |
prāṇāgnyapānān sandūṣya janayantyudaraṃ nṛṇām ||2||
(ca| ci| a| 13) |
The dosas undergoing increase and accumulation obstruct the channels of sweat and other body fluids, vitiate prāna, apāna and agni (pitta) and produce Udararoga (enlargement of abdomen).(2)

Udara Samanya Lakshana – General symptoms

ādhmānaṃ gamane'śaktirdaurbalyaṃ durbalāgnitā |
śothaḥ sadanamaṅgānāṃ saṅgo vātapurīṣayoḥ ||3||
dāhastandrā ca sarveṣu jaṭhareṣu bhavanti hi | (su| ni| a| 7) |
The symptoms generally seen in all kinds of udara roga are –

- distension of the abdomen,
- inability to walk,
- weakness,
- weakness of digestive fire (capacity)
- swelling / oedema
- looseness / debility in the body parts (extremities)
- obstruction to the movement (expulsion) of flatus and faeces
- burning sensation
- stupor (3-4)

Udara Samkhya – Types of Udara Roga

pṛthagdoṣaiḥ samastaiśca plīhabaddhakṣatodakaiḥ ||4||
sambhavantyudarāṇyaṣṭau teṣāṃ liṅgaṃ pṛthak śṛṇu |5|
Udara is of eight kinds. They are –

1-3. one from each doşha – vataja udara (vatodara), pittaja udara (pittodara) and kaphaja udara (shleshmodara / kaphodara)

4. one from the combination of all three vitiated doshas – sannipatodara
5. plīhodara,
6. baddhodara,
7. kşatodara and
8. udakodara / jalodara

The symptoms of each of these 8 types of udara will be described separately further on. (4)

Vatodara Symptoms

tatra vātodare śothaḥ pāṇipānnābhikukṣiṣu ||5||
kukṣipārśvodarakaṭīpṛṣṭharuk parvabhedanam |
śuṣkakāso'ṅgamardo'dhogurutā malasaṅgrahaḥ ||6||
śyāvāruṇatvagāditvamakasmādvṛddhihrāsavat |
satodabhedamudaraṃ tanukṛṣṇasirātatam ||7||
ādhmātadṛtivacchabdamāhataṃ prakaroti ca |
vāyuścātra sarukśabdo vicaret sarvato gatiḥ ||8||
(vā| ni| a| 12) |

The symptoms of Vatodara are – swelling (oedema) of the hands, feet, umbilicus and lower abdomen; pain in the cavity of the abdomen, flanks, abdomen, waist (pelvis), and back and splitting pain in the joints, mainly small joints of the hands and feet (fingers and toes); dry cough, body aches, feeling of heaviness of the lower parts of the body, accumulation of wastes products (excreta) in the body, dark brown (bluish) or reddish-brownish (golden yellow) discolouration of skin, etc. (nails, eyes, face, teeth etc), sudden increase or decrease of size of the abdomen without any apparent reason, pricking, throbbing and other types of pain in the abdomen, appearance of thin, black network of veins on the abdomen, highly resonant sound elicited on percussion (sound resembling that coming when you tap on a bag / sac filled with air) and the vayu (gases) move all round inside the abdomen (intestines) producing gurgling noises and pain. (5-8)

Pittodara Symptoms

pittodare jvaro mūrchā dāhastṛṭ kaṭukāsyatā |
bhramo'tisāraḥ pītatvaṃ tvagādāvudaraṃ harit ||9||
pītatāmrasirānaddhaṃ sasvedaṃ soṣma dahyate |
dhūmāyate mṛdusparśaṃ kṣiprapākaṃ pradūyate ||10||
(vā| ni| a| 12) |
The symptoms of Pittodara are – fever, loss of consciousness (fainting), burning sensation, thirst, manifestation of bitter taste in the mouth, giddiness, diarrhoea, yellowish discolouration of skin (nails, eyes, teeth, face) etc., and greenish colour of the abdomen, network of veins of yellow or coppery colour spread out over the abdomen, sweating, feeling of excessive heat and burning sensation, sensation of hot smoke or fumes from the surface of the abdomen, abdomen is soft to touch and the condition (pittaja udara) undergoes quick suppuration (quickly progresses towards ascites) and there will be severe pain in the abdomen. (9-10)

Kaphodara Symptoms

śleṣmodare'ṅgasadanaṃ svāpaśvayathugauravam |
nidrotkleśo'ruciḥ śvāsaḥ kāsaḥ śuklatvagāditā ||11||
udaraṃ stimitaṃ snigdhaṃ śuklarājītataṃ mahat |

cirābhivṛddhaṃ kaṭhinaṃ śītasparśaṃ guru sthiram ||12||
(vā| ni| a| 12) |
The symptoms of Kaphodara are - debility, loss of activity, oedema and heaviness of the body parts, excessive sleep, nausea, loss of taste, dyspnoea (difficulty in breathing), cough, whitish discolouration of skin (nails, eyes, teeth, face) etc. The abdomen is tense (loss of movements), unctuous, having white striae (covered by long white marks / streak), large in size, increasing slowly, hard, cold to touch, heavy and without movement. (11-12)

Sannipatodara Symptoms

striyo'nnapānaṃ nakhalomamūtraviḍārtavairyuktamasādhuvṛttāḥ |
yasmai prayacchantyarayo garāṃśca duṣṭāmbudūṣīviṣasevanādvā ||13||
tenāśu raktaṃ kupitāśca doṣāḥ kuryuḥ sughoraṃ jaṭharaṃ triliṅgam |
tacchītavāte bhṛśadurdine ca viśeṣataḥ kupyati dahyate ca ||14||
sa cāturo muhyati hi prasaktaṃ pāṇḍuḥ kṛśaḥ śuṣyati tṛṣṇayā ca |
dūṣyodaraṃ kīrtitametadeva ||
(su| ni| a| 7) |
Causative factors of Sannipatodara are –

- Ingestion of harmful foods containing (mixed with) nails, body hairs, urine, faeces and menstrual blood etc by women of bad or unappreciable nature (wicked women) or by wicked men or enemies, or
- consumptions of foods mixed with (artificial) poisons served by enemies,
- drinking polluted water
- consumption of slow poisons etc

Pathogenesis – Due to the consumption of the above said etiological factors, the blood along with the three doshas will get aggravated in quick time and cause tridoshaja udara roga. In this condition the symptoms of all the three doshas will be present together.
Symptoms - This symptom of this condition exacerbates in cold breeze (on days of cold breeze) and overcast conditions (when the sky is enveloped by clouds), and there is severe burning sensation. The person faints frequently,

is pale, emaciated, and his mouth gets dried due to severe thirst. This condition is also called as Dusyodara also. (13-14)

Plihodara Symptoms

.... plīhodaraṃ kīrtayato nibodha ||15||
vidāhyabhiṣyandiratasya jantoḥ praduṣṭamatyarthamasṛk kaphaśca |
plīhābhivṛddhiṃ kurutaḥ pravṛddhau plīhotthametajjaṭharaṃ vadanti ||16||
tadvāmapārśve parivṛddhimeti viśeṣataḥ sīdati cāturo'tra |
mandajvarāgniḥ kaphapittaliṅgairupadrutaḥ kṣīṇabalo'tipāṇḍuḥ |
Understand the symptoms of Plīhodara (which has been explained) further In persons who indulge in foods which produce burning sensation during digestion and those which block the tissue pores by greasy material, the rakta (blood) and kapha undergo severe aggravation. They in turn cause enlargement of the spleen and produce plihodara (splenomegaly). In this condition the abdomen is enlarged more towards the left side. The patient is very much debilitated, will have mild fever, poor digestion, symptoms of increased kapha and pitta, loss of strength and severe form of anaemia. (15-16)

Yakrutodaram / Yakruddalyudaram

savyānyapārśve yakṛti pravṛddhe jñeyaṃ yakṛddālyudaraṃ tadeva ||17||
(su| ni| a| 7) |
If there is such an enlargement on the right side of the abdomen (just like in plihodara) involving the liver, the disease shall be named as Yakrtodara (hepatomegaly). (17)

Dosha symptoms in both Plihodara and Yakrtodara

udāvartarujānāhairmohatṛḍdahanajvaraiḥ |
gauravārucikāṭhinyairvidyāttatra malān kramāt ||18||
(vā| ni| a| 12) |
In both these conditions i.e., plihodara and yakrtodara, the dosha involvement should be understood on seeing the associated dosha symptoms –

- in association of vata, the symptoms of vata are seen, they are – upward movement of vata, pain in the abdomen and flatulence (distension of abdomen)
- in association of pitta, the symptoms of pitta are seen, they are – delusion (loss of consciousness), thirst, burning sensation and fever
- in association of kapha, the symptoms of kapha are seen, they are – heaviness in the abdomen, loss of taste in food, and hardness of the abdomen (18)

Baddhagudodara

yasyāntramannairupalepibhirvā bālāśmabhirvā pihitaṃ yathāvat |
sañcīyate tasya malaḥ sadoṣaḥ śanaiḥ śanaiḥ saṅkaravacca nāḍyām ||19||
nirudhyate tasya gude purīṣaṃ nireti kṛcchrādapi cālpamalpam |
hṛnnābhimadhye parivṛddhimeti tasyodaraṃ baddhagudaṃ vadanti ||20||
(su| ni| a| 7) |

Due to the obstruction of the intestines by food materials which are sticky in nature, hairs, stones, etc. the wastes (faeces) along with the three doshas gradually accumulates inside the intestines just like a mixture of dirt (just like the dirt gradually accumulates in a tube or pipe and prevents free flow of water within). The waste materials thus accumulated in the anus (intestines) get eliminated in small quantities (in the form of small pellets) with great difficulty. In this condition the abdomen is enlarged between the chest and umbilicus. This condition is called Baddhagudodara (intestinal obstruction). (19-20)

Parisravyudara Symptoms

śalyaṃ tathā'nnopahitaṃ yadantraṃ bhuktaṃ bhinattyāgatamanyathā vā |
tasmātsruto'ntrātsalilaprakāśaḥ srāvaḥ sravedvai gudatastu bhūyaḥ ||21||
nābheradhaścodarameti vṛddhiṃ nistudyate dālyati cātimātram |
etat parisrāvyudaraṃ pradiṣṭaṃ ||| |22| (su| ni| a| 7) |

When the foreign bodies (objects) are ingested along with the food or otherwise damages and tears the walls of the intestine or if there is perforation of the wall of the intestine due to any other cause, it will lead to exudation of watery material in large quantities. This watery fluid will accumulate in the abdominal cavity and produce enlargement of the abdomen. Later this fluid will get discharged through the anal route. In this condition the enlargement of the abdomen takes place below the umbilicus. The person will experience pricking or crushing (tearing, bursting) pain in the abdomen. This type of udara is called Parisrāviudara (intestinal perforation and peritonitis). (21-22)

Jalodara symptoms

… dakodaraṃ kīrtayato nibodha ||22||
yaḥ snehapīto'pyanuvāsito vā vānto virikto'pyathavā nirūḍhaḥ |
pibejjalaṃ śītalamāśu tasya srotāṃsi dūṣyanti hi tadvahāni ||23||
snehopalipteṣvathavā'pi teṣu dakodaraṃ pūrvavadabhyupaiti |
snigdhaṃ mahattatparivṛttanābhisamātataṃ pūrṇamivāmbunā ca |
yathā dṛtiḥ kṣubhyati kampate ca śabdāyate cāpi dakodaraṃ tat ||24|| (su| ni| a| 7) |
sUnderstand the type of udara called as Dakodara now –
When a patient drinks cold water immediately after he has undergone (administered with) therapies like oleation – oral consumption of medicated lipids (oil or ghee) as part of therapy, unctuous (oil or ghee) enema, emesis, purgation or decoction enema, it would cause contamination of the channels of water / fluids. Also when the interior of the water / fluid conveying channels get coated and obstructed by unctuous material (oily material), the fluid gets accumulated in the abdominal cavity as explained in Chidrodara and causes dakodara (ascites).
The abdomen is unctuous (oily appearance) and is greatly enlarged with the umbilicus protruding out. The abdomen trembles (shakes), produces movements and sounds just like a leather bag filled with water. This condition is called Dakodara (enlargement of the abdomen due to the accumulation of the fluid, ascites). (23-24)

Symptoms of incurability of Udara

janmanaivodaraṃ sarvaṃ prāyaḥ kṛcchratamaṃ matam |
balinastadajātāmbu yatnasādhyaṃ navotthitam ||25||
pakṣādbaddhagudaṃ tūrdhvaṃ sarvaṃ jātodakaṃ tathā |
prāyo bhavatyabhāvāya chidrāntraṃ codaraṃ nṛṇām ||26||
(ca| ci| a| 13)0 |27|

Generally, all kinds of udara rogas are difficult to cure right from the time of their onset. This condition can only be cured with great effort in persons who are strong (strong constitution), before the formation of fluid (before fluid accumulates in the abdominal cavity) and when it is of recent onset. Baddha Gudodara will become incurable after the lapse of 15 days (if it cannot be cured within a fortnight it cannot be cured at all). All other types of abdominal enlargements which have progressed to the stage of ascites (accumulation of fluid in the abdominal cavity) are incurable. Parisravi Udara – wherein there is perforation of intestines are going to be fatal and hence incurable. (25-26)

Other symptoms of incurability of udara roga

śūnākṣaṃ kuṭilopasthamupaklinnatanutvacam |
balaśoṇitamāṃsāgniparikṣīṇaṃ ca varjayet ||27|| (ca| ci| a| 13) |
pārśvabhaṅgānnavidveṣaśothātīsārapīḍitam |
viriktaṃ cāpyudariṇaṃ pūryamāṇaṃ vivarjayet ||28|| (su| sū| a| 33) |
iti śrīmādhavakaraviracite mādhavanidāne udaranidānaṃ samāptam ||35||

Patients of udara who have developed oedema of the eyes, abnormal curvature of the penis, wet and thin skin, and loss of strength, blood, muscles and digestive capacity are to be refused treatment.

Similarly, when there is compression of the ribs (compression or pain in the flanks), aversion to food, oedema, diarrhoea and fluid accumulating quickly in spite of administering repeated purgation (therapy) are to be rejected. (27-28)

iti śrīmādhavakaraviracite mādhavanidāne udaranidānaṃ samāptam ||35||

Thus ends the chapter on Udara.

CHAPTER THIRTY-SIX

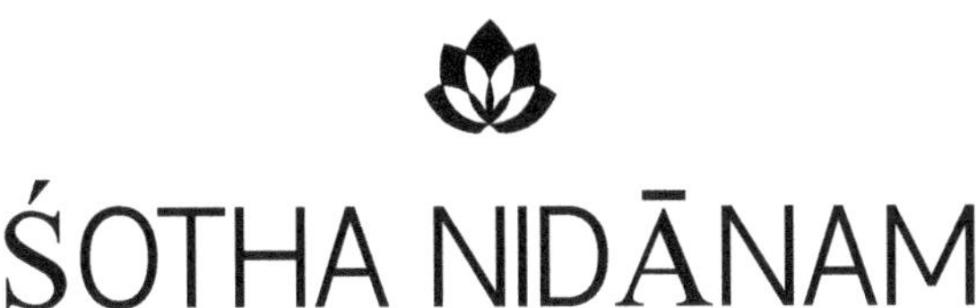

ŚOTHA NIDĀNAM

Sotha Samprapti, Bheda – Pathogenesis and types of Sotha

raktapittakaphān vāyurduṣṭo duṣṭān bahiḥsirāḥ |
nītvā ruddhagatistairhi kuryāttvaṅmāṃsasaṃśrayam ||1||
utsedhaṃ saṃhataṃ śothaṃ tamāhurnicayādataḥ |
sarvaṃ hetuviśeṣaistu rūpabhedānnavātmakam ||2||
doṣaiḥ pṛthagdvayaiḥ sarvairabhighātādviṣādapi |3| (vā| ni| a| 13) |
Vāta undergoing increase due to its own etiological factors pushes the vitiated rakta (blood), pitta and kapha into the superficial veins. Therein (inside the veins) the vata gets obstructed by the same blood, pitta and kapha. These three doshas along with the vitiated blood gets accumulated between the skin and muscles and cause swelling. This swelling is called as Sotha.
Types of Sotha – All sothas are of one type seeing that they all present with swelling. But due to different causative factors and symptoms (caused due to different causative factors), sotha is classified into nine types. They are – one each from each dosha (vataja, pittaja and kaphaja), one each from combination of two doshas (vata-pittaja, vata-kaphaja and pitta-kaphaja), one type from the combination of all three doshas (tridoshaja, sannipataja), one from injury (abhighataja) and one from the effect of poisons (vishaja). (1-2)

Sotha Purvarupa – Premonitory symptoms of Sotha

tatpūrvarūpaṃ davathuḥ sirāyāmo'ṅgagauravam ||3||
(vā| ni| a| 13) |
Premonitory symptoms of sotha are mild burning sensation of the skin

(eyes, nose, etc.), appearance of venous network (engorgement of veins) and feeling of heaviness of the body parts. (3)

Sotha Nidana – General etiological factors of Sotha

śuddhyāmayābhuktakṛśābalānāṃ kṣārāmlatīkṣṇoṣṇagurūpasevā |
dadhyāmamṛcchākavirodhiduṣṭagaropasṛṣṭānnaniṣevaṇaṃ ca ||4||
arśāṃsyaceṣṭā na ca dehaśuddhirmarmopaghāto viṣamā prasūtiḥ |
mithyopacāraḥ pratikarmaṇāṃ ca nijasya hetuḥ śvayathoḥ pradiṣṭaḥ ||5|| (ca| ci| a| 12) |
Below mentioned are the general etiological factors of Sotha –
Causes for Nija Sotha (Sotha caused by doshas) –

- Excessive administration of foods which are alkaline, sour, strong / deep penetrating, hot (heat producing) or heavy foods (difficult to digest foods), to those who have got emaciated due to (excessive or improper) administration of purificatory therapies (panchakarma therapies like emesis, purgation etc), long standing diseases (fever etc), not eating food / lack of food (starvation) or foods of low quality (and nutrition) and to the weakened persons will cause sotha (by causing aggravation of doshas).
- Excessive consumption of curds, uncooked foods, mud, leafy vegetables, mutually incompatible (having opposite qualities and nature) foods, spoilt (contaminated) foods, and gara visha (combination of poisons or foods poisoned by such poisons)
- Haemorrhoids
- Absence of physical activities
- Not administering purificatory measures (panchakarma treatments) in spite of their requirement
- Damage to the marmas (vital organs and tissues) by aggravated doshas (disorders of marmas caused by aggravated doshas)
- Abnormal delivery in women (miscarriage, abortion)
- Improper administration of purificatory therapies (4-5)

Sotha Samanya Lakshana – General Symptoms of Sotha

sagauravaṃ syādanavasthitatvaṃ sotsedhamūṣmā'tha sirātanutvam |
salomaharṣaśca vivarṇatā ca sāmānyaliṅgaṃ śvayathoḥ pradiṣṭam ||6||
The general symptoms of sotha are - swelling associated with feeling of heaviness, inconsistency i.e., increasing or decreasing frequently, warmth, thinning of the veins, horripilation (hairs standing on ends), and discolouration. (6)

Vataja Sotha

calastanutvak paruṣo'ruṇo'sitaḥ suṣuptiharṣārtiyuto'nimittataḥ |
praśāmyati pronnamati prapīḍito divābalī ca śvayathuḥ samīraṇāt ||7|| (ca| ci| a| 12) |
The symptoms of vataja sotha (oedema caused due to increase of vata) are –

- the skin over the oedema is movable, thin, rough, golden yellow / brown (reddish brown) or black in colour,
- loss of sensation or feeling of pins and needles, horripilations / hyperesthesia,
- oedema subsides temporarily without any apparent cause
- pits on pressure and when the pressure is released the pit fills up quickly
- the swelling increases during daytime (7)

Pittaja Sotha

mṛduḥ sagandho'sitapītarāgavān bhramajvarasvedatṛṣāmadānvitaḥ |
ya uṣyate spaṣṭarugakṣirāgakṛt sa pittaśotho bhṛśadāhapākavān ||8|| (ca| ci| a| 12) |
The symptoms of pittaja sotha (oedema caused due to increase of pitta) are –

- the swelling (skin over the swelling) is soft
- swelling emits peculiar type of smell
- is black, yellow or red in colour
- the patient has giddiness, fever, excessive sweating and thirst, intoxication

- will have peculiar type of burning sensation in the affected part, clear pain,
- redness of the eyes
- there will be severe burning sensation and quick suppuration of the swelling (8)

Kaphaja Sotha

guruḥ sthiraḥ pāṇḍurarocakānvitaḥ prasekanidrāvamivahnimāndyakṛt |
sa kṛcchrajanmapraśamo nipīḍito na connamedrātribalī kaphātmakaḥ ||9|| (ca| ci| a| 12) |
The symptoms of pittaja sotha (oedema caused due to increase of pitta) are –

- the swelling is heavy and immovable (fixed) and pale
- the patient has loss of taste, excessive salivation, excessive sleep, poor digestion (weakness of digestive fire or capacity)
- the swelling manifests and subsides slowly
- the swelling pits on pressure and doesn't fill up quickly after the pressure is released
- the swelling is profound (increases) during night time (9)

Dwidoshaja, Tridoshaja Sotha – Swelling caused by two and three doshas

nidānākṛtisaṃsargācchvayathuḥ syāddvidoṣajaḥ |
sarvākṛtiḥ sannipātācchotho vyāmiśralakṣaṇaḥ ||10|| (ca| sū| a| 18) |
In dvidosaja sotha there will be presence of combined etiological factors and symptoms of two dosas. On the other hand, in sannipataja sotha the symptoms of all the three doshas are collectively present together. (10)

Abhighataja Sotha

abhighātena śastrādicchedabhedakṣatādibhiḥ |
himānilodadhyanilairbhallātakapikacchujaiḥ ||11||

rasaiḥ śūkaiśca saṃsparśācchvayathuḥ syādvisarpavān |
bhṛśoṣmā lohitābhāsaḥ prāyaśaḥ pittalakṣaṇaḥ ||12||
(vā| ni| a| 13) |
Assault by weapons causing cutting, breaking or tearing of the parts, assault by snow (frost), breeze, or winds coming from sea (cyclone); contact with fumes or oil of bhallātaka (marking nut) and fine thorns of the pod of kapikacchu (Mucuna pruriens), irritating juices of herbs, etc., bring about an oedema which spreads quickly all around. This condition is associated with severe burning sensation, redness and other symptoms of pitta increase. (11-12)

Vishaja Sotha

viṣajaḥ saviṣaprāṇiparisarpaṇamūtraṇāt |
daṃṣṭrādantanakhāghātādaviṣaprāṇināmapi ||13||
viṇmūtraśukropahatamalavadvastrasaṅkarāt |
viṣavṛkṣānilasparśādgarayogāvacūrṇanāt ||14||
mṛduścalo'valambī ca śīghro dāharujākaraḥ |15| (vā| ni| a| 13) |
Poisonous animals crawling or urinating on the body, stinging, biting with teeth, scratching with nails by non-poisonous animals, contact with faeces, urine, or semen of poisonous animals or coverings / contact with contaminated cloth, contact with poisonous trees, air (gases) and sprinkling or application of artificial poisonous materials also produce oedema. The skin over she swollen part is soft, movable, moves (spreads) quickly in downward direction (to the lower parts of the body) and is associated with burning sensation and pain which manifests quickly. (13-14)

Seat of doshas and sotha

doṣāḥ śvayathumūrdhvaṃ hi kurvantyāmāśayasthitāḥ ||15||
pakvāśayasthā madhye tu varcaḥsthānagatāstvadhaḥ |
kṛtsnadehamanuprāptāḥ kuryuḥ sarvasaraṃ tathā ||16||
(su| ci| a| 23) |
Doṣas residing in the stomach produce oedema in the upper part of the body. Doshas residing in the colon (large intestine) produces oedema / swelling in the trunk. The doshas residing in the rectum produce oedema in the lower parts of the body. The doshas which are spread out in the entire

body produces swelling / oedema in the entire body (all parts of the body). (15-16)

Symptoms of incurability of Sotha

yo madhyadeśe śvayathuḥ sa kaṣṭaḥ sarvagaśca yaḥ |
ardhāṅge riṣṭabhūtaḥ syādyaścordhvaṃ parisarpati ||17||
śvāsaḥ pipāsā chardiśca daurbalyaṃ jvara eva ca |
yasya cānne rucirnāsti śvayathuṃ taṃ vivarjayet ||18|| (su| ci| a| 23) |
navo'nupadravaḥ śothaḥ sādhyo'sādhyaḥ pureritaḥ ||19|| (vā| ni| a| 13) |
vivarjayet kukṣyudarāśritaṃ ca tathā gale marmaṇi saṃśritaṃ ca |
sthūlaḥ kharaścāpi bhavedvivarjyo yaścāpi bālasthavirābalānām ||20||
Oedema manifesting in the trunk and that which has spread to involve the entire body (all parts of the body) is difficult to cure.
Oedema / swelling occurring in half of the body and also spreads to involve the upper parts of the body are considered to be equal to arista (ominous signs which indicate that the person is going to die shortly) i.e., it is incurable.
The patients in whom the oedema / swelling is associated with dyspnoea (difficulty in respiration), thirst, vomiting, debility, fever and lack of desire in food should be refused treatment i.e., such a condition of shotha is incurable.
Oedema caused by its own complications which begins in the feet in men should be considered as fatal. Likewise, the swelling which begins in the face and spreads downwards in women should be considered as fatal in women. When the swelling begins in the genitals is considered as fatal in both men and women.
Oedema of recent onset which is not associated with complications is curable and the other type of oedema (explained above) are said to be incurable.
Oedema occurring in the abdominal cavity, abdomen, and neck and located in the vital organs is considered incurable. Similarly, the oedema occurring in children, old aged people and weak (women) people is incurable and hence should not be treated. (17-20)

iti śrīmādhavakaraviracite mādhavanidāne śothanidānaṃ samāptam ||36||
Thus ends the chapter on Sotha.

CHAPTER THIRTY-SEVEN

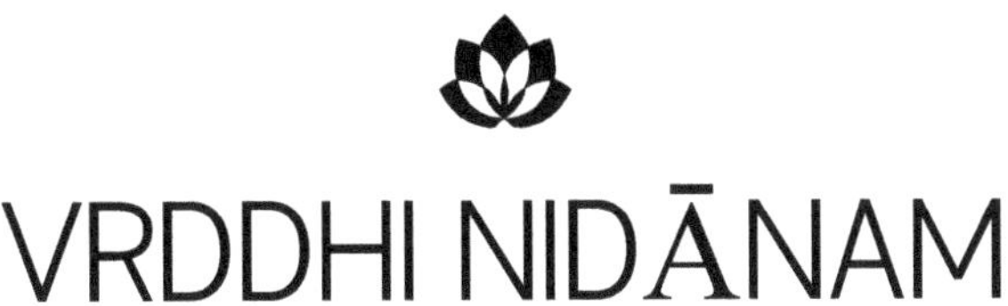

VRDDHI NIDĀNAM

Vrddhi Samprapti, bheda – Pathogenesis and types of Vrddhi

kruddho'nūrdhvagatirvāyuḥ śothaśūlakaraścaran |
muṣkau vaṅkṣaṇataḥ prāpya phalakoṣābhivāhinīḥ ||1||
prapīḍya dhamanīrvṛddhiṃ karoti phalakoṣayoḥ |
doṣāsramedomūtrāntraiḥ sa vṛddhiḥ saptadhā gadaḥ ||2||
mūtrāntrajāvapyanilāddhetubhedastu kevalam |3| (vā| ni| a| 11) |
Pathogenesis - Vāta undergoing increase moves downwards through the groins to the scrotum and causes derangement of the vessels of the scrotum and produces enlargement of the scrotum. This condition is associated with oedema and pain and is called vrddhi.
Types of Vrddhi – Vrddhi is said to be of 7 types – one from each of the three doshas, one from rakta (blood), one from meda (fat), one from mutra (urine) and the seventh one from antra (intestines).
Even the mūtraja and āntraja are mainly due to vāta, though named separately after their causes. (1-2)

Vrddhi Lakshanas – Symptoms of types of Vrddhi

vātapūrṇadṛtisparśo rūkṣo vātādaheturuk ||3||
pakvodumbarasaṅkāśaḥ pittāddāhoṣmapākavān
kaphācchīto guruḥ snigdhaḥ kaṇḍūmān kaṭhino'lparuk ||4||
kṛṣṇasphoṭāvṛtaḥ pittavṛddhiliṅgaśca raktajaḥ |
kaphavanmedasā vṛddhirmṛdustālaphalopamaḥ ||5||
mūtradhāraṇaśīlasya mūtrajaḥ sa tu gacchataḥ |
ambhobhiḥ pūrṇadṛtivat kṣobhaṃ yāti saruṅmṛduḥ ||6||
mūtrakṛcchramadhaḥ syācca cālayan phalakoṣayoḥ |7| (vā| ni| a| 11) |

Vataja Vrddhi - In vātaja vrddhi, the scrotum resembles a bag filled with air on touch and is rough. There will be pain without any apparent reason.
Pittaja Vrddhi - In pittaja víddhi, the scrotum resembles a ripe udumbara (wild fig, Ficus glomerata) fruit. The swelling is accompanied with burning sensation, increased heat and tendency to undergo suppuration quickly.
Kaphaja Vrddhi - In kaphaja vrddhi, the scrotum is cold to touch, heavy and unctuous. There is itching, the scrotum is hard on touch and is accompanied with very little pain.
Raktaja Vrddhi – In raktaja vrddhi caused by vitiated blood, the swelling of the scrotum is surrounded by (studded with) black coloured eruptions (blisters). This condition will have all the symptoms of pittaja vrddhi.
Medoja Vrddhi – In Medaja vrddhi caused by vitiated fat, all symptoms of kaphaja vrddhi are seen. The scrotal swelling is soft and resembles (big) a tala fruit (wild palm).
Mutraja Vrddhi – This type of vrddhi occurs in persons who are habituated in suppressing the natural urge of urination. The scrotum is filled with fluid and resembles a water bag filled with fluid and fluctuates while walking. The swelling of the scrotum is soft and is painful. When the scrotum is moved it produces pain similar to that of mutrakrchra (dysuria – difficulty in urination). (3-6)

Antra Vrddhi

vātakopibhirāhāraiḥ śītatoyāvagāhanaiḥ ||7||
dhāraṇeraṇabhārādhvaviṣamāṅgapravartanaiḥ |
kṣobhaṇaiḥ kṣobhito'nyaiśca kṣudrāntrāvayavaṃ yadā ||8||
pavano viguṇīkṛtya svaniveśādadho nayet |
kuryādvaṅkṣaṇasandhistho granthyābhaṃ śvayathuṃ tadā ||9||
upekṣyamāṇasya ca muṣkavṛddhimādhmānarukstambhavatīṃ sa vāyuḥ |
prapīḍito'ntaḥsvanavān prayāti pradhmāpayanneti punaśca muktaḥ ||10||
yasyāntrāvayavāśleṣānmuṣkayorvātasambhavāt |
antravṛddhirasādhyo'yaṃ vātavṛddhisamākṛtiḥ ||11|| (vā| ni| a| 11) |
Etiological Factors – Below mentioned are the etiological factors of antra vrddhi –

- Excessive consumption of foods which increase (or tends to increase) vata

- Sitting in a tub of cold water regularly and for prolonged periods (tub bath)
- Withholding (forcibly controlling) the impending natural body urges or forcibly trying to create the urges which are not present
- Carrying heavy loads
- Excessive walking for long distances
- Abruptly moving the body parts (like doing acrobatics) and such other tiresome activities

Pathogenesis – The vata gets aggravated due to the above said etiological factors. This aggravated vata would constrict a part of the intestine and brings it down into the scrotum causing its enlargement. A swelling resembling a cyst is formed in the groin. When this condition is neglected the vata further gets aggravated and moves the intestine even downwards and causes distension, pain and stiffness in the scrotum. On pressing, the intestine produces sounds and moves back into its position but soon come back into the scrotum once the pressure is released. This condition is called as antraja vrddhi. The symptoms of antra vrddhi are similar to those of vataja vrddhi and this condition is incurable. (7-10)

iti śrīmādhavakaraviracite mādhavanidāne vṛddhinidānaṃ samāptam ||37||
Thus ends the chapter on Vrddhirog

CHAPTER THIRTY-EIGHT

GALAGANDA-GANDAMALA-APACI-GRANTHI-ARBUDA NIDANAM

Galaganda Paribhasha – Word derivation and meaning of the term Galaganda

nibaddhaḥ śvayathuryasya muṣkavallambate gale |
mahān vā yadi vā hrasvo galagaṇḍaṃ tamādiśet ||1||
(su| ni| a| 11) |
Galaganda is defined as a swelling (tumour) in the neck, big or small in size, and hanging like the scrotum. (1).

Galaganda Samprapti – pathogenesis of galaganda

vātaḥ kaphaścāpi gale praduṣṭo manye ca saṃśritya tathaiva medaḥ |
kurvanti gaṇḍaṃ kramaśaḥ svaliṅgaiḥ samanvitaṃ taṃ galagaṇḍamāhuḥ ||2||
(su| ni| a| 11) |
Vāta, kapha and medas (fat) get aggravated in the neck (throat) and reach manya (nape of the neck / side of the neck) and produce ganda i.e., a knot like swelling which grows in size gradually. This condition is called galaganda. In this the symptoms of the involved doshas would manifest (depending on their predominance in the disease). (2)

Vataja Galaganda Symptoms

todānvitaḥ kṛṣṇasirāvanaddhaḥ śyāvo'ruṇo vā pavanātmakastu |
pāruṣyayuktaściravṛddhyapāko yadṛcchayā pākamiyātkadācit ||3||
vairasyamāsyasya ca tasya jantorbhavettathā tālugalapraśoṣaḥ |4|
(su| ni| a| 11) |
In Vataja Galaganda there will be pricking pain and the swelling will be

surrounded by a network of black coloured veins, is blackish brown or golden-brown colour, rough on touch, which grows gradually and doesn't undergo suppuration. By chance if suitable etiological factors are available the swelling may even go suppuration. The patient will also experience bad (opposite) tastes in his mouth and also dryness of the throat and palate. (3)

Kaphaja Galaganda Symptoms

sthiraḥ savarṇo gururugrakaṇḍūḥ śīto mahāṃścāpi kaphātmakastu ||4||
cirābhivṛddhiṃ bhajate cirādvā prapacyate mandarujaḥ kadācit |
mādhuryamāsyasya ca tasya jantorbhavettathā tālugalapralepaḥ ||5|| (su| ni| a| 11) |
In Kaphaja Galaganda, the swelling is immovable, having the same colour as the skin, is heavy, with severe itching, cold to touch, big in size, will grow slowly, will occasionally undergo suppuration slowly, and will be associated with mild pain. The person would experience a sweet taste in the mouth and coating (furring) of the palate and throat. (4-5)

Medoja Galaganda Symptoms

snigdho guruḥ pāṇḍuraniṣṭagandho medobhavaḥ kaṇḍuyuto'lparuk ca |
pralambate'lābuvadalpamūlo dehānurūpakṣayavṛddhiyuktaḥ ||6||
snigdhāsyatā tasya bhavecca jantorgale'nuśabdaṃ kurute ca nityam |7|
(su| ni| a| 11) |
In Medoja Galaganda the swelling will be unctuous, heavy, pale (yellowish white), emit an unpleasant smell, associated with itching and mild pain (one will experience mild pain on scratching). The swelling hangs like an alabu (pitcher gourd) and is attached very loosely. It keeps undergoing increase and decrease (in size) in accordance to the body (health of the body). The inside of the mouth of the patient in this condition will be unctuous (will produce copious salivation) and the patient will make cooing sounds or indistinct sounds from the throat. (6-7)

Symptoms of incurability of Galaganda

kṛcchrācchvasantaṃ mṛdusarvagātraṃ saṃvatsarātītamarocakārtam ||7||
kṣīṇaṃ ca vaidyo galagaṇḍayuktaṃ bhinnasvaraṃ cāpi vivarjayecca |8|

(su| ni| a| 11) |
The patient of galaganda who has difficulty in breathing, very soft (looseness of) body parts, his swelling persisting for more than one year, is associated with loss of taste, emaciation and broken voice (hoarseness of voice) should be rejected treatment (should not be treated since this condition is incurable). (7-8)

Gandamala

karkandhukolāmalakapramāṇaiḥ kakṣāṃsamanyāgalavaṅkṣaṇeṣu ||8||
medaḥkaphābhyāṃ ciramandapākaiḥ syādgaṇḍamālā bahubhiśca gaṇḍaiḥ |9|
(su| ni| a| 11) |
More than one ganda (swelling) caused by kapha and medas (fat), appearing in the regions of axilla, shoulders (scapular region), sides of the neck (nape of the neck), front of neck or the groin, varying in size from that of karkandhu and kola (fruit of jujube) to that of amalaka (gooseberry, Phyllanthus Emblica), and undergoing suppuration after long period of time is known as Gandamala (chain of swellings). (8)

Apaci

te granthayaḥ kecidavāptapākāḥ sravanti naśyanti bhavanti cānye ||9||
kālānubandhaṃ ciramādadhāti saivāpacīti pravadanti tajjñāḥ |
sādhyāḥ smṛtāḥ pīnasapārśvaśūlakāsajvaracchardiyutāstvasādhyāḥ ||10||
Some of the swellings undergo suppuration, some more burst open and discharge their contents, some get destroyed or disappear, and some new ones appear. This process continues for a long time. Experts call such conditions as Apaci. This condition is curable. On the other hand, apaci associated with complications like running from the nose, pain in the flanks, cough, fever and vomiting will become incurable. (9-10)

Granthi

vātādayo māṃsamasṛk praduṣṭāḥ sandūṣya medaśca tathā sirāśca |
vṛttonnataṃ vigrathitaṃ ca śothaṃ kurvantyato granthiriti pradiṣṭaḥ ||11||
(su| ni| a| 11) |
Vāta and other two doṣhas (pitta and kapha) undergoing increase,

contaminate (bring about abnormalities in the) mamsa (muscles), asrk (blood), meda (fat) and siras (veins) produce round, elevated and cystic swelling. Therefore, these swellings (masses) are called granthi (cyst, tumour). (11)

Vatika Granthi

āyamyate vṛścyati tudyate ca pratyasyate mathyati bhidyate ca |
kṛṣṇo mṛdurbastirivātataśca bhinnaḥ sraveccānilajo'sramaccham ||12||
(su| ni| a| 11) |
In vataja granthi different kinds of pains are manifested – like pulling / stretching, tearing, throbbing (pricking), pulling, churning, and splitting (cutting) types of pains. The cyst is black in colour, soft, resembles and bulged like a water bag and discharges thin, clear (thin) blood when pricked. (12)

Pittaja Granthi

dandahyate dhūpyati vṛścyate ca pāpacyate prajvalatīva cāpi |
raktaḥ sapīto'pyathavā'pi pittādbhinnaḥ sraveduṣṇamatīva cāsram ||13||
(su| ni| a| 11) |
The symptoms of pittaja granthi include severe burning sensation as if burnt by fire, feeling as if smoke is being eliminated from the swelling / body (raised temperature), pain as if that part of the body is excised, undergoes quick suppuration as if burnt by alkali, and feeling as if the body is burnt into ash. The colour of the cyst is either red or yellow in colour. When the cysts burst open (or pricked), they discharge (exude) large amounts of warm blood. (13)

Kaphaja Granthi

śīto'vivarṇo'lparujo'tikaṇḍuḥ pāṣāṇavat saṃhananopapannaḥ |
cirābhivṛddhaśca kaphaprakopādbhinnaḥ sravecchuklaghanaṃ ca pūyam ||14||
(su| ni| a| 11) |
In kaphaja granthi, the cyst is cold to touch, will not have any discolouration (or have slight discolouration), will have mild pain and severe itching. The

cyst has stone like consistency (hard), grows slowly and when it breaks open it discharges thick and white coloured pus. (14)

Medoja Granthi

śarīravṛddhikṣayavṛddhihāniḥ snigdho mahān kaṇḍuyuto'rujaśca |
medaḥkṛto gacchati cātra bhinne piṇyākasarpiḥpratimaṃ tu medaḥ ||15||
(su| ni| a| 11) |
The cyst of medaja granthi (caused due to vitiated fat) will increase or decrease in size in accordance with that of the body. It is unctuous, big in size, is associated with itching and is painless. When pricked (bursts open), it will discharge thick fatty exudates which resembles the paste of sesame seeds or ghee. (15)

Siraja Granthi

vyāyāmajātairabalasya taistairākṣipya vāyustu sirāpratānam |
saṅkucya sampiṇḍya viśoṣya cāpi granthiṃ karotyunnatamāśu vṛttam ||16||
granthiḥ sirājaḥ sa tu kṛcchrasādhyo bhavedyadi syāt sarujaścalaśca |
sa cāruja ścāpyacalo mahāṃśca marmotthitaścāpi vivarjanīyaḥ ||17||
(su| ni| a| 11) |
In persons who are weakened but do excessive indulgence in various kinds of strenuous activities / exercises, vata undergoing increase invades the network of veins, making them constricted, condensed and dried and quickly rolls them into a round big mass. This is known as siraja granthi (cysts or tumours of veins). When there is pain and movement in these granthis it will become difficult to cure. If these cysts are bigger in size and appear on or around the vital organs of the body they are considered as incurable in spite of them being devoid of pain and immobile (fixed). (16-17)

Arbuda

gātrapradeśe kvacideva doṣāḥ sammūrchitā māṃsamasṛk pradūṣya |
vṛttaṃ sthiraṃ mandarujaṃ mahāntamanalpamūlaṃ ciravṛddhyapākam ||18||
kurvanti māṃsocchrayamatyagādhaṃ tadarbudaṃ śāstravido vadanti |

vātena pittena kaphena cāpi raktena māṃsena ca medasā vā ||19||
tajjāyate tasya ca lakṣaṇāni grantheḥ samānāni tadā bhavanti |20|
(su| ni| a| 11) |
Pathogenesis of Arbuda - Doshas undergoing increase in any particular part of the body, invade and contaminate the muscle and blood and produce round, immobile, slightly painful, big, deep-seated, slowly increasing tumours which do not suppurate. They appear like balls of muscles (big muscular mass) and are termed by the learned experts as Arbuda (cancer).
Types of Arbuda – Arbuda is of six types. They are – Vataja, Pittaja, Kaphaja, Raktaja, Mamsaja and Medaja. Each of these arbudas will have the symptoms similar to the granthis (granthis formed by the same doshas respectively).
Example – Vataja arbuda will have symptoms similar to vataja granthi, pittaja arbuda will have symptoms similar to pittaja granthi etc. (18-19)

Raktarbuda

doṣaḥ praduṣṭo rudhiraṃ sirāśca saṅkucya sampiṇḍya tatastvapākam ||20||
sāsrāvamunnahyati māṃsapiṇḍaṃ māṃsāṅkurairācitamāśuvṛddham |
karotyajasraṃ rudhirapravṛttimasādhyametadrudhirātmakaṃ tu ||21||
raktakṣayopadravapīḍitatvāt pāṇḍurbhavedarbudapīḍitastu |
(su| ni| a| 11) |
The doshas which have undergone increase will contaminate (constrict) and compress the blood and veins. By doing so they would produce a big sized muscular mass (tumour) which does not undergo suppuration (or undergoes less suppuration), is surrounded by (studded all over) many muscular sprouts, grows quickly and has little discharges. Bleeding takes place constantly from such a mass. This is called as raktaja arbuda and it is incurable. Since there is excessive bleeding from the rakta arbuda there would occur severe loss of blood in this condition which would eventually lead to many complications. Due to this the person would quickly become victim of anaemia. (20-21)

Mamsa Arbuda

muṣṭiprahārādibhirardite'ṅge māṃsaṃ praduṣṭaṃ janayeddhi śotham ||22||
avedanaṃ snigdhamananyavarṇamapākamaśmopamamapracālyam |

praduṣṭamāṃsasya narasya gāḍhametadbhavenmāṃsaparāyaṇasya ||23||
māṃsārbudaṃ tvetadasādhyamuktaṃ||| | (su| ni| a| 11) |
Assault on the body by the fist, etc.; leads to contamination (derangement) of the muscles. This leads to causation of a swelling (tumour) which is painless, unctuous, has colour of the skin, does not undergo suppuration, is hard like a stone, and fixed. This condition is called mamsa arbuda. This condition occurs commonly in those who are accustomed and habituated to eating excessive (contaminated) meat (flesh) in their food. This condition should be considered as incurable. (22-23)

Incurability / prognosis of arbuda

.... sādhyeṣvapīmāni tu varjayecca ||
samprasrutaṃ marmaṇi yacca jātaṃ srotaḥsu vā yacca bhavedacālyam ||24||
(su| ni| a| 11) |
Even among the curable forms of arbuda, the following are to be rejected –

- that which has heavy discharges (exudation)
- that occurring on or around the vital organs
- that occurring on or around the channels including nasal passage etc (and hence imparting pressure on them and obstructing their functioning)
- that which is immobile (24)

Adyarbuda / Dwirarbuda

yajjāyate'nyat khalu pūrvajāte jñeyaṃ tadaddhyarbudamarbudajñaiḥ |
yaddvandvajātaṃ yugapat kramādvā dvirarbudaṃ tacca bhavedasādhyam ||25||
(su| ni| a| 11) |
Adyarbuda - A second arbuda developing over an already existing arbuda (superseding) or after the course of an earlier one (the earlier one being removed) is called Adhyarbuda by the specialists of arbuda.
Dwirarbuda – Arbuda developing alongside yet another arbuda simultaneously or after some time at the same place or at some other place of the body is called as Dvirarbuda.

Both these conditions are incurable. (25)

Why arbudas do not suppurate?

na pākamāyānti kaphādhikatvānmedobahutvācca viśeṣatastu |
doṣasthiratvādgrathanācca teṣāṃ sarvārbudānyeva nisargatastu ||26||
(su| ni| a| 11) |
All arbudas do not suppurate when –

- there is predominance of kapha and medas (fat) in them
- by the hardness and immobility of doshas
- by the very nature of the disease (26)

iti śrīmādhavakaraviracite mādhavanidāne galagaṇḍagaṇḍamālāpacīgranthyarbudanidānaṃ samāptam ||38||
Thus ends the chapter on Galaganda etc.

CHAPTER THIRTY-NINE

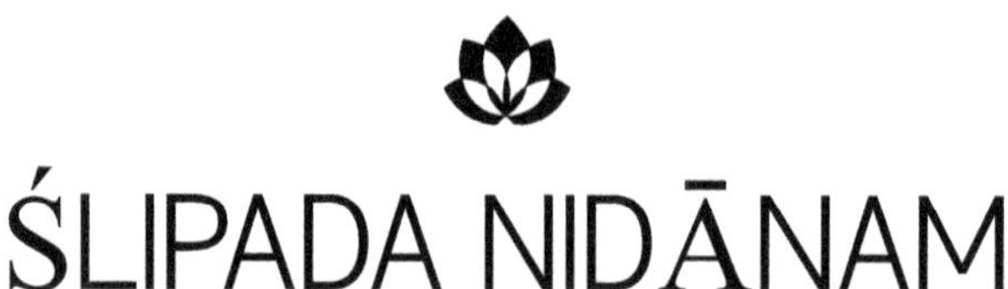

ŚLIPADA NIDĀNAM

Slipada Samanya Lakshana – General Symptoms

yaḥ sajvaro vaṅkṣaṇajo bhṛśārtiḥ śotho nṛṇāṃ pādagataḥ krameṇa |
tacchlīpadaṃ syāt karakarṇanetraśiśnauṣṭhanāsāsvapi kecidāhuḥ ||1||
A swelling starting in the groins and gradually moving towards (involving) the leg, associated with fever and severe pain is known as Ślīpada. According to the opinion of others (experts) slipada may occur even in the hands, ears, eyes, penis, lips and nose. (1)

Symptoms of Doshaja Slipada

vātajaṃ kṛṣṇarūkṣaṃ ca sphuṭitaṃ tīvravedanam |
animittarujaṃ tasya bahuśo jvara eva ca ||2||
pittajaṃ pītasaṅkāśaṃ dāhajvarayutaṃ mṛdu |
ślaiṣmikaṃ snigdhavarṇaṃ ca śvetaṃ pāṇḍu guru sthiram ||3||
Vataja Slipada - In this condition the swelling is black, dry and has fissures, (cracks). There is severe pain which appears without any apparent reason and is covered with fever.
Pittaja Slipada – In this condition there is yellowish discolouration. It is associated with burning sensation and fever and the swelling is soft to touch.
Kaphaja Slipada – Here the swelling is unctuous (oily). It is white or pale in colour, is heavy and fixed (immobile). (2-3)

Asadhya Lakshana – symptoms of incurability

valmīkamiva sañjātaṃ kaṇṭakairupacīyate |

abdātmakaṃ mahattacca varjanīyaṃ viśeṣataḥ ||4||
The swelling of slipada growing upwards like an ant-hill with many small hill-like projections and sprouts (knots), that which exists for more than one year, and that which is very big in size are to be rejected (should not be treated because such slipada is incurable). (4)

Kapha predominance in all types of Slipada

trīṇyapyetāni jānīyācchlīpadāni kaphocchrayāt |
gurutvaṃ ca mahattvaṃ ca yasmānnāsti kaphaṃ vinā ||5||
(su| ni| a| 12) |
In all the three varieties of ślīpada, kapha is the predominant doşha, because heaviness and increase in size cannot be caused without kapha.(5)

Places where Slipada is prevalent

purāṇodakabhūyiṣṭhāḥ sarvartuṣu ca śītalāḥ |
ye deśāsteṣu jāyante ślīpadāni viśeṣataḥ ||6||
(su| ni| a| 12) |
Ślīpada is generally prevalent in such places (areas) where there is stagnation of water for a long period of time, in places wherein there is excessive cold in all the seasons of the year. (6)

Other symptoms of incurability of Slipada

yacchleṣmalāhāravihārajātaṃ puṃsaḥ prakṛtyā'pi kaphātmakasya |
sāsrāvamatyunnatasarvaliṅgaṃ sakaṇḍuraṃ śleṣmayutaṃ vivarjyam ||7||
Slipada should be rejected (should not be treated) when it is caused due to excessive indulgence in foods and habits which increase kapha, in those who are of kapha prakriti (whose birth constitution is predominantly kapha) and when the disease presents with exudation, is very big in size, is associated with all the signs and symptoms and has itching. (7)

iti śrīmādhavakaraviracite mādhavanidāne ślīpadanidānaṃ samāptam ||39|||
Thus ends the chapter on ślīpada.

CHAPTER FORTY

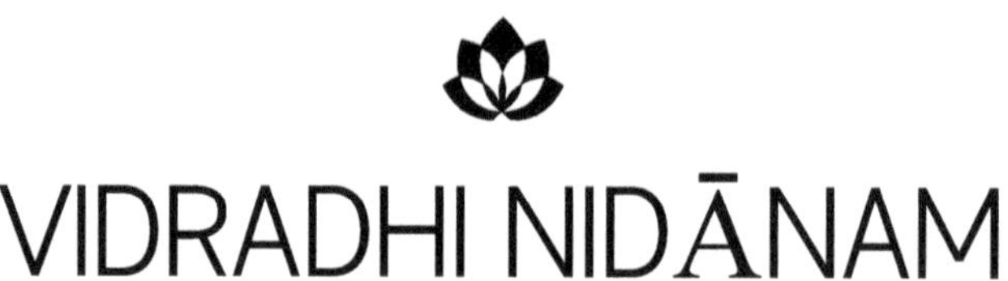

VIDRADHI NIDĀNAM

Vidradhi Samprapti, Bheda – Pathogenesis and types of vidradhi

tvagraktamāṃsamedāṃsi sandūṣyāsthisamāśritāḥ |
doṣāḥ śothaṃ śanairghoraṃ janayantyucchritā bhṛśam ||1||
mahāmūlaṃ rujāvantaṃ vṛttaṃ vā'pyathavā''yatam |
sa vidradhiriti khyāto vijñeyaḥ ṣaḍvidhaśca saḥ ||2||
pṛthagdoṣaiḥ samastaiśca kṣatenāpyasṛjā tathā |
ṣaṇṇāmapi hi teṣāṃ tu lakṣaṇaṃ sampravakṣyate ||3||
(su| ni| a| 9) |
The doshas which have undergone abnormal increase get lodged in the bones and contaminate (bring about abnormal change) skin, blood, muscles and fat gradually (slowly increasing in size) causing localized swelling which is deep seated, painful, round or broad (elongated) in shape. This is known as vidradhi.
This vidradhi is of six types – one from each dosha (vataja, pittaja and kaphaja), one from the combination of all the three doshas (tridoshaja), one from injury (ksataja) and the other one from blood (raktaja). Their features will be described further on. (1-3)

Vatika (Vataja) Vidradhi

kṛṣṇo'ruṇo vā viṣamo bhṛśamatyarthavedanaḥ |
citrotthānaprapākaśca vidradhirvātasambhavaḥ ||4||
(su| ni| a| 9) |
The vidradhi caused due to increase of vata is black or red (reddish brown) in colour, often increasing or decreasing in size, associated with severe pain, gets manifests and suppurates in many ways (variations are seen in the

duration of onset and time of suppuration). (4)

Paittika (Pittaja) Vidradhi

pakvodumbarasaṅkāśaḥ śyāvo vā jvaradāhavān |
kṣiprotthānaprapākaśca vidradhiḥ pittasambhavaḥ ||5||
The vidradhi caused due to increase of pitta resembles a ripened fruit of udumbara (wild fig) or is blackish (bluish black) in colour, associated with fever and burning sensation, quickly manifests and suppurates quickly. (5)

Shlaishmika (Kaphaja) Vidradhi

śarāvasadṛśaḥ pāṇḍuḥ śītaḥ snigdho'lpavedanaḥ |
cirotthānaprapākaśca vidradhiḥ kaphasambhavaḥ ||6||
(su| ni| a| 9) |
The vidradhi caused due to increase of kapha resembles a big saucer, is pale (yellowish white in colour), cold, unctuous (smooth), associated with mild pain, and is slow in manifesting and suppurating. (6)

Nature of secretions (pus) in the doshaja types of vidradhi

tanupītasitāścaiṣāmāsrāvāḥ kramaśaḥ smṛtāḥ |7|
The pus exuding from the above-mentioned types of doshaja vidradhi will be thin, yellow and white respectively i.e., thin in vataja, yellow in pittaja and white in kaphaja vidradhi.

Sannipataja Vidradhi

nānāvarṇarujāsrāvo ghāṭālo viṣamo mahān ||7||
viṣamaṃ pacyate cāpi vidradhiḥ sānnipātikaḥ |
(su| ni| a| 9) |
Sannipātajavidradhi(due to increase of all the three doṣas) will be having different kinds of colours,pain and exudation,with elevated sprout, unsteady in nature, very troublesome and with irregular time of suppuration.(7)

Agantuja Vidradhi

taistairbhāvairabhihate kṣate vā'pathyakāriṇaḥ ||8||
kṣatoṣmā vāyuvisṛtaḥ saraktaṃ pittamīrayet |
jvarastṛṣṇā ca dāhaśca jāyate tasya dehinaḥ ||9||
āganturvidradhirhyeṣa pittavidradhilakṣaṇaḥ |10|
(su| ni| a| 9) |
In persons who are subjected to injury by canes (baton), stones etc (and other weapons) and also get indulged in unwholesome foods, the heat of the wound being stimulated by vata will also vitiate the blood and pitta. The vidradhi formed as a result of this is called as agantuja vidradhi (abscess caused by external agents / injury). In this condition the person will have fever, thirst and burning sensation. The other symptoms of pittaja vidradhi are also seen in this type of vidradhi. (8-9)

Raktaja Vidradhi

kṛṣṇasphoṭāvṛtaḥ śyāvastīvradāharujākaraḥ ||10||
pittavidradhiliṅgastu raktavidradhirucyate |11|
(su| ni| a| 9) |
In raktaja vidradhi (abscess caused by aggravated blood) the abscess is enveloped on all sides by black coloured eruptions (boils, blisters), is of blackish blue in colour, causes severe burning sensation and pain and has other symptoms of pittaja vidradhi. (10)

Antarvidradhi (internal abscess)

pṛthak sambhūya vā doṣāḥ kupitā gulmarūpiṇam ||11||
valmīkavat samunnaddhamantaḥ kurvanti vidradhim |
gude bastimukhe nābhyāṃ kukṣau vaṅkṣaṇayostathā ||12||
vṛkkayoḥ plīhni yakṛti hṛdi vā klomni vā'pyatha |
teṣāmuktāni liṅgāni bāhyavidradhilakṣaṇaiḥ ||13||
adhiṣṭhānaviśeṣeṇa liṅgaṃ śṛṇu viśeṣataḥ |
The doshas undergoing abnormal increase due to their etiological factors, either individually or in combination, produce vidradhis inside the body, in different organs, resembling a spreading shrub / bush or anthill. Since these abscesses happen inside the body they are called as antarvidradhi.
Places of the body where antarvidradhi develops – The seats of internal

abscess include the rectum, opening of urinary bladder, umbilicus, lower part of the abdomen (abdominal cavity), groins, kidneys, spleen, liver, heart, pancreas or any other place in the body i.e., abscesses can occur in these organs or any other organ which has not been mentioned.
General Symptoms – The general symptoms of internal abscesses are similar to the symptoms of external abscesses. Apart from these, the internal abscesses have special symptoms related to the seat in which they get manifested. They will be described here now. (11-14)

Symptoms of Antarvidradi based on the organs in which they get manifested

gude vātanirodhaśca bastau kṛcchrālpamūtratā ||14||
nābhyāṃ hikkā tathā''ṭopaḥ kukṣau mārutakopanam |
kaṭīpṛṣṭhagrahastīvro vaṅkṣaṇotthe tu vidradhau ||15||
vṛkkayoḥ pārśvasaṅkocaḥ plīhnyucchvāsāvarodhanam |
sarvāṅgapragrahastīvro hṛdi kāsaśca jāyate |
śvāso yakṛti hikkā ca klomni pepīyate payaḥ ||16||
(su| ni| a| 9) |
If the abscess is in the rectum, it causes obstruction to movement of the flatus.
If the abscess occurs in the urinary bladder, it would cause difficulty in urination and scanty urination.
The abscess occurring in the umbilicus would cause hiccough and gurgling sounds in the abdomen.
If the abscess occurs in the abdomen, it would cause the symptoms of vata increase like pain, distension of the abdomen etc.
If the abscess happens in the groins, it would cause severe stiffness or gripping (catching) pain in the waist or back.
If the abscess occurs in the kidney, there would be constriction of the flanks.
If the abscess occurs in the spleen, there will be obstruction or difficulty in breathing.
If the abscess is found occurring in the heart (region of the heart), there will be catching pain in all the parts of the body and cough.
If the abscess occurs in the liver it would cause dyspnoea and hiccough.
If the abscess occurs in the pancreas the person would drink large quantities

of water often because in this condition there will be severe thirst. (14-16)

Prognosis of Vidradhi

nābheruparijāḥ pakvā yāntyūrdhvamitare tvadhaḥ |17| (su| ni| a| 9) |
adhaḥsruteṣu jīvettu sruteṣūrdhvaṃ na jīvati ||17||
hṛnnābhibastivarjyā ye teṣu bhinneṣu bāhyataḥ |
jīvet kadācit puruṣo netareṣu kadācana ||18||
(su| ni| a| 9) |

When the vidradhis occurring above the level of umbilicus (organs placed above the level of umbilicus) burst open, they discharge (expel) their contents through an upward route (mouth). On the other hand, when the vidradhis below the level of the umbilicus (organs below the level of umbilicus) burst open, they discharge their content through a downward route (anus or urinary passage – urethra). (The discharges may be in the form of pus or blood).

When the discharges come out in the downward direction the patient will survive. On the other hand, if the discharges occur from the upward routes he will not survive (will die).

The patient in whom the internal abscess, other than those occurring in the region of the heart, umbilicus and urinary bladder burst open towards outside of the body may sometimes survive. (The abscess occurring in the heart, umbilicus and urinary bladder are incurable). Even if the abscess occurring in the region of the heart, umbilicus and urinary bladder open towards outside of the body, the patient would not survive. (17-18)

sādhyā vidradhayaḥ pañca vivarjyaḥ sānnipātikaḥ |
āmapakvavidagdhatvaṃ teṣāṃ śothavadādiśet ||19||
(vā| ni| a| 11) |
ādhmātaṃ baddhaniṣyandaṃ chardihikkātṛṣānvitam |
rujāśvāsasamāyuktaṃ vidradhirnāśayennaram ||20||
(su| sū| a| 33) |

Apart from the tridoshaja vidradhi (abscess caused by simultaneous aggravation of all three doshas) the other five kinds of vidradhis are curable. Tridoshaja Vidradhi is incurable. The unripe, ripening and ripened stages of vidradhi are similar to those explained in the context of sotha (inflammatory oedema explained in the next chapter). If the patient of antarvidradhi also has distension of abdomen, obstruction of urination, vomiting, hiccough, thirst, severe pain and difficulty in respiration, the patient will die. (19-20)

iti śrīmādhavakaraviracite mādhavanidāne vidradhinidānaṃ samāptam ||40||
Thus ends the chapter on Vidradhi.

CHAPTER FORTY-ONE

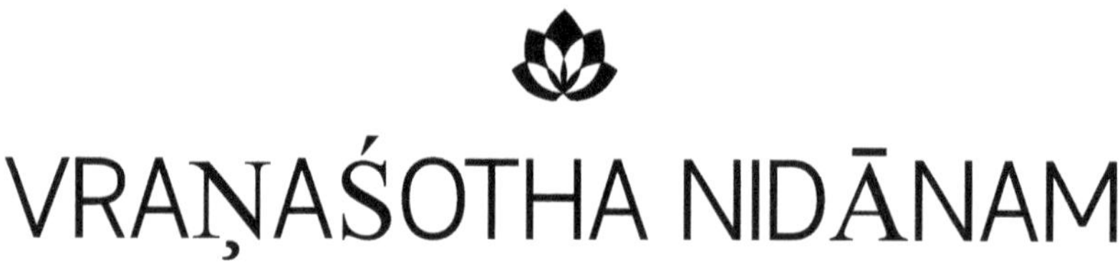

VRAṆAŚOTHA NIDĀNAM

ekadeśotthitaḥ śotho vraṇānāṃ pūrvalakṣaṇam |
ṣaḍvidhaḥ syāt pṛthaksarvaraktāgantunimittajaḥ ||1||
śothāḥ ṣaḍete vijñeyāḥ prāguktaiḥ śothalakṣaṇaiḥ |
viśeṣaḥ kathyate caiṣāṃ pakvāpakvādiniścaye ||2||
A swelling which is localized (and limited to a particular area of the body) becomes the premonitory symptom (stage) of an ulcer and is called as vranasotha. In short, vranasotha is a localized swelling which occurs prior to the formation of an ulcer.
Vranasotha is of six kinds – one each from each dosha (vataja, pittaja and kaphaja), one caused by combination of all three doshas, one from rakta (blood) and one from external causes (agantu).
The symptoms of all these six kinds of vranasotha are similar to those explained in the context of the types of sotha previously.
Now, the special features of unripe and ripened stages of vranasotha will be described ahead. (1-2)

Specific symptoms of the types of vranasotha

viṣamaṃ pacyate vātāt pittotthaścāciraācciram |
kaphajaḥ pittavacchotho raktāgantusamudbhavaḥ ||3||
Vātaja type of vranasotha undergoes ripening inconsistently. Pittaja type of vranasotha will undergo quick suppuration. Kaphaja vranasotha will undergo suppuration very slowly. The raktaja and agantuja vranasothas will have symptoms similar to those of pittaja vranasotha. (3)

Ama (unripe) and Pacyamana (ripening) Vranasotha Symptoms

mandoṣmatā'lpaśothatvaṃ kāṭhinyaṃ tvaksavarṇatā |
mandavedanatā caitacchothānāmāmalakṣaṇam ||4||
dahyate dahaneneva kṣāreṇeva ca pacyate |
pipīlikāgaṇeneva daśyate chidyate tathā ||5||
bhidyate caiva śastreṇa daṇḍeneva ca tāḍyate |
pīḍyate pāṇinevāntaḥ sūcībhiriva tudyate ||6||
soṣācoṣo vivarṇaḥ syādaṅgulyevāvaghaṭyate |
āsane śayane sthāne śāntiṃ vṛścikaviddhavat ||7||
na gacchedātataḥ śotho bhavedādhmātabastivat |
jvarastṛṣṇā'ruciścaiva pacyamānasya lakṣaṇam ||8||
Ama Vranasotha Symptoms – In the unripe stage of vranasotha the swelling is slightly warm. There is also mild swelling. The swelling is hard, has normal colour of the skin and mild pain.
Pacyamana Vranasotha Symptoms – In the ripening stage of vranasotha there will be a severe burning sensation as if being burnt by fire or being corroded by strong alkali. The person will feel as if the region of swelling is being bitten by a swarm of ants, being cut or torn by sharp instruments, beaten by a baton, being pressed or squeezed by hands, pricked by (pierced by) needles, is being burnt and as if being burnt in the flanks, discolouration, pain as if being pressed by fingers.
The patient would not find comfort either by sitting, sleeping or standing and will experience continuous pain similar to that of a scorpion sting. The swelling is distended and expanded similar to a urinary bladder filled and distended by urine.
This condition is associated with fever, thirst and loss of taste. (4-8)

Pakva (ripened) Vranasotha Symptoms

vedanopaśamaḥ śotho'lohito'lpo na connataḥ |
prādurbhāvo valīnāṃ ca todaḥ kaṇḍūrmuhurmuhuḥ ||9||
upadravāṇāṃ praśamo nimnatā sphuṭanaṃ tvacām |
bastāvivāmbusañcāraḥ syācchothe'ṅgulipīḍite ||10||
pūyasya pīḍayatyekamantamante ca pīḍīte |
bhaktākāṅkṣā bhaveccaitacchothānāṃ pakvalakṣaṇam ||11||
Pakva Vranasotha Symptoms - Reduction in the severity of pain, reduction in the size of swelling, reduction or absence of redness, absence of elevation, appearance of wrinkles on the swelling, repeated episodes of

pricking pain and itching, and reduction of complications are seen in the ripened vranasotha. The swelling easily pits on pressure with the fingers, cracks appear on the skin, and the movements resembling the movement of water in the bladder or in a water bag are perceived in the swelling when it is pressed with the finger. When the swelling is pressed on one of its edges (side), the pressure of the pus is experienced on the other side of the swelling. The patient would develop a desire for food. (9-11)

Dosha relation during suppuration

narte'nilādruṅna vinā ca pittaṃ pākaḥ kaphaṃ cāpi vinā na pūyaḥ |
tasmāddhi sarve paripākakāle pacanti śothāṃstraya eva doṣāḥ ||12||
(su| sū| a| 17) |
There is no pain without the involvement of aggravated vata. There will be no suppuration without the involvement of aggravated pitta. There will be no formation of pus without the involvement of aggravated kapha. So, all the three doshas are actively involved during the period of ripening. (12)

Effect of pus which has not been drained

kālāntareṇābhyuditaṃ tu pittaṃ kṛtvā vaśe vātakaphau prasahya |
pacatyataḥ śoṇitameṣa pāko mataḥ pareṣāṃ viduṣāṃ dvitīyaḥ ||13||
kakṣaṃ samāsādya yathaiva vahnirvāyvīritaḥ sandahati prasahya |
tathaiva pūyo hyaviniḥsṛto hi māṃsaṃ sirāḥ snāyu ca khādatīha ||14||
(su| sū| a| 17) |
Just as a small fire hidden inside a haystack (or hearth) activated by the wind burns up the whole mass of hay, the pus too which has not been drained properly would destroy the muscles, veins, tendons etc. (13)

A true physician should know the stages of vranasotha

āmaṃ vidahyamānaṃ ca samyak pakvaṃ ca yo bhiṣak |
jānīyāt sa bhavedvaidyaḥ śeṣāstaskaravṛttayaḥ ||15||
Only he who can recognise the unripe, ripening and ripened stages (of the inflammatory swellings) deserves to be called as a physician. All others are only imposters. (14)

yaśchinattyāmamajñānādyo vā pakvamupekṣate |
śvapacāviva mantavyau tāvaniścitakāriṇau ||16||
(su| sū| a| 17) |
He who cuts open the swelling in its unripe stage with ignorance or he who delays its opening though fully ripened-both are to be considered as very mean persons, because they are uncertain in their act.(15)

iti śrīmādhavakaraviracite mādhavanidāne vraṇaśothanidānaṃ samāptam ||41||
Thus ends the chapter on Vranaśotha.

CHAPTER FORTY-TWO

ŚĀRĪRA VRAṆA NIDĀNAM

Vrana Bheda – Types of Vrana

dvidhā vraṇaḥ sa vijñeyaḥ śārīrāgantubhedataḥ |
doṣairādyastayoranyaḥ śastrādikṣatasambhavaḥ ||1||
Vraṇas (ulcers)are of two kinds. They are –

- Śārīra Vrana – physical or organic ulcers and
- Āgantuja Vrana – traumatic ulcers

The first one i.e., saririka vrana is caused by the doshas. The second type i.e., agantuja vrana is caused by injury caused by weapons, sharp instruments etc. (1)

Lakshanas – symptoms of types of sarira vranas

stabdhaḥ kaṭhinasaṃsparśo mandasrāvo mahārujaḥ |
tudyate sphurati śyāvo vraṇo mārutasambhavaḥ ||2||
tṛṣṇāmohajvarakledadāhaduṣṭyavadāraṇaiḥ |
vraṇaṃ pittakṛtaṃ vidyādgandhaiḥ srāvaiśca pūtikaiḥ ||3||
bahupiccho guruḥ snigdhaḥ stimito mandavedanaḥ |
pāṇḍuvarṇo'lpasaṅkledaścirapākī kaphavraṇaḥ ||4|| (ca| ci| a| 25) |
rakto raktasrutī raktāddvitrijaḥ syāttadanvayaiḥ |5|
Vataja Vrana – The ulcer caused by vitiated vata is immobile (stiff), hard on touch, has less discharges (scanty exudation) and severe pain. The pain is of pricking or pulsating type. The ulcer is of bluish black colour.
Pittaja Vrana – The ulcer caused by vitiated pitta is associated with thirst,

delusion (fainting, unconsciousness), fever, wetness (due to secretions), burning sensation, dirty, pain as if being torn (cracking of skin or tendency to burst open quickly), emits bad smell and discharges foul smelling secretions.
Kaphaja Vrana – The ulcer caused by vitiated kapha is excessively sticky, heavy, unctuous (oily), and feels as if covered by wet leather or cloth. The ulcer will be slightly painful, pale (yellowish white) in appearance, less moist, and suppurates slowly.
Raktaja Vrana – The ulcer caused by vitiated blood will be red in colour and will discharge only blood.
Dwija / Dwidoshaja Vraṇa – This is caused by combination of two doshas and will have combined symptoms of those two doshas involved.
Trija / Tridoshaja Vrana – This is caused by a combination of all three vitiated doshas and will have combined symptoms of all three doshas together. (2-4)

Sadhyasadhyata – Prognosis of Sarira Vrana

tvaṅmāṃsajaḥ sukhe deśe taruṇasyānupadravaḥ ||5||
dhīmato'bhinavaḥ kāle sukhe sādhyaḥ sukhaṃ vraṇaḥ |
Ulcers are curable when they –

- are located in the skin or muscles,
- are located in a convenient place (places of the body other than marmas – vital spots),
- occur in a young person,
- are not associated with complications,
- occur in intelligent persons (those who can discriminate between good and bad)
- are of recent origin,
- occur in appropriate time i.e., favourable season, age etc (mainly Hemanta and Sisira – late and early winter) (5)

guṇairanyatamairhīnastataḥ kṛcchro vraṇaḥ smṛtaḥ ||6||
sarvairvihīno vijñeyastvasādhyo bhūryupadravaḥ |
(ca| ci| a| 25) |

Those (physical ulcers) which possess a few of the above qualities (few qualities less than those mentioned above – in the curable category) are difficult to cure. On the other hand, those which are devoid of any of the above-mentioned qualities (of curable ulcers) and also associated with many severe complications are incurable. (6)

Dusta Vrana (bad, contaminated ulcer) Symptoms

pūtiḥ pūyātiduṣṭāsṛksrāvyutsaṅgī cirasthitiḥ ||7||
duṣṭo vraṇo'tigandhādiḥ śuddhaliṅgaviparyayaḥ |8|
Duṣṭavraṇa (bad, intractable ulcer) is one which discharges the blood heavily contaminated with foul smelling pus, has sinuses inside it, remains for long periods, has excessive foul smell, discolouration, discharges and pain and possesses opposite qualities of a clean ulcer. (7)

Shuddha Vrana (clean ulcer) Symptoms

jihvātalābho'timṛduḥ ślakṣṇaḥ snigdho'lpavedanaḥ ||8||
suvyavastho nirāsrāvaḥ śuddho vraṇa iti smṛtaḥ |9|
A śuddhavraṇa (clean ulcer) is one which is very soft like the upper surface of the tongue, smooth, unctuous (moist), with mild pain, even (without sprouts and sinuses) and without excessive discharges (exudation). (8)

Ruhyamana Vrana (ulcer in the stage of healing) Symptoms

kapotavarṇapratimā yasyāntāḥ kledavarjitāḥ ||9||
sthirāśca piḍakāvanto rohatīti tamādiśet | (su| sū| a| 23) |
The edges of a ruhyamana vraṇa (ulcer) i.e., the ulcer in the stage of healing has the colour of a pigeon (slightly blackish white) and is devoid of moistness. The ulcer is fixed and is studded all around by granulations. (9)

Samyak Rudha (ulcer which has healed) Symptoms

rūḍhavartmānamagranthimaśūnamarujaṃ vraṇam ||10||
tvaksavarṇaṃ samatalaṃ samyagrūḍhaṃ vinirdiśet | (su| sū| a| 23) |
The ulcers in which the edges have closed up (ulcer is filled up with granulation tissue indicating that it is healed), which does not have knots

(elevations), which is devoid of swelling or pain, which has attained the normal colour of the skin, and that which is levelled is considered to be a samyak rudha vrana i.e., the ulcer which has healed up. (10)

Prognosis of Vranas

kuṣṭhināṃ viṣajuṣṭānāṃ śoṣiṇāṃ madhumehinām ||11||
vraṇāḥ kṛcchreṇa sidhyanti yeṣāṃ cāpi vraṇe vraṇāḥ |
vasāṃ medo'tha majjānaṃ mastuluṅgaṃ ca yaḥ sravet ||12||
āgantujo vraṇaḥ siddhyenna siddhyeddoṣasambhavaḥ |
(su| sū| a| 23) |
Vranas (ulcer) heals with great difficulty in persons who are suffering from leprosy, poisons, tuberculosis and diabetes mellitus. The ulcers in which ulcers develop should also be considered as difficult to cure.
The ulcers which are caused by trauma and discharge muscle fat, fat, bone marrow or brain tissues (brain matter) etc are curable. On the other hand, if this is caused due to the aggravation of doshas, it is incurable. (11-12)

Arista Lakshanas - signs of ulcer indicating bad prognosis

madyāgurvājyasumanaḥpadmacandanacampakaiḥ ||13||
sagandhā divyagandhāśca mumūrṣūṇāṃ vraṇāḥ smṛtāḥ |
(su| sū| a| 28) |
Vranas (ulcers) which emit a smell similar to alcohol, aguru (Aquilaria agallocha), ghee, flower of jasmine or lotus, sandalwood, campaka flower and such other pleasant / divine smells are going to kill the patient. (13)

Other symptoms of incurability of ulcers

ye ca marmasvasambhūtā bhavantyatyarthavedanāḥ ||14||
dahyante cāntaratyarthaṃ bahiḥśītāśca ye vraṇāḥ |
dahyante bahiratyarthaṃ bhavantyantaśca śītalāḥ ||15||
prāṇamāṃsakṣayaśvāsakāsārocakapīḍitāḥ |
pravṛddhapūyarudhirā vraṇā yeṣāṃ ca marmasu ||16||
kriyābhiḥ samyagārabdhā na sidhyanti ca ye vraṇāḥ |
varjayedapi tān vaidyaḥ saṃrakṣannātmano yaśaḥ ||17|| (su| sū| a| 28) |
Below mentioned are the other symptoms of incurability of ulcers –

- Vranas (ulcers) having severe pain in spite of not manifesting on vital organs,
- Ulcers having severe burning sensation inside and are cold outside
- Ulcers having severe burning sensation outside but are cold inside
- Ulcers manifesting in those having loss of strength, loss of muscles (emaciation), dyspnoea, cough, and loss of taste (appetite)
- Ulcers discharging large quantities of pus or blood
- Ulcers occurring on the vital spots of the body
- Ulcers which are not responding to any kind of treatment (ulcers not getting healed in spite of administering best of well-planned treatments)

All these kinds of ulcers shall be rejected (should not be treated) by a physician who does not want his reputation to be damaged. (14-17)

iti śrīmādhavakaraviracite mādhavanidāne śārīravraṇanidānaṃ samāptam ||42||
Thus ends the chapter on SārīraVrana.

CHAPTER FORTY-THREE

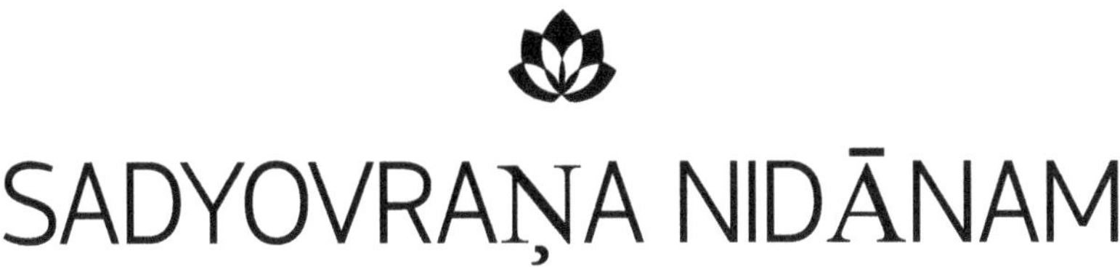

SADYOVRAṆA NIDĀNAM

Sadyo Vrana Hetu – Causative factors

nānādhāramukhaiḥ śastrairnānāsthānanipātitaiḥ |
bhavanti nānākṛtayo vraṇāstāṃstānnibodha me ||1||
Different kinds of ulcers having different shapes, caused by assault with different types of sharp weapons having different kinds of edges, in different places of the body are described further on. (1)

Types of ulcers based on the shapes (appearance)

chinnaṃ bhinnaṃ tathā viddhaṃ kṣataṃ piccitameva ca |
ghṛṣṭamāhustathā ṣaṣṭhaṃ teṣāṃ vakṣyāmi lakṣaṇam ||2||
(su| ci| a| 2) |
Below mentioned are the six kinds of ulcers –

- Chinna - incised wound)
- Bhinna - puncture wound
- Viddha – stabbed wound
- Ksata - lacerated wound
- Piccita - crushed wound and
- Ghrsta – excoriated

The features of these ulcers shall be henceforth explained. (2)

Chinna Vrana

tiryak chinna ṛjurvā'pi yo vraṇastvāyato bhavet |
gātrasya pātanaṃ taddhi chinnamityabhidhīyate ||3||
(su| ci| a| 2) |
In Chinnavraṇa the wound is either curved or straight and also wide. The organ or the part of the body which has been mutilated hangs from the wound or even may fall off. (3)

Bhinna Vrana

śaktidanteṣu khaḍgāgraviṣāṇairāśayo hataḥ |
yatkiñcit prasravettaddhi bhinnalakṣaṇamucyate ||4||
(su| ci| a| 2) |
Bhinna vraṇa is a puncture wound. It is caused by pointed javelin, teeth / tusk, arrow / spear, the pointed end of the sword or horns of animals. When these enter and damage the interiors of different visceral organs, ulcers (punctured) are formed. This would lead to discharge of various materials depending on the organ which has been punctured. (4)

Definition of Koshta (hollow viscera which would hold many visceral organs) and symptoms of puncture of various visceral organs

sthānānyāmāgnipakvānāṃ mūtrasya rudhirasya ca |
hṛduṇḍukaḥ phupphusaśca koṣṭha ityabhidhīyate ||5||
tasmin bhinne raktapūrṇe jvaro dāhaśca jāyate |
mūtramārgagudāsyebhyo raktaṃ ghrāṇācca gacchati ||6||
mūrchā śvāsastṛṣā''dhmānamabhaktacchanda eva ca |
viṇmūtravātasaṅgaśca svedāsrāvo'kṣiraktatā ||7||
lohagandhitvamāsyasya gātradaurgandhyameva ca |
hṛcchūlaṃ pārśvayoścāpi viśeṣaṃ cātra me śṛṇu ||8||
The organs or seats of āma (undigested food i.e., stomach), agni (digestive juices / enzymes i.e., duodenum, liver, gallbladder and pancreas together), pakva ahara (digested food i.e., intestines / colon), mutra (urine i.e., urinary bladder), and rudhira (blood i.e., liver and spleen), along with hrdaya (heart), unduka (caecum), phuppusa / fupfusa (lungs) are known as kostha (abdominal viscera / visceral space which lodges the mentioned organs).
A Puncture wound into the kostha will cause accumulation of blood in the injured organs which leads to manifestation of fever and burning sensation.

Bleeding will occur through urethra, anus or nose.
The other general symptoms of puncture to the koshta are fainting (losing consciousness), dyspnoea (increased / difficult respiration), thirst, distension of the abdomen, loss of taste (aversion towards food), obstruction to the movement (expulsion) of urine, faeces and flatus, excessive sweating, redness of the eyes, smell of iron from the mouth, foul smell emitted from the body and pain in the heart and flanks. (5-8)

Symptoms of puncture of specific organs

āmāśayasthe rudhire rudhiraṃ chardayatyapi |
ādhmānamatimātraṃ ca śūlaṃ ca bhṛśadāruṇam ||9||
pakvāśayagate cāpi rujā gauravameva ca |
adhaḥkāye viśeṣeṇa śītatā ca bhavediha ||10||
(su| ci| a| 2) |
If ámāśaya (stomach) is punctured, blood accumulates in the stomach and there will be vomiting of blood, severe distension of abdomen and severe pain in the abdomen.
If pakvāśaya (small and large intestines, mainly colon) is punctured there will be severe pain, heaviness and coldness of the lower extremities. (9-10)

Viddha Vrana

sūkṣmāsyaśalyābhihataṃ yadaṅgaṃ tvāśayaṃ vinā |
uttuṇḍitaṃ nirgataṃ vā tadviddhamiti nirdiśet ||11||
(su| ci| a| 2) |
Viddha vrana (stab / puncture wound) is that caused by a pointed instrument, on other body parts, away from any viscera (viscera not involved). Viddha vrana is of two types – uttundita which presents with swelling around the opening of the wound (due to the instrument lodged inside the wound) or nirgata which presents without swelling, the opening of the wound being depressed (because the instrument causing the wound is not lodged inside the swelling i.e. it has gone out or is extracted). (11)

Ksata Vrana

nāticchinnaṃ nātibhinnamubhayorlakṣaṇānvitam |

viṣamaṃ vraṇamaṅge yattat kṣataṃ tvabhidhīyate ||12||
(su| ci| a| 2) |
Kṣata vrana (lacerated wound) is that which is neither deeply incised nor punctured but it does have symptoms of both of them and is irregular in shape. (12)

Piccita Vrana

prahārapīḍanābhyāṃ tu yadaṅgaṃ pṛthutāṃ gatam |
sāsthi tat piccitaṃ vidyānmajjaraktapariplutam ||13||
(su| ci| a| 2) |
Piccita vrana (crushed wound) is caused by a blow (by a baton, hammer etc) or pressure (by a blunt weapon). Due to this, a part of the body is flattened, the bones also get crushed and blood mixed with bone marrow flows out. (13)

Ghrsta Vrana

gharṣaṇādabhighātādvā yadaṅgaṃ vigatatvacam |
uṣāsrāvānvitaṃ tacca ghṛṣṭamityabhidhīyate ||14||
(su| ci| a| 2) |
Ghrsta vrana (abrasion) is caused by friction with some object or any other kind of trauma / injury. In this condition the skin is peeled off from the body parts. Discharges consistingof hot watery fluids will flow out. (There will be burning sensation and flow of watery fluids). (14)

Ulcers with foreign body

śyāvaṃ saśothaṃ piḍakācitaṃ ca muhurmuhuḥ śoṇitavāhinaṃ ca |
mṛdūdgataṃ budbudatulyamāṃsaṃ vraṇaṃ saśalyaṃ sarujaṃ vadanti ||15||
A wound in which the foreign body is hidden inside is bluish black in colour, swollen, studded with eruptions, bleeds frequently, surrounding muscular appearing like soft bubbles (frothy) and is very painful. (15)

Foreign body lodged inside the abdomen

tvaco'tītya sirādīni bhittvā vā parihṛtya vā |

koṣṭhe pratiṣṭhitaṃ śalyaṃ kuryāduktānupadravān ||16|| (su| ci| a| 2) |
tatrāntarlohitaṃ pāṇḍuśītapādakarānanam |
śītocchvāsaṃ raktanetramānaddhaṃ ca vivarjayet ||17||
A foreign body getting lodged inside the abdomen, after piercing all the layers of the skin and injuring or destroying the veins (blood vessels), muscles, ligaments (and tendons), bones and joints, if not removed at proper time, would cause severe complications like gurgling sounds in the abdomen, flatulence etc explained in pranastashalya vijnaniya chapter.
When the blood is filled in the abdomen it would cause pallor and coldness of the feet, hands and face. Such a patient and those having cold breath and redness of the eyes shall be refused treatment. (16-17)

General symptoms of Ksata in muscles, blood vessels (veins), ligaments, bones and joints

bhramaḥ pralāpaḥ patanaṃ pramoho viceṣṭanaṃ glānirathoṣṇatā ca |
srastāṅgatā mūrchanamūrdhvavātastīvrā rujā vātakṛtāśca tāstāḥ ||18||
māṃsodakābhaṃ rudhiraṃ ca gacchet sarvendriyārthoparamastathaiva |
daśārdhasaṅkhyeṣvatha vikṣateṣu sāmānyato marmasu liṅgamuktam ||19|| (su| sū| a| 25) |
General symptoms of wounds to the five structures (muscles, veins, tendons bony joints and vital organs) are - giddiness, delirium, falling on the ground, unconsciousness (fainting), undesirable movements of the hands and feet, exhaustion, feeling of warmth, laxity or looseness (drooping) of the body parts, perversion of sense organs (abnormal functions), upward movements of vata (inside the abdomen) and severe and many types of pains characteristic of vāta, discharge of blood resembling mutton washed water, and loss of functions of the sense organs. (18-19)

Viddha Lakshanas of Veins etc

surendragopapratimaṃ prabhūtaṃ raktaṃ sravettatkṣayajaśca vāyuḥ |
karoti rogān vividhān yathoktān sirāsu viddhāsvatha vā kṣatāsu ||20||
kaubjyaṃ śarīrāvayavāvasādaḥ kriyāsvaśaktistumulā rujaśca |
cirādvraṇo rohati yasya cāpi taṃ snāyuviddhaṃ puruṣaṃ vyavasyet ||21||
Special symptoms manifesting due to injury of particular structures are as follows -

If śirās (blood vessels) are injured or punctured, there will be heavy discharge of blood resembling indragopa insects (bright red in colour). The vāta undergoing increase due to the injury (destruction of tissues caused due to injury and subsequent vata increase) would cause a wide array of disorders in later time.
Snayu viddha lakshana – The symptoms of injury / puncture to the tendons (nerves) are - decrease in height (hunchback), looseness or weakness (drooping) of the body parts, loss of functions, very severe pain and wound taking long time to heal.

Sandhi viddha lakshana

śophābhivṛddhistumulā rujaśca balakṣayaḥ sarvata eva śothaḥ |
kṣateṣu sandhiṣvacalācaleṣu syāt sarvakarmoparamaśca liṅgam ||22||
Increase of the swelling, severe pain, loss of strength, oedema in other parts of the body and total loss of functions – are the symptoms of injury to mobile or immobile bony joints of the body. (22)

Asthi Viddha Lakshanas

ghorā rujo yasya niśādineṣu sarvāsvavasthāsu ca naiti śāntim |
bhiṣagvipaścidviditārthasūtrastamasthividdhaṃ puruṣaṃ vyavasyet ||23|| (su| sū| a| 25) |
The symptoms which would enable an intelligent physician who is well conversant with science (of wounds) to recognize and diagnose that the person is having injury to the bones include very severe pain which is continuously present throughout the day and night (entire day) and not being able to find relief in any posture. (23)

Injury to the Marmas

yathāsvametāni vibhāvayecca liṅgāni marmasvabhitāḍiteṣu |24| (su| sū| a| 25) |
pāṇḍurvivarṇaḥ spṛśitaṃ na vetti yo māṃsamarmaṇyabhipīḍitaḥ syāt ||24|| (su| sū| a| 25) |
Similar symptoms will be found in persons whose vital organs are injured. In case or injury to the vital spots, the same symptoms (mentioned above)

should be understood in accordance with the seat of injury (wherein the marma is located).
When the mamsa marmas (vital spots predominantly made up of muscle tissue) are injured, there will be anaemia (pallor) or discoloration. The patient would not appreciate touch sensation (loss of tactile sensation). (24)

Upadrava - complications

visarpaḥ pakṣaghātaśca sirāstambho'patānakaḥ |
mohonmādavraṇarujo jvarastṛṣṇā hanugrahaḥ ||25||
kāsaśchardiratīsāro hikkā śvāsaḥ savepathuḥ |
ṣoḍaśopadravāḥ proktā vraṇānāṃ vraṇacintakaiḥ ||26|| (ca| ci| a| 25) |
According to the specialists in the knowledge of wounds the sixteen complications or sequelae of wounds are - erysipelas, hemiplegia, stiffness of the veins, tetanus, delusion, insanity, severe pain in the wound, fever, thirst, lockjaw, cough, vomiting, diarrhoea, hiccough, dyspnoea (difficulty in breathing) and tremors. (25-26)

iti śrīmādhavakaraviracite mādhavanidāne sadyovraṇanidānaṃ samāptam ||43||
Thus ends the chapter on SadhyoVrana

CHAPTER FORTY-FOUR

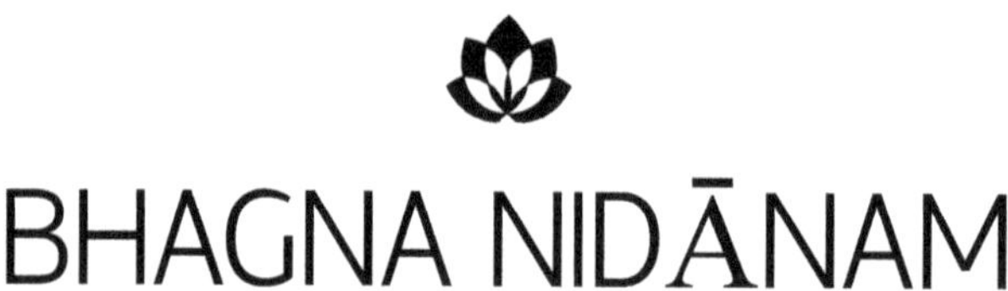

BHAGNA NIDĀNAM

Bhagna Bheda – Types of fractures

bhagnaṃ samāsāddvividhaṃ hutāśa kāṇḍe ca sandhau ca hi tatra sandhau |
utpiṣṭaviśliṣṭavivartitaṃ ca tiryaggataṃ kṣiptamadhaśca ṣaṭ ca ||1||
Bhagna (fracture) is, in brief, of two kinds;

- Kanda Bhagna – that which occurs at the shaft or body of the bones and
- Sandhi Bhagna – that which occurs at the sandhi – bony joints (meeting place of two bones)

Types of Sandhi Bhagna (fracture at the meeting place of two bones or sutures) – Sandhi Bhagnas are of six types, they are –

- Utpista
- Vislista
- Vivartita
- Tiryak Ksipta
- Ksipta and
- Adhah Ksipta (1)

Sandhi Bhagna Samanya Lakshana – General Symptoms of Sandhi Bhagna

prasāraṇākuñcanavartanogrā ruk sparśavidveṣaṇametaduktam |
sāmānyataḥ sandhigatasya liṅgam||| |2|
The general symptoms of sandhi bhagna are – severe pain during extension,

contraction and rotation, and tenderness.

Symptoms of types of Sandhi Bhagna / Sandhi Vislesa

...utpiṣṭasandheḥ śvayathuḥ samantāt ||2||
viśeṣato rātribhavā rujā ca, viśliṣṭaje tau ca rujā ca nityam |
vivartite pārśvarujaśca tīvrāstiryaggate tīvrarujo bhavanti ||3||
kṣipte'tiśūlaṃ viṣamatvamasthnoḥ kṣipte tvadho rugvighaṭaśca sandheḥ |
Utpista – In this condition there will be swelling all around the joint and severe pain at nights.
Vislista – This condition will also have the above mentioned two symptoms (swelling around the joint and severe pain at night) but the pain will be constantly present all through the day (day and night), but the swelling will be less
Vivartita – In this type severe pain will be present on both sides of the fracture site (joint)
Tiryak Ksipta – In this type there will be severe pain.
Ksipta – In this type there will be overlapping (overriding) of the bones involved in the fracture leading to curvature of the bones and pain.
Adhah Ksipta – In this type there will be severe pain and abnormal activities (functions) in the joints. According to yet another opinion, the bones at the seat of fracture of joints will slip / slide downwards. (2-3)

Kanda Bhagna – fracture of the bone shaft

kāṇḍe tvataḥ karkaṭakāśvakarṇavicūrṇitaṃ piccitamasthichallikā ||4||
kāṇḍeṣu bhagnaṃ hyatipātitaṃ ca majjāgataṃ ca sphuṭitaṃ ca vakram |
chinnaṃ dvidhā dvādaśadhā'pi kāṇḍe srastāṅgatā śotharujātivṛddhiḥ ||5||
sampīḍyamāne bhavatīha śabdaḥ sparśāsahaṃ spandanatodaśūlāḥ |
sarvāsvavasthāsu na śarmalābho bhagnasya kāṇḍe khalu cihnametat ||6||
bhagnaṃ tu kāṇḍe bahudhā prayāti samāsato nāmabhireva tulyam ||7||
Kānda Bhagna (fracture of shafts or body of bones) is of twelve kinds namely - Karkataka, Aśvakarna, Vicūrnita, Piccita, Asthichallikā, Kāndabhagna, Atipātita, Majjāgata, Sphutita, Vakra, and two types of Chinna.
In all these kinds, the general features are – looseness / laxity of the body parts (drooping of the part), swelling and severe pain, crackling sounds

at the site of fracture, tenderness, pulsations, pricking pain, pain, and not feeling comfort in any position.
Apart from these twelve types of fractures there might also occur many other types of kanda bhagna i.e., fracture of shafts. They are either included in these types or shall be understood by similarity with its meaning. (4-7)

Symptoms of incurability of Bhagna

alpāśino'nātmavato jantorvātātmakasya ca |
upadravairvā juṣṭasya bhagnaṃ kṛcchreṇa sidhyati ||8||
(su| ci| a| 3) |
Fractures heal with difficulty in persons who take very little (non-nutritious) quantity of food, in those who do not have self control or those who are habitually indulged in unsuitable foods and activities, in those of vata constitution and in the fractures associated with complications. (8)

Other symptoms of incurability of fractures

bhinnaṃ kapālaṃ kaṭyāṃ tu sandhimuktaṃ tathā cyutam |
jaghanaṃ pratipiṣṭaṃ ca varjayeddhi vicakṣaṇaḥ ||9||
asaṃśliṣṭakapālaṃ ca lalāṭe cūrṇitaṃ ca yat |
bhagnaṃ stanāntare pṛṣṭhe śaṅkhe mūrdhni ca varjayet ||10|| (su| ni| a| 15) |
Fracture of the skull / hip bone, fracture of the hip bone, dislocation, Cyuta or Adhahksipta type of fractures, Utpista fracture of hip / pelvic bones (at the sutures of the hip bones), fracture / dislocation of cranial sutures, crushing / cracking of forehead, fracture occurring between the breasts (centre of the chest), fracture of the back, temples and head (skull, vault of the head) are to be rejected considering them as incurable. (9-10)

samyak sandhitamapyasthi durnikṣepanibandhanāt |
saṅkṣobhādvā'pi yadgacchedvikriyāṃ tacca varjayet ||11||
(su| ni| a| 15) |
Fractures which have once healed but happening again and again due to bad positioning, bandaging or violent activity and creating loss of functions should also be refused treatment since it is incurable. (11)

Fractures presenting in different forms (presentation) in different bones

taruṇāsthīni namyante bhidyante nalakāni ca |
kapālāni vibhajyante sphuṭanti rucakāni ca ||12|| (su| ni| a| 15) |
Young bones (cartilages) bend and the long bones break in the middle. Flat bones crack in their body while the teeth (which are also considered as bones in Ayurveda) splinter off. (12)

iti śrīmādhavakaraviracite mādhavanidāne bhagnanidānaṃ samāptam ||44||
Thus ends the chapter on Bhagna.

CHAPTER FORTY-FIVE

NĀDĪ VRANA NIDĀNAM

Nadivrana Nidana, Samprapti – Etiological Factors and Pathogenesis of Nadivrana

yaḥ śothamāmamatipakvamupekṣate'jño yo vā vraṇaṃ pracurapūyamasādhuvṛttaḥ |
abhyantaraṃ praviśati pravidārya tasya sthānāni pūrvavihitāni tataḥ sapūyaḥ ||1||
(su| ni| a| 10) |
When the ignorant physician who cuts open an unripe swelling or delays draining of a fully ripened swelling (in which the pus has formed completely) or an unscrupulous physician who does not drain out the pus from an ulcer completely, the pus which has been formed makes way into the deeper structures / tissues by making a sinus and piercing into the vrana sthanas (seats of ulcer like skin, muscles etc mentioned by Master Sushruta). (This leads to the formation of nadi vrana) (1).

Nadivrana Nirukti, Bheda – Definition of the word Nadivrana, types of nadivrana

tasyātimātragamanādgatiriṣyate tu nāḍīva yadvahati tena matā tu nāḍī |2|
(su| ni| a| 10) |
doṣaistribhirbhavati sā pṛthagekaśaśca sammūrchitairapi ca śalyanimittato'nyā ||2|| (su| ni| a| 10) |
Gati – Since there is excessive movement of pus inside the sinus it is called as gati. (gati = movement).
Nadivrana - Since it is in the form of a tube or hollow pipe (because of the formation of hollow passage or sinus) and carries pus in it, this condition is

called as nadi vrana.
Types of Nadivrana – Nadivrana is of five types, one from each of the three doshas (caused by single dosha predominance – vataja, pittaja and kaphaja), one from the combined vitiation of all the three doshas (tridoshaja, sannipataja) and the other one due to the presence of a foreign body (shalyaja). (2)
Note – The five types of nadivrana are –

1. Vataja Nadivrana
2. Pittaja Nadivrana
3. Kaphaja Nadivrana
4. Sannipataja Nadivrana
5. Shalyaja Nadivrana

Symptoms of types of nadivrana

tatrānilāt paruṣasūkṣmamukhī saśūlā phenānuviddhamadhikaṃ sravati kṣapāsu |3|
(su| ni| a| 10) |
pittāttṛṣājvarakarī paridāhayuktā pītaṃ sravatyadhikamuṣṇamahaḥsu cāpi ||3||
(su| ni| a| 10) |
jñeyā kaphādbahughanārjunapicchilāsrā stabdhā sakaṇḍurarujā rajanīpravṛddhā |4|
(su| ni| a| 10) |
dāhajvaraśvasanamūrchanavaktraśoṣā yasyāṃ bhavantyabhihitāni ca lakṣaṇāni ||4||
tāmādiśet pavanapittakaphaprakopādghorāmasukṣayakarīmiva kālārātrim |
(su| ni| a| 10) |
naṣṭaṃ kathañcidanumārgamudīriteṣu sthāneṣu śalyamacireṇa gatiṃ karoti ||5||
Vataja Nadivrana – In this type, the nadi is rough, will have small orifice (opening), is painful, and will have exudation of frothy material especially during cold times and at night.
Pittaja Nadivrana – In this type, the person will have thirst, fever and burning sensation. The sinus will discharge yellowish material (exudates)

especially during hot time i.e., daytime (midday).
Kaphaja Nadivrana – In this type, the discharge is copious, excessively thick, white and sticky. The ulcer is hard, has more itching and the pain increases during night time.
Tridoshaja Nadivrana – In this type, there is burning sensation, fever, difficulty in breathing, fainting (loss of consciousness), dryness of the mouth and all symptoms of doshaja nadivranas (vataja, pittaja and kaphaja) explained above mixed together. This condition is said to be fatal and should be considered similar to Kalaratri i.e., sister of God of death in terms of taking away life. (2-5)

Shalyaja Nadivrana

sā phenilaṃ mathitamuṣṇamasṛgvimiśraṃ srāvaṃ karoti sahasā sarujā ca nityam |
(su| ni| a| 10) |
A foreign body somehow reaching and gettingembedded and hidden in the skin, muscle and other seats of vrana (ulcer) will make way into the deeper tissues creating a passage (sinus) and quickly cause nadivrana. From this sinus there is exudation of frothy, as if churned, hot and blood mixed material spontaneously accompanied with pain. This is called as shalyaja nadivrana. (5)

Symptoms of incurability of Nadivrana

nāḍī tridoṣaprabhavā na sidhyeccheṣāścatasraḥ khalu yatnasādhyāḥ ||6||
(su| ci| a| 17) |
Nadi Vrana (sinus ulcer) of the tridoṣhaja kind does not respond to treatment (it is incurable). The other four types of nadivrana can be treated with difficulty. (6)

iti śrīmādhavakaraviracite mādhavanidāne nāḍīvraṇanidānaṃ samāptam ||45||
Thus ends the chapter on Nädī Vran

CHAPTER FORTY-SIX

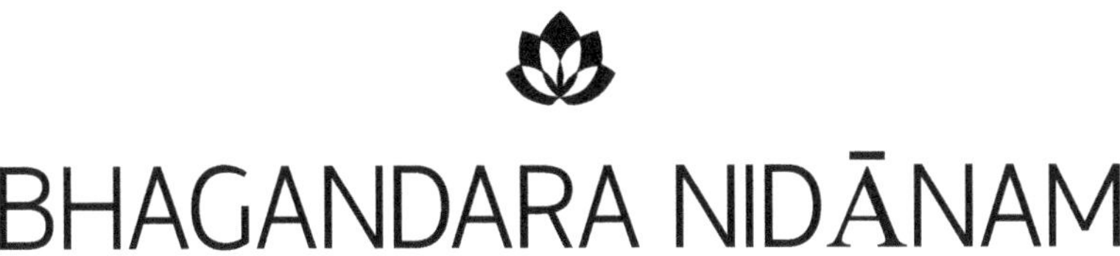

BHAGANDARA NIDĀNAM

Bhagandara rupa, sankhya – meaning and types of bhagandara

gudasya dvyaṅgule kṣetre pārśvataḥ piḍakā''rtikṛt |
bhinnā bhagandaro jñeyaḥ sa ca pañcavidho mataḥ ||1||
A papule (boil, blister) developing on either side of the anus, within a radius of two angulas accompanied with pain and exudation is known as Bhagandara (fistula-in-ano). It is of five kinds. (1)

Vatika Bhagandara (Shataponaka Bhagandara)

kaṣāyarūkṣaistvatikopito'nilastvapānadeśe piḍakāṃ karoti yām |
upekṣaṇātpākamupaiti dāruṇaṃ rujā ca bhinnā'ruṇaphenavāhinī ||2||
tatrāgamo mūtrapurīṣaretasāṃ vraṇairanekaiḥ śataponakaṃ vadet |3|
Due to excessive indulgence in foods predominant in astringent taste and dry in nature leads to aggravation of vata.
This aggravated vata causes a papule in the anal region. When it is neglected, it undergoes suppuration and produces severe pain. Many ulcers are formed around the papule. Through these orifices of multiple ulcers, urine, faeces and semen are discharged. Due to multiple ulcers / openings (orifices) vataja bhagandara is also called as sataponaka. (2-3)

Pittaja Bhagandara (Ushtragriva)

prakopaṇaiḥ pittamatiprakopitaṃ karoti raktāṃ piḍakāṃ gudāśritām ||3||
tadā''śupākā'himapūtivāhinīṃ bhagandaraṃ tūṣṭraśirodharaṃ vadet ||4||
Pitta undergoing severe increase in a person who has indulged in pitta aggravating etiological factors produces a red coloured pustule in the anal

region. This pustule quickly undergoes suppuration. The discharges coming from it are hot and foul smelling. This type of bhagandara is called Ustraśirodhara (ustragrīvā). (4)
Note – Since its shape resembles the neck of the camel, it is called as Ustragriva.

Kaphaja Bhagandara (Parisravi)

kaṇḍūyano ghanasrāvī kaṭhino mandavedanaḥ |
śvetāvabhāsaḥ kaphajaḥ parisrāvī bhagandaraḥ ||5||
The bhagandara which is produced by aggravated kapha has itching, thick discharges (exudates), is hard, slightly painful and whitish in colour. This is also called as Parisravi Bhagandara. (5)

Note – Since there are continuous thick discharges taking place from this type of bhagandara it is called parisravi bhagandara.

Sannipataja Bhagandara (Sambukavarta)

bahuvarṇarujāsrāvā piḍakā gostanopamā |
śambūkāvartavannāḍī śambūkāvartako mataḥ ||6||
These pustules have different kinds of colours and discharges (exudates) which resemble the teeth of the cow, creating spiral sinuses inside resembling that of seashell or whirls in a river. This is known as Śambūkavārtā (this is produced by increase of all the three doshas together and is associated with many types of pain). (6)

Agantuja Bhagandara (Unmargini)

kṣatādgatiḥ pāyugatā vivardhate hyupekṣaṇāt syuḥ krimayo vidārya te |
prakurvate mārgamanekadhā mukhairvraṇaistadunmārgibhagandaraṃ vadet ||7||
Injury caused by any foreign object like thorns, etc. at the anus, causes formation of sinus which goes on increasing in size (depth). When this condition is neglected worms (germs) are formed in these sinuses (sinuses get infected with worms / germs). These worms later form many small ulcers with many openings inside the sinuses. This condition is called as

unmargi bhagandara. (7)

Symptoms of incurability of Bhagandara

ghorāḥ sādhayituṃ duḥkhāḥ sarva eva bhagandarāḥ |
teṣvasādhyastridoṣotthaḥ kṣatajaśca viśeṣataḥ ||8||
(su| ni| a| 4) |
All kinds of bhagandara - fistula are dreadful and difficult to cure. Those caused by all the three doshas and injury (by external agents / foreign objects) are mainly incurable. (8)

Other symptoms of incurability of Bhagandara

vātamūtrapurīṣāṇi krimayaḥ śukrameva ca |
bhagandarāt sravantastu nāśayanti tamāturam ||9||
(su| sū| a| 33) |
When gas (fart), urine, faeces, worms and semen begin to come out of the fistula, it is going to kill the patient (such fistula is incurable). (9)

iti śrīmādhavakaraviracite mādhavanidāne bhagandaranidānaṃ samāptam ||46||
Thus ends the chapter on Bhagandara.

CHAPTER FORTY-SEVEN

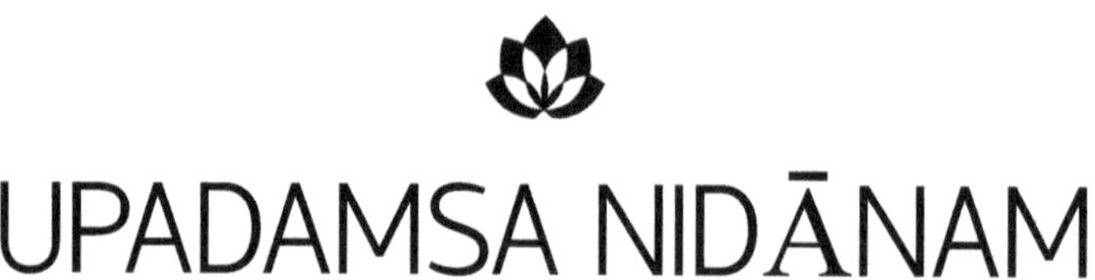

UPADAMSA NIDĀNAM

Upadamsa Nidana – Etiological Factors of Upadamsa

hastābhighātānnakhadantapātādadhāvanādratyatisevanādvā |
yonipradoṣācca bhavanti śiśne pañcopadaṃśā vividhāpacāraiḥ ||1||
Below mentioned are the etiological factors of upadamsa –

- injury to the penis by the hand (masturbation), nails and teeth;
- keeping it dirty without washing,
- indulging in excessive sexual intercourse,
- contact (sexual intercourse) with contaminated or diseased vagina and
- indulgence in such other bad habits

The above-mentioned etiological factors lead to the causation of the disease upadamsa (venereal disease). Upadamsa is of five types. (1)

Upadamsa Lakshanas – Symptoms of upadamsa and its types

satodabhedaiḥ sphuraṇaiḥ sakṛṣṇaiḥ sphoṭairvyavasyet pavanopadaṃśam |
pītairbahukledayutaiḥ sadāhaiḥ pittenaraktāt piśitāvabhāsaiḥ ||2||
sphoṭaiḥ sakṛṣṇai rudhiraṃ sravantaṃ raktātmakaṃ pittasamānaliṅgam |
sakaṇḍuraiḥ śothayutairmahadbhiḥ śuklairghanaiḥ srāvayutaiḥ kaphena ||3||
nānāvidhasrāvarujopapannamasādhyamāhustrimalopadaṃśam
viśīrṇamāṃsaṃ krimibhiḥ prajagdhaṃ muṣkāvaśeṣaṃ parivarjayecca ||4||
Vataja Upadamsa – In this type of upadamsa, there will be pricking, cutting and pulsating type of pain. Small papules (eruptions) which are black in colour appear on the penis.

Pittaja Upadamsa – In this type, the papules discharge yellowish fluid, the fluid is large in quantity and the person will also experience a burning sensation.
Raktaja Upadamsa – In this type, the papules resemble muscle, black in colour, bleeds and will have all other symptoms of pittaja upadamsa.
Kaphaja Upadamsa – In this type, the papules are big in size, swollen, have itching and discharges thick white fluid.
Tridoshaja Upadamsa – The upadamsa caused by all the three doshas together will present with different kinds of discharges (exudates) and pains. This condition is incurable.

Symptoms of incurability of Upadamsa

A condition of upadamsa in which the entire fleshy part of the penis has been eroded or eaten away by germs leaving only the scrotum is to be refused treatment (this condition is incurable). (2-4)

Consequence of not treating Upadamsa at right time

sañjātamātre na karoti mūḍhaḥ kriyāṃ naro yo viṣaye prasaktaḥ |
kālena śothakrimidāhapākairviśīrṇaśiśno mriyate sa tena ||5||
Foolish people who are engrossed in excessive sex and do not seek treatment soon after the onset of upadamsa and neglect it, the penis of such a person becomes swollen and gets infected by bacteria. There is also burning sensation, pus formation and destruction (falling off) of penis which eventually leads to the death of the person. (5)

Lingarsa, Lingavarti

aṅkurairiva saṅghātairuparyuparisaṃsthitaiḥ |
krameṇa jāyate vartistāmracūḍaśikhopamā ||6||
koṣasyābhyantare sandhau sarvasandhigatā'pi vā |
(savedanā picchilā ca duścikitsyā tridoṣajā) |
liṅgavartirabhikhyātā liṅgārśa iti cāpare ||7||
Sprouts of muscular tissue lying one over the other (superimposed), resembling the crown of a cock, developing inside the prepuce of the penis or at its junction with the penis or nearby, accompanied by pain, discharges which are sticky (sticky exudates) and caused by the combined vitiation of

all the tridoshas is called as lingavarti or lingarsa. This condition is difficult to treat. (6-7)

iti śrīmādhavakaraviracite mādhavanidāne upadaṃśanidānaṃ samāptam ||47||
Thus ends the chapter on Upadamśa.

CHAPTER FORTY-EIGHT

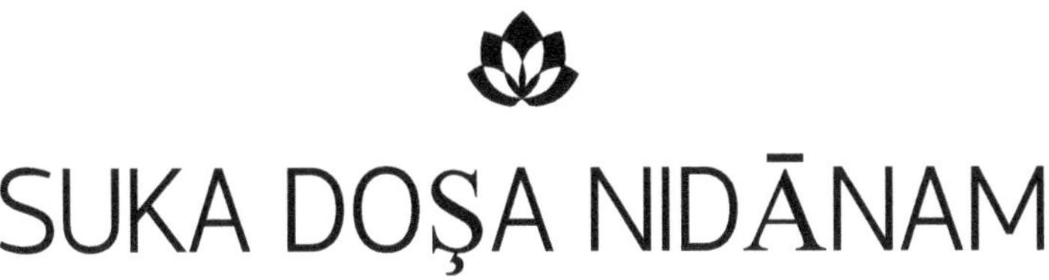

SUKA DOṢA NIDĀNAM

Nidana – Etiological factors

akramācchephaso vṛddhiṃ yo'bhivāñchati mūḍhadhīḥ |
vyādhayastasya jāyante daśa cāṣṭau ca śūkajāḥ ||1||
Foolish people who try to increase the size of their penis by unnatural methods (by application of paste of poisonous insects and other materials to the penis) become afflicted with eighteen kinds of diseases (of penis), caused by şükas (poisonous worms and other substances). These diseases are called as suka dosa or suka janya vyadhi. (1)

Sarsapika

gaurasarṣapasaṃsthānā śūkadurbhugnahetukā |
piḍakā śleṣmavātābhyāṃ jñeyā sarṣapikā tu sā ||2||
(su| ni| a| 14) |
Sarsapa means mustard. In Sarsapika, vesicles the size of white mustard appear on the penis. This happens due to indiscriminate application of pastes (as mentioned above in the etiological factors). Such pastes cause aggravation of kapha and vata and cause Sarsapika. (12)

Asthilika

kaṭhinā viṣamairbhugnairvāyunā'ṣṭhīlikā bhavet |3|
(su| ni| a| 14) |
Application of bad and unsuitable suka on the penis indiscriminately leads to abnormal increase of vata. This produces asthilika which is hard and irregular in shape.

Gratita

śūkairyat pūritaṃ śaśvadgrathitaṃ nāma tat kaphāt ||3||
The eruptions / vesicles which are caused by aggravated vata and appear like nodules (cysts) filled with sukas are called as Gratita Suka Dosha. (3)

Kumbhika

kumbhikā raktapittotthā jāmbavāsthinibhā'śubhā |4|
(su| ni| a| 14) |
Kumbhika is produced by abnormally increased rakta (blood) and pitta. It resembles the seeds of jambū fruit (Eugenia jambolina) and is black in colour.

Alaji

tulyajāṃ tvalajīṃ vidyādyathāproktāṃ vicakṣaṇaḥ ||4||
(su| ni| a| 14) |
According to Ayurveda experts Alaji Suka Dosa is a condition which resembles a disease of the same name which has been described earlier in the context of prameha pidaka – diabetic carbuncles. (One of the types of prameha pidaka is also named as Alaji. The alaji explained here will have the similar causative factors and symptoms like that of the alaji prameha pidaka). (4)

Mrudita & Sammudha Pidaka

mṛditaṃ pīḍitaṃ yacca saṃrabdhaṃ vātakopataḥ |5| (su| ni| a| 14) |
pāṇibhyāṃ bhṛśasammūḍhe sammūḍhapiḍakā bhavet ||5|| (su| ni| a| 14) |
Mrdita is a swelling of the penis. It is caused by the aggravation of vata caused by rubbing of the penis after application of suka.
Sammudha piḍakā is appearance of papules by rubbing the penis briskly after the application of suka. (This should also be considered as caused by aggravated vata). (5)

In ancient times some kinds of molluscs, shrimps, crabs were made into a

paste along with some herbs and applied over the penis to make it big and strong. Many of them were poisonous and so caused sepsis. (This is an extra explanation which was not found in this context. Think of retaining it or removing it. It was not added by me.)

Adhimanta

dīrghā bahvyaśca piḍakā dīryante madhyatastu yāḥ |
so'dhimanthaḥ kaphāsṛgbhyāṃ vedanāromaharṣakṛt ||6||
(su| ni| a| 14) |
In Adhimanta, multiple vesicles which are long are manifested. These vesicles burst open at their centre and are accompanied with pain and horripilation. This condition is caused by increased kapha and rakta (blood). (6)

Puskarika

piḍakā piḍakāvyāptā pittaśoṇitasambhavā |
padmakarṇikasaṃsthānā jñeyā puṣkarikā tu sā ||7||
(su| ni| a| 14) |
Vesicles caused by increased pitta and rakta, many in number and resembling the sprouts of a lotus flower is known as Puskarika.(7)

Sparsahani

sparśahāniṃ tu janayecchoṇitaṃ śūkadūṣitam |8|
(su| ni| a| 14) |
Sparsahani is a condition caused by rakta infected by suka poison. This infected blood causes loss of (tactile) sensation or sense of touch in the penis.

Uttama

mudgamāṣopamā raktā raktapittodbhavā tu yā ||8||
vyādhireṣottamā nāma śūkājīrṇanimittajā |
(su| ni| a| 14) |
Uttama is the name of the disease in which papules of the size of green gram

or black gram appear on the penis. They are red in colour and are caused by vitiated rakta (blood) and pitta. This is caused by repeated application of suka – poisonous paste over the penis. (8)

Sataponaka

chidrairaṇumukhairliṅgaṃ citaṃ yasya samantataḥ ||9||
vātaśoṇitajo vyādhiḥ sa jñeyaḥ śataponakaḥ |
(su| ni| 14) ||11||
The disease in which the penis is studded (enveloped) by many small openings (holes) all around and is caused by vitiated vata and rakta (blood) is called as Sataponaka. (9)

Tvakpaka

vātapittakṛto jñeyastvakpāko jvaradāhakṛt ||10|| (su| ni| a| 14) |
Vata and pitta which are abnormally increased cause ulceration (suppuration) of the skin of the penis, accompanied by fever and burning sensation. This condition is called as Tvakpaka. (10)

Sonitarbuda

kṛṣṇaiḥ sphoṭaiḥ saraktābhiḥ piḍakābhirnipīḍitam |
yasya vāsturujaścogrā jñeyaṃ tacchoṇitārbudam ||11||
(su| ni| a| 14) |
The condition in which black coloured vesicles / blisters or reddish coloured eruptions (papules) appear all over the penis, associated with severe pain is called as Sonitarbuda. (11)

Mamsarbuda, Mamsapaka and Vidradhi

māṃsadoṣeṇa jānīyādarbudaṃ māṃsasambhavam |12| (su| ni| a| 14) |
śīryante yasya māṃsāni yasya sarvāśca vedanāḥ ||12||
vidyāttaṃ māṃsapākaṃ tu sarvadoṣakṛtaṃ bhiṣak | (su| ni| a| 14) |
vidradhiṃ sannipātena yathoktamiti nirdiśet ||13|| (su| ni| a| 14) |
Mamsarbuda should be recognised by involvement of muscle tissue. The muscles are contaminated due to the application of suka poisons leading to

the manifestation of this condition.
Mamaspaka is a condition in which the fleshy part of the penis falls off. A wise physician should consider this condition as caused by the vitiation of all the three doshas. As a result, mamsapaka is accompanied by severe kinds of pains caused by all three doshas.
Vidradhi is another condition caused by vitiation of all the three doshas. The signs and symptoms resemble those of sannipataja vidradhi described earlier and presents with different kinds of colours, pains and discharges. (12-13)

Tilakalaka

kṛṣṇāni citrāṇyathavā śūkāni saviṣāṇi vā |
pātitāni pacantyāśu meḍhraṃ niravaśeṣataḥ ||14||
kālāni bhūtvā māṃsāni śīryante yasya dehinaḥ |
sannipātasamutthāṃstu tān vidyāttilakālakān ||15|| (su| ni| a| 14) |
When the paste of the highly poisonous insects which are of black colour or of many colours is applied over the penis, it causes quick suppuration of the penis and the entire penis would get detached and fall off without any residue. The muscular part of the penis becomes black in colour and these parts would fall off. This condition is known as Tilakalaka and is caused due to the abnormal increase of all the three doshas together. (It is called as tilakalaka also due to the appearance of warts resembling the black moles of the skin). (14-15)

Asadhyata – Symptoms of incurability of suka dosha

tatra māṃsārbudaṃ yacca māṃsapākaśca yaḥ smṛtaḥ |
vidradhiśca na siddhyanti ye ca syustilakālakāḥ ||16|| (su| ni| a| 14) |
Among the above suka dosha diseases, mamsarbuda, mamsapaka, vidradhi and tilákalaka do not respond to treatment i.e. they are incurable. (16)

iti śrīmādhavakaraviracite mādhavanidāne śūkadoṣanidānaṃ samāptam ||48||
Thus ends the chapter on Sukadoṣa,

CHAPTER FORTY-NINE

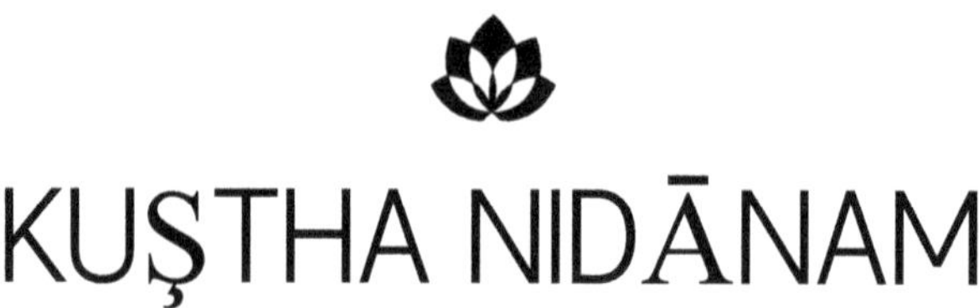

KUṢTHA NIDĀNAM

Nidana, Samprapti – Etiological Factors and Pathogenesis of Kustha

virodhīnyannapānāni dravasnigdhagurūṇi ca |
bhajatāmāgatāṃ chardiṃ vegāṃścānyān pratighnatām ||1||
vyāyāmamatisantāpamatibhuktvā niṣeviṇām |
gharmaśramabhayārtānāṃ drutaṃ śītāmbusevinām ||2||
ajīrṇādhyaśināṃ caiva pañcakarmāpacāriṇām |
navānnadadhimatsyātilavaṇāmlaniṣeviṇām ||3||
māṣamūlakapiṣṭānnatilakṣīraguḍāśinām |
vyavāyaṃ cāpyajīrṇe'nne nidrāṃ ca bhajatāṃ divā ||4||
viprān gurūn dharṣayatāṃ pāpaṃ karma ca kurvatām |
vātādayastrayo duṣṭāstvagraktaṃ māṃsamambu ca ||5||
dūṣayanti sa kuṣṭhānāṃ saptako dravyasaṅgrahaḥ |
ataḥ kuṣṭhāni jāyante sapta caikādaśaiva ca ||6||
(ca| ci| a| 7) |
Etiological Factors of Kustha –

- indulgence in incompatible (mutually opposite or antagonistic) foods and drinks,
- excessive intake of foods which are very watery, fatty (unctuous) and heavy (hard to digest),
- suppressing the urges of vomiting and other natural bodily urges,
- doing heavy and excessive physical exercises immediately after taking food and
- too much of exposure to heat (immediately after taking food),
- consuming cold water (immersing in cold water) immediately after exposure to the sunlight (heat of the sun), after doing hard (strenuous)

works and after incidents which have caused fear
- use of uncooked foods and over-eating,
- improper methods of administering panchakarma (five purifactory) therapies (emesis, purgation, enema, errhines and bloodletting)
- excessive consumption of fresh grains, curds, fishes, and foods are very salty and sour,
- excessive consumption of black-gram, radish, flours, sesame, milk and jaggery
- indulgence in sexual intercourse while having indigestion
- excessive sleeping during day time (though suffering from indigestion),
- showing disrespect and abusing gods and teachers
- committing many kinds of sinful acts etc

The above-mentioned etiological factors cause abnormal increase of all the three doshas and derangement (contamination) of skin, blood, muscular tissue and body fluids and produce kustha (leprosy, skin diseases). These seven substances (three doshas and four tissues – skin, blood, muscles and fluid components) together cause seven (major, greater) and eleven (minor, lesser) skin diseases. (1-6)

Seven types of Kustha

kuṣṭhāni saptadhā doṣaiḥ pṛthagdvandvaiḥ samāgataiḥ |
sarveṣvapi tridoṣeṣu vyapadeśo'dhikastvataḥ ||7||
(vā| ni| a| 14) |
Kustha (leprosy and other skin disorders) is of seven kinds, one from each dosha, three from the combination of two doshas, and one from the combination of all the three doshas together. Though all the kushtas are tridoshaja (caused due to involvement of all the three doshas), the types of kustha are named as vataja, pittaja etc based on the predominance of any one or two doshas in those types of kustha. (The varieties are named to indicate the predominance of a dosha or doshas in the kustha). (7)

Kustha Purvarupa – Premonitory symptoms of Kustha

atiślakṣṇakharasparśasvedāsvedavivarṇatāḥ |

dāhaḥ kaṇḍūstvaci svāpastodaḥ koṭhonnatirbhramaḥ ||8||
vraṇānāmadhikaṃ śūlaṃ śīghrotpattiściracsthitiḥ |
rūḍhānāmapi rūkṣatvaṃ nimitta'lpe'tikopanam ||9||
romaharṣo'sṛjaḥ kārṣṇyaṃ kuṣṭhalakṣaṇamagrajam |
(vā| ni| a| 14) |
Below mentioned are the premonitory symptoms of Kustha –

- the skin is either very smooth or rough,
- presence or absence of sweating,
- discolouration,
- burning sensation,
- itching,
- loss of sensation in the skin,
- pricking pain,
- appearance of elevated patches,
- giddiness,
- severe pain in the ulcers,
- ulcers form quickly and remain for long periods (does not heal for long periods of time),
- dryness in those ulcers which have healed,
- severe aggravation (re-appearance) of ulcer with trivial (simplest of or feeble) causes,
- horripilation,
- blackish discolouration of the blood (8-9)

Mahakustha – Seven types of major skin disorders and their symptoms

kṛṣṇāruṇakapālābhaṃ yadrūkṣaṃ paruṣaṃ tanu ||10||
kāpālaṃ todabahulaṃ tatkuṣṭhaṃ viṣamaṃ smṛtam |
rugdāharāgakaṇḍūbhiḥ parītaṃ romapiñjaram ||11||
udumbaraphalābhāsaṃ kuṣṭhamaudumbaraṃ vadet |
śvetaṃ raktaṃ sthiraṃ styānaṃ snigdhamutsannamaṇḍalam ||12||
kṛcchramanyonyasaṃyuktaṃ kuṣṭhaṃ maṇḍalamucyate |
karkaśaṃ raktaparyantamantaḥśyāvaṃ savedanam ||13||
yadṛṣyajihvasaṃsthānamṛṣyajihvaṃ taducyate |
saśvetaṃ raktaparyantaṃ puṇḍarīkadalopamam ||14||

sotsedhaṃ ca sarāgaṃ ca puṇḍarīkaṃ taducyate |
śvetaṃ tāmraṃ tanu ca yadrajo ghṛṣṭaṃ vimuñcati ||15||
prāyaścorasi tat sidhmamalābukusumopamam |
yat kākaṇantikāvarṇaṃ sapākaṃ tīvravedanam ||16||
tridoṣaliṅgaṃ tat kuṣṭhaṃ kākaṇaṃ naiva sidhyati |
(ca| ci| a| 7) |

Kapala Kustha – In this condition, the skin resembles a blackish or reddish-brown coloured piece of potsherd (kapala); is dry and rough (coarse) and thin; has severe pricking pain and is intractable.

Udumbara Kustha – This type of kustha resembles the fruit of udumbara (Ficus infectoria) and hence the name. It presents with pain, burning sensation, redness, itching and hairs turned to pink colour.

Mandala Kustha – In this condition, the skin is white or red in colour, tight (hard), moist (wet) and unctuous (oily). It has round and elevated patches which are joined to one another and is difficult to treat.

Rsyajihva Kustha – In this type of Mahakustha, the skin is very rough, is red in colour outside and black inside, and is associated with pain. It resembles the tongue of a black deer (Rsya) and hence the name.

Pundarika Kustha – In this, the skin is white at the centre and red at the edges resembling the petals of the lotus flower, with elevated patches which are red in colour.

Sidhma Kustha – The skin in this condition is white or coppery red in colour. It has thin scales which come off on scratching and are found mainly on the chest. They resemble the flowers of pitcher gourd.

Kakana Kustha – This type of mahakustha has the colour of guñja (Abrus precatorius), undergoing suppuration (pus formation), very painful and caused by all the three doshas and which does not respond to any kind of treatment (incurable). (10-16)

Ksudra kustha – Seven types of minor skin disorders and their symptoms

asvedanaṃ mahāvāstu yanmatsyaśakalopamam ||17||
tadekakuṣṭhaṃ, carmākhyaṃ bahalaṃ hasticarmavat |
śyāvaṃ kiṇakharasparśaṃ paruṣaṃ kiṭibhaṃ smṛtam ||18||
vaipādikaṃ pāṇipādasphuṭanaṃ tīvravedanam |
kaṇḍūmadbhiḥ sarāgaiścaḥ gaṇḍairalasakaṃ citam ||19||

sakaṇḍūrāgapiḍakaṃ dadrumaṇḍalamudgatam |
raktaṃ saśūlaṃ kaṇḍūmat sasphoṭaṃ yadgalatyapi |
taccarmadalamākhyātaṃ saṃsparśāsahamucyate ||20|| (ca| ci| a| 7) |
sūkṣmā bahvyaḥ piḍakāḥ srāvavatyaḥ pāmetyuktāḥ kaṇḍumatyaḥ sadāhāḥ |
saiva sphoṭaistīvradāhairupetā jñeyā pāṇyoḥ kacchurugrā sphicośca ||21||
sphoṭāḥ śyāvāruṇābhāsā visphoṭāḥ syustanutvacaḥ |
raktaṃ śyāvaṃ sadāhārti śatāruḥ syādbahuvraṇam ||22||
sakaṇḍūḥ piḍakā śyāvā bahusrāvā vicarcikā |
(ca| ci| a| 7) |

Ekakustha – In this, there is no sweating, the area of skin involved is large, and the skin resembles the scales of a fish.

Carmakhya Kustha – In this condition, the skin becomes thick like that of an elephant skin.

Kitibha Kustha – The skin in this condition is blackish, rough and coarse just like the scar of a wound (granulation).

Vaipadika Kustha – This type of ksudra kustha presents with cracks and fissures formed on the hands and feet associated with severe pain.

Alasaka Kustha – This presents with nodules which are red in colour and associated with itching.

Dadru Mandala Kustha – In this condition there are raised patches studded with small, itching, reddish papules.

Carmadala Kustha – It is a condition in which the skin is studded with red coloured nodules in which there is pain and itching. They burst open and fall off and are sensitive to touch (do not tolerate when touched).

Pama – It presents in the form of small and plentiful pustules from which discharges (exudates) take place. Itching and burning sensation are also present.

Kacchu – This is a condition in which the same pustules (as explained in pama) appear on the hands and on the buttocks associated with burning sensation.

Visphota – This condition presents with boils on the skin which are bluish black or brownish red in colour. It is called Visphota in which the skin becomes thin.

Sataru – This type of kshudra kustha presents with innumerable small ulcers which are red or blackish blue in colour and are associated with severe burning sensation and pain.

Vicarcika – In this condition, black coloured nodules are found from which

plenty of copious exudates are discharged. This condition is also associated with itching. (17-22)
(The above eleven kinds are known as Ksudra kusthas i.e. minor leprosies / skin diseases).

Symptoms of Kustha based on the predominance of dosha

kharaṃ śyāvāruṇaṃ rūkṣaṃ vātāt kuṣṭhaṃ savedanam ||23||
pittāt prakvathitaṃ dāharāgasrāvānvitaṃ matam |
kaphāt kledi ghanaṃ snigdhaṃ sakaṇḍūśaityagauravam ||24||
dviliṅgaṃ dvandvajaṃ kuṣṭhaṃ, triliṅgaṃ sānnipātikam |25|
Symptoms of vata predominance in all kinds of Kustha include – manifestation of roughness, bluish black or brownish red colour, dryness and pain.
Symptoms of pitta predominance in all kinds of Kustha include – manifestation of putrefaction, burning sensation, redness and exudation (discharges).
Symptoms of kapha predominance in all kinds of Kustha include – manifestation of moistness (wetness), thickness, unctuousness (greasiness), itching, coldness and heaviness.
In dwandwaja Kustha – symptoms of two doshas are manifested together.
In sannipataja Kustha – symptoms of all three doshas are present together. (23-24)

Dhatugata Kustha Symptoms

tvaksthe vaivarṇyamaṅgeṣu kuṣṭheraukṣyaṃ ca jāyate ||25||
tvaksvāpo romaharṣaśca svedasyātipravartanam |
kaṇḍūrvipūyakaścaiva kuṣṭhe śoṇitasaṃśrite ||26||
bāhulyaṃ vaktraśoṣaśca kārkaśyaṃ piḍakodgamaḥ |
todaḥ sphoṭaḥ sthiratvaṃ ca kuṣṭhe māṃsasamāśrite ||27||
kauṇyaṃ gatikṣayo'ṅgānāṃ sambhedaḥ kṣatasarpaṇam |
medaḥsthānagate liṅgaṃ prāguktāni tathaiva ca ||28||
nāsābhaṅgo'kṣirāgaśca kṣateṣu krimisambhavaḥ |
svaropaghātaśca bhavedasthimajjasamāśrite ||29||
dampatyoḥ kuṣṭhabāhulyādduṣṭaśoṇitaśukrayoḥ |
yadapatyaṃ tayorjātaṃ jñeyaṃ tadapi kuṣṭhitam ||30||

(su| ni| a| 5) |

Twakgata Kustha – When kustha is located in the skin (rasa tissue) there will be discolouration of the skin, roughness, loss of sensation, horripilation and profuse sweating.

Raktagata Kustha – When kustha is located in the blood, there will be itching and the appearance of pustules in large numbers / foul smelling pus formation.

Mamsagata Kustha – When kustha is located in the muscle tissue, there will be the appearance of thick elevated patches, dryness of the mouth, roughness, appearance of nodules, pricking pain, boils / blisters and tightness of the skin.

Medogata Kustha – When kustha is located in the fat tissue, the fingers will fall off, and there will be loss of movements in the body parts (inability to walk), splitting pain and spreading of ulcer.

Asthi-Majjagata Kustha – When kustha is located in the bones and bone marrow, there is loss of / falling of nose, redness of the eyes, appearance of worms in the ulcers and loss of voice.

Shukragata Kustha – When the couple suffer from kustha, the child produced by them will also be born with kustha since both sperm (of the man) and ovum (of the woman) are both affected by kustha. (25-30)

Prognosis of Kustha

sādhyaṃ tvagraktamāṃsasthaṃ vātaśleṣmādhikaṃ ca yat |
medasi dvandvajaṃ yāpyaṃ varjyaṃ majjāsthisaṃśritam ||31||

Kustha is located (invading) in skin, blood and muscle tissues and those varieties which are caused by the predominance of vata and kapha are easy to cure.

Kushta located (invading) the fat tissue and those caused by combination of two doshas together become manageable (chronic – curable but needs treatment throughout the life).

Kustha is located (invading) in the bone marrow and bones should not be treated (because they are incurable). (31)

Symptoms which are fatal in Kustha

krimitṛḍdāhamandāgnisaṃyuktaṃ yattridoṣajam |
prabhinnaṃ prasrutāṅgaṃ ca raktanetraṃ hatasvaram ||32||

pañcakarmaguṇātītaṃ kuṣṭhaṃ hantīha mānavam |
(su| sū| a| 33) |
Kustha is going to kill the patient in the presence of the below mentioned symptoms / conditions –

- presence of worms in the ulcers,
- thirst,
- burning sensation,
- poor digestive capacity
- involvement of all the three doshas together (in the causation of kustha – tridoshaja kustha)
- mutilation, loss of and decaying of body parts
- redness of the eyes
- loss of voice
- if the cure is beyond the capacity of panchakarma (cannot be cured in spite of administering the five purifactory therapies or the patients not suitable to undergo these therapies which are otherwise highly beneficial) (32)

Dosha relation in each kustha

vātena kuṣṭhaṃ kāpālaṃ pittenaudumbaraṃ kaphāt ||33||
maṇḍalākhyaṃ vicarcī ca ṛṣyākhyaṃ vātapittajam |
carmaikakuṣṭhaṃ kiṭibhaṃ sidhmālasavipādikāḥ ||34||
vātaśleṣmodbhavāḥ śleṣmapittāddadruśatāruṣī |
puṇḍarīkaṃ savisphoṭaṃ pāmā carmadalaṃ tathā ||35||
sarvaiḥ syāt kākaṇaṃ pūrvatrikaṃ dadru sakākaṇam |
puṇḍarīkarṣyajihve ca mahākuṣṭhāni sapta tu ||36|| (vā| ni| a| 14) |
Kapala kustha is produced by vata predominance.
Udumbara Kustha is caused by pitta predominance.
Mandala Kustha and Vicarcika Kustha are caused by kapha predominance.
Rsyajihva Kustha is caused by predominance of vata and pitta together.
Carmakhya Kustha, Eka Kustha, Kitibha Kustha, Sidhma Kustha, Alasa Kustha, Vipadika Kustha – all these are caused by predominant vitiation of both vata and kapha together.
Dadru Kustha, Sataru Kustha, Pundarika Kustha, Visphota Kustha, Pama

Kustha and Carmadala Kustha – all these are caused by predominance of both kapha and pitta together.
Kakana Kustha is caused by vitiation of all the three doshas together.
The first three types of Kustha i.e. Kapala, Udumbara and Mandala and Dadru, Kakana, Pundarika and Rsyajihva – these seven types are called as Mahakusthas. (33-36)

Kilasa Kustha

kuṣṭhaikasambhavaṃ śvitraṃ kilāsaṃ vāruṇaṃ bhavet |
nirdiṣṭamaparisrāvi tridhātūdbhavasaṃśrayam ||37||
vātādrūkṣāruṇaṃ, pittāttāmraṃ kamalapatravat |
sadāhaṃ romavidhvaṃsi kaphācchvetaṃ ghanaṃ guru ||38||
sakaṇḍūraṃ kramādraktamāṃsamedaḥsu cādiśet |
varṇenaivedṛgubhayaṃ kṛcchraṃ taccottarottaram ||39||
(vā| ni| a| 14) |
Svitra, Kiläsa and Aruna are the variants of Kustha. They are produced by the same causative factors which cause kustha (leprosy).
There is no production of exudates in this condition (no discharges) and are caused by vitiation of all the three doshas together.
Vata predominance in these conditions causes roughness and pinkish discolouration.
Pitta predominance would present with lesions which are red like the petals of a lotus, associated with burning sensation and destruction (loss) of body hairs.
Kapha predominance in these conditions causes whitish discolouration, thickness, feeling of heaviness and itching.
Kilasa is of three types – Aruna, Tamra and Sveta. They are manifested in the blood, muscles and fat tissues respectively. (Involvement of blood causes aruna with pinkish or brownish red or golden yellow discolouration, Involvement of muscles causes tamra i.e., coppery discoloration and involvement of fat tissue will cause sveta i.e., whitish discoloration). The successive kinds are more dreadful than their preceding ones. Kilasa caused by ulcers and doshas will become incurable in successive (deeper) tissues. (37-39)

Prognosis of Svitra / Kilasa

śuklaromā'bahulamasaṃśliṣṭamatho navam |
anagnidagdhajaṃ sādhyaṃ śvitraṃ varjyamato'nyathā ||40||
guhyapāṇitalauṣṭheṣu jātamapyacirantanam |
varjanīyaṃ viśeṣeṇa kilāsaṃ siddhimicchatā ||41||
(a| saṃ| ni| a| 14) |
Svitra (leucoderma) in which the hairs are not white; the skin is not thick, the patches are not joined together, which is of recent origin and that which has not been caused by burns are curable. Those having symptoms opposite to these are said to be incurable.
The physician desirous of success should refuse treating kilasa which has been manifested over the genitals, palms of the hands, soles of the food and lips and those which have persisted for a long time (chronic cases). (40-41)

Aupasargika Roga

prasaṅgādgātrasaṃsparśānniḥśvāsāt sahabhojanat |
ekaśayyāsanāccaiva vastramālyānupalenāt ||42||
kuṣṭhaṃ jvaraśca śoṣaśca netrābhiṣyanda eva ca |
aupasargikarogāśca saṅkrāmanti narānnaram ||43||
(su| ni| a| 5) |
Sexual intercourse, physical contact, contact with expired air, dining together, sleeping together, and sharing the dress and garlands / ornaments, diseases like leprosy (skin diseases), fever, tuberculosis and conjunctivitis and many other diseases are transmitted from one person to the other. These diseases are called Aupasargika Rogas (infectious / contagious diseases). (42-44)

iti śrīmādhavakaraviracite mādhavanidāne kuṣṭhanidānaṃ samāptam ||49||
Thus ends the chapter on Kustha.

CHAPTER FIFTY

SITAPITTA UDARDA KOTHA NIDANAM

Sitapitta, Udarda, Kotha Samanya Nidana – General etiological factors for all three conditions

śītamārutasaṃsparśāt praduṣṭau kaphamārutau |
pittena saha sambhūya bahirantarvisarpataḥ ||1||
By contact with a very cold breeze, kapha and väta get increase. These doshas get associated with pitta (increased by its etiological factors) spreads out externally (towards the skin) and internally (into blood and other tissues) and produces sitapitta, udarda and kotha. (1)

Purvarupa – Premonitory symptoms

pipāsārucihṛllāsadehasādāṅgagauravam |
raktalocanatā teṣāṃ pūrvarūpasya lakṣaṇam ||2||
The premonitory symptoms of the above-mentioned conditions are – thirst, loss of taste, nausea, debility in the body parts, and feeling of heaviness in the body and redness of the eyes. (2)

Udarda Lakshana – Symptoms of Udarda

varaṭīdaṣṭasaṃsthānaḥ śothaḥ sañjāyate bahiḥ |
sakaṇḍūstodabahulaśchardijvaravidāhavān ||3||
udardamiti taṃ vidyācchītapittamathāpare |
vātādhikaṃ śītapittamudardastu kaphādhikaḥ ||4||
Swelling / elevated patches (rashes) resembling the rashes produced by

the sting of the wasp produced on the skin, associated with itching and severe pricking pain, vomiting, fever and feeling of burning sensation are the characteristic features of Udarda. This condition is called Sitapitta by other experts. The difference in these two conditions is that in Sitapitta, vata is predominant and in udarda, kapha is predominant. (3-4)

Other form and presentation of Udarda

sotsaṅgaiśca sarāgaiśca kaṇḍūmadbhiśca maṇḍalaiḥ |
śaiśiraḥ kaphajo vyādhirudarda iti kīrtitaḥ ||5||
A condition manifesting with elevated patches which are reddish, have severe itching, caused by vitiated kapha during sisira rtu (late winter) is also known as udarda. (5)

Kotha

asamyagvamanodīrṇapittaśleṣmānnanigrahaiḥ |
maṇḍalāni sakaṇḍūni rāgavanti bahūni ca |
utkoṭhaḥ sānubandhaśca koṭha ityabhidhīyate ||6||
Incomplete / inadequate or erroneous administration of emesis therapy (improper administration of emetics and other treatments), and suppression (obstruction) of the movement of pitta, kapha and anna (food) leads to the appearance of innumerable rashes, red in colour and highly itching is called as Kotha. If the same condition repeats (relapses) again and again, many times, it is called as Utkotha. (6)

iti śrīmādhavakaraviracite mādhavanidāne śītapittodardakoṭhānidānaṃ samāptam ||50||
Thus ends the chapter on Śītapitta etc.

CHAPTER FIFTY-ONE

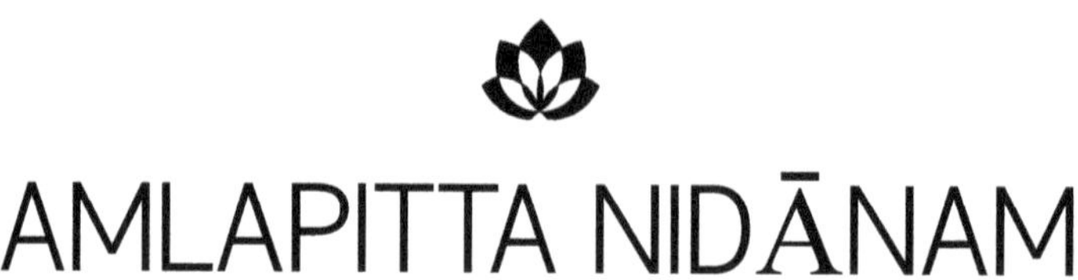

AMLAPITTA NIDĀNAM

Nidana, Samprapti – Etiological Factors and Pathogenesis of Amlapitta

viruddhaduṣṭāmlavidāhipittaprakopipānānnabhujo vidagdham |
pittaṃ svahetūpacitaṃ purā yattadamlapittaṃ pravadanti santaḥ ||1||
In persons in whom pitta has already undergone increase and excessive sourness; excessive indulgence in foods which are of incompatible combinations, spoiled, very sour, those causing burning sensation inside and such other foods and drinks which cause increase of pitta, produce Amlapitta, so say the wise. (1)

Amlapitta Lakshana – symptoms of amlapitta

avipākaklamotkleśatiktāmlodgāragauravaiḥ |
hṛtkaṇṭhadāhārucibhiścāmlapittaṃ vadedbhiṣak ||2||
The disease in which the patient has indigestion, exhaustion without any exertion, nausea, eructation (belching) with bitter or sour taste, feeling of heaviness of the body, burning sensation in the chest and throat and loss of taste - is to be called as Amlapitta. (2)

Adhoga Amlapitta Symptoms

tṛḍdāhamūrchābhramamohakāri prayātyadho vā vividhaprakāram |
hṛllāsakoṭhānalasādaharṣasvedāṅgapītatvakaraṃ kadācit ||3||
The symptoms of adhoga (downward) amlapitta are - thirst, burning sensation, fainting, giddiness, delusion, movement downwards of different kinds (of diarrhoea), nausea (occasional oppression in the chest), rashes on the skin, poor digestion, horripilation, excessive perspiration and yellowish

skin (of parts of the body). (3)

Urdhwaga Amlapitta Symptoms

vāntaṃ haritpītakanīlakṛṣṇamāraktaraktābhamatīva cāmlam |
māṃsodakābhaṃ tvatipicchilācchaṃ śleṣmānujātaṃ vividhaṃ rasena ||4||
bhukte vidagdhe tvathavā'pyabhukte karoti tiktāmlavamiṃ kadācit |
udgāramevaṃvidhameva kaṇṭhahṛtkukṣidāhaṃ śiraso rujaṃ ca ||5||
karacaraṇadāhamauṣṇyaṃ mahatīmaruciṃ jvaraṃ ca kaphapittam |
janayati kaṇḍūmaṇḍalapiḍakāśatanicitagātrarogacayam ||6||
Symptoms of ūrdhvaga (upward) amlapitta are - vomiting of green, yellow, blue, black, slightly red or bright red coloured very sour materials, resembling mutton wash, very sticky, thin, followed by kapha (expulsion of kapha) and of different tastes (salty, pungent, bitter etc). Vomiting having a bitter or sour taste occurs during digestion of food or even on an empty stomach, occasionally.
Belching is also of similar nature (as that of vomiting). Burning sensation in the throat, chest and upper abdomen and headache are also present. Apart from this there is burning sensation in the palms and soles, feeling of great heat, severe loss of taste, fever of kapha-pitta type, itching, appearance of circular rashes, studded with numerous small vesicles on the skin, indigestion, watery secretions in the mouth and other troubles of the body. (4-6)

Prognosis of Amlapitta

rogo'yamamlapittākhyo yatnāt saṃsādhyate navaḥ |
cirotthito bhavedyāpyaḥ, kṛcchrasādhyaḥ sa kasyacit ||7||
This disease amlapitta - which is of recent onset, responds to treatment with difficulty. The amlapitta which is of long duration will be chronic or curable with difficulty in a few people. (7)

Amlapitta Samsarga

sānilaṃ sānilakaphaṃ sakaphaṃ tacca lakṣayet |
doṣaliṅgena matimān bhiṣaṅmohakaraṃ hi tat ||8||
kampapralāpamūrchācimicimigātrāvasādaśūlāni |
tamaso darśanavibhramavimohaharṣāṇyanilakopāt ||9||

kaphaniṣṭhīvanagauravajaḍatāruciśītasādavamilepāḥ |
dahanabalasādakaṇḍūnidrāścihnaṃ kaphānugate ||10||
ubhayamidameva cihnaṃ mārutakaphasambhave bhavatyamle |
tiktāmlakaṭukodgārahṛtkukṣikaṇṭhadāhakṛt ||11||
bhramo mūrchāruciśchardirālasyaṃ ca śirorujā |
praseko mukhamādhuryaṃ śleṣmapittasya lakṣaṇam ||12||
The physician should clearly recognise the symptoms of amlapitta caused by vata, vata kapha and kapha as they are likely to create confusion to him (and hence the mastery in understanding these conditions is a must).
Vata symptoms – Symptoms caused by vata are - tremors, delirium, fainting, feeling of pins and needles, weakness of the body parts, pain, appearance of darkness before the eyes, giddiness, delusion, horripilation.
Kapha symptoms – Symptoms of kapha are - expectoration of thick phlegm, feeling of heaviness, lassitude, loss of taste, coldness, weakness, vomiting, and coating on the tongue, decrease of digestive strength, itching and excessive sleep.
Appearance of both the above symptoms together is seen in amlapitta in which both vata and kapha are associated.
(Eructation / belching having bitter, sour and pungent tastes, burning sensation in the chest, upper abdomen and throat, giddiness, fainting, loss of taste, vomiting, lassitude, headache, excessive salivation, sweet taste in the mouth are the symptoms of amla-pitta caused by kapha and pitta together.(8-12)

iti śrīmādhavakaraviracite mādhavanidāne'mlapittanidānaṃ samāptam ||51||
Thus ends the chapter on Amlapitta.

CHAPTER FIFTY-TWO

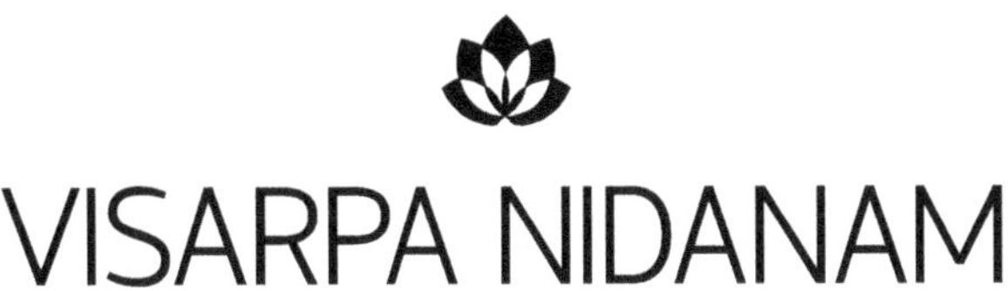

VISARPA NIDANAM

Visarpa Nidana – Etiological factors of Visarpa

lavaṇāmlakaṭūṣṇādisaṃsevādoṣakopataḥ |
visarpaḥ saptadhā jñeyaḥ sarvataḥ parisarpaṇāt ||1||
Ingestion of too much of salty, sour, pungent and hot foods and such other factors would lead to abnormal increase of all the three doshas. These vitiated doshas produce seven types of visarpa. Visarpa is called so because of its nature of spreading all over the body. (1)

Types of Visarpa

pṛthak trayastribhiścaiko visarpā dvandvajāstrayaḥ |
vātikaḥ paittikaścaiva kaphajaḥ sānnipātikaḥ ||2||
catvāra ete vīsarpā vakṣyante dvandvajāstrayaḥ |
āgneyo vātapittābhyāṃ granthyākhyaḥ kaphavātajaḥ ||3||
yastu kardamako ghoraḥ sa pittakaphasambhavaḥ |4|
(ca| ci| a| 21) |
There are seven kinds of visarpa – one from each dosha, one from all three doshas mixed together and three from combination of two doshas. They are –

1. Vataja Visarpa
2. Pittaja Visarpa
3. Kaphaja Visarpa
4. Sannipataja Visarpa
5. Agneya Visarpa – from the combination of vata and pitta
6. Granthi Visarpa – from the combination of kapha and vata

7. Kardama Visarpa – from the combination of pitta and kapha, which is considered dreadful (2-3)

Hetu – Sapta Dhatu (7 body components involved in the causation of visarpa)

raktaṃ lasīkā tvaṅmāṃsaṃ dūṣyaṃ doṣāstrayo malāḥ ||4||
visarpāṇāṃ samutpattau vijñeyāḥ sapta dhātavaḥ |
(ca| ci| a| 21)
The seven factors involved in the causation of visarpa are –

- Dushyas / tissues (4 in number) - Rakta (blood), Lasīkā (lymph), Tvak (skin) and Mamsa (muscles) are the düsyas (tissues involved) and
- Doshas (3 in number) – all the three doshas are involved in the causation of visarpa

The 4 tissues and 3 doshas put together form the seven important (and mandatory) factors responsible for causation of visarpa. (4)

Symptoms of Doshaja Visarpa

tatra vātāt sa vīsarpo vātajvarasamavyathaḥ ||5||
śothasphuraṇanistodabhedāyāsārtiharṣavān |
pittāddrutagatiḥ pittajvaraliṅgo'tilohitaḥ ||6||
kaphāt kaṇḍūyutaḥ snigdhaḥ kaphajvarasamānaruk | (vā| ni| a| 13) |
sannipātasamutthaśca sarvaliṅgasamanvitaḥ ||7||
Vataja visarpa – This type of visarpa has identical symptoms as found in vāta jwara (fever). Along with these there will also be the presence of swelling, pulsations, pricking or splitting (cutting) types of pain, tiredness, body aches and horripilation.
Pittaja visarpa – This type of visarpa would progress quickly and has similar symptoms to those of pittaja jwara and the lesions are dark red in colour.
Kaphaja visarpa – This type of visarpa would have itching and unctuousness of the lesions and its symptoms will be similar to those of kaphaja jwara.
Sannipataja Visarpa – In this type of visarpa caused by aggravation of all the

three doshas, all the symptoms of individual doshaja visarpa will be seen together. (5-7)

Ajgneya Visarpa (Vata-Pittaja Visarpa)

vātapittājjvaracchardimūrchātīsāratṛḍbhramaiḥ |
granthibhedāgnisadanatamakārocakairyutaḥ ||8||
karoti sarvamaṅgaṃ ca dīptāṅgārāvakīrṇavat |
yaṃ yaṃ deśaṃ visarpaśca visarpati bhavet sa saḥ ||9||
śāntāṅgārāsito nīlo rakto vā''śu ca cīyate |
agnidagdha iva sphoṭaiḥ śīghragatvāddrutaṃ sa ca ||10||
marmānusārī vīsarpaḥ syādvāto'tibalastataḥ |
vyathate'ṅgaṃ haret sañjñāṃ nidrāṃ ca śvāsamīrayet ||11||
hikkāṃ ca sa gato'vasthāmīdṛśīṃ labhate na nā |
kvaciccharmāratigrasto bhūmiśayyāsanādiṣu ||12||
ceṣṭamānastataḥ kliṣṭo manodehapramohavān |
duṣprabodho'śnute nidrāṃ so'gnivīsarpa ucyate ||13||
(vā| ni| a| 13) |
Visarpa caused by combination of increased väta and pitta will have the following symptoms –

- fever, vomiting, fainting, diarrhoea, thirst, giddiness,
- bursting pain in the glands or joints
- poor digestion capacity
- experiencing darkness before the eyes
- loss of taste
- feeling as if the whole body, mainly the affected part of the body has been covered by and is in contact with burning charcoal,
- the skin of the part or parts of the body to which visarpa spreads becomes black or blue just like burning coal which has calmed down and that area quickly gets covered by blebs resembling fire burns, the lesions quickly spread out to other places,
- visarpa gets located in the vital spots or organs (marma) quickly due to the quick spreading nature of the disease,
- (due to this) the vata gets aggravated and produces pain and trouble in the affected parts, and causes loss of consciousness and sleep, hiccough and dyspnoea (difficulty in breathing)

- the patient having reached this condition does not find even slightest of relief with anything and anywhere, he becomes restless sleeps (lays) or sits on the ground repeatedly, while doing so he would faint becoming severely distressed and would enter into a deep sleep (which is equivalent to death) from which he cannot wake up again (dies). This type of visarpa is known as Agni Visarpa. (8-13)

Granthi Visarpa (Vata-Kaphaja Visarpa)

kaphena ruddhaḥ pavano bhittvā taṃ bahudhā kapham |
raktaṃ vā vṛddharaktasya tvaksirāsnāyumāṃsagam ||14||
dūṣayitvā tu dīrghāṇuvṛttasthūlakharātmanām |
granthīnāṃ kurute mālāṃ saraktāṃ tīvrarugjvarām ||15||
śvāsakāsātisārāsyaśoṣahikkāvamibhramaiḥ |
mohavaivarṇyamūrchāṅgabhaṅgāgnisadanairyutām ||16||
ityayaṃ granthivīsarpaḥ kaphamārutakopajaḥ |17|
(vā| ni| a| 13) |
Visarpa caused by combination of increased väta and kapha will have the following symptoms –
Väta getting obstructed by kapha in turn spreads the kapha immensely in the body. Or in a person in whom the blood has already undergone abnormal increase, vata would vitiate the blood located in the skin, veins, ligaments (and tendons) and muscles. Following these events vata would produce chains of tumours (cystic swellings) which are elongated, small, round, hard or rough. These cysts are red in colour, painful and associated with fever. Other symptoms include dyspnoea (difficulty in breathing), cough, diarrhoea, dryness of the mouth, hiccough, vomiting, giddiness, delusion, discolouration, fainting, pain all over the body and poor digestion. This disease caused by vitiated vata and kapha together is called as Granthi Visarpa. (14-16)

Kardama Visarpa (Kapha-Pittaja Visarpa)

kaphapittājjvaraḥ stambho nidrā tandrā śirorujā ||17||
aṅgāvasādavikṣepau pralepārocakabhramāḥ |
mūrchāgnihānirbhedo'sthnāṃ pipāsendriyagauravam ||18||

āmopaveśanaṃ lepaḥ srotasāṃ sa ca sarpati |
prāyeṇāmāśayaṃ gṛhṇannekadeśaṃ na cātiruk ||19||
piḍakairavakīrṇo'tipītalohitapāṇḍuraiḥ |
snigdho'sito mecakābho malinaḥ śothavān guruḥ ||20||
gambhīrapākaḥ prājyoṣmā spṛṣṭaḥ klinno'vadīryate |
paṅkavacchīrṇamāṃsaśca spaṣṭasnāyusirāgaṇaḥ ||21||
śavagandhī ca vīsarpaḥ kardamākhyamuśanti tam |22| (vā| ni| a| 13) |
Visarpa caused by combination of increased kapha and pitta will have the following symptoms –

- fever, stiffness of the body parts, stupor, sleep, headache,
- weakness of the body parts, involuntary movements of the body parts, coating of the tongue, loss of taste, giddiness,
- fainting, destruction of digestive fire (loss of digestive functions), splitting pain in the bones, thirst, dullness (heaviness) of the sense organs,
- excretion of faeces mixed with ama (inadequately formed faeces or faeces mixed with undigested portions of foods)
- coating of thick material which leads to obstruction in the channels of the body (orifices, cell pores, tissue spaces, passages of transportation etc)
- this type of visarpa probably invades the stomach or one side of the body and presents with mild pain,
- it is surrounded by small tumours which are of deep yellow, red, pale, unctuous, black, dark black like collyrium and dirty
- they are swollen, heavy, undergoes suppuration deep within (pus is formed inside) and excessively hot,
- since the lesions are filled with fluids, they mostly burst out discharging the pus on touching them
- the muscles become loose, semi-liquid like silt and fall off exposing the network of tendons and veins and emits smell resembling that of a dead body

This type of visarpa is called as Kardama Visarpa. (17-21)

Ksata Visarpa

bāhyahetoḥ kṣatāt kruddhaḥ saraktaṃ pittamīrayan ||22||
vīsarpaṃ mārutaḥ kuryāt kulatthasadṛśaiścitam |
sphoṭaiḥ śothajvararujādāhāḍhyaṃ śyāvaśoṇitam ||23|| (vā| ni| a| 13) |
Another variety of visarpa is caused by ksata (external injury).
Vata aggravated due to external injury would provoke blood along with pitta and cause visarpa. In this, vesicles of the size of horse gram appear all over the body and are associated with swelling, fever, pain and burning sensation. The lesions have blackish blue or blood colour. (22-23)

Complications of Visarpa

jvarātisārau vamathustvaṅmāṃsadaraṇaṃ klamaḥ |
arocakāvipākau ca visarpāṇāmupadravāḥ ||24||
The complications of visarpa are Fever, diarrhoea, vomiting, cracking / fissuring of skin and muscles, exhaustion, loss of taste and indigestion are the complications of visarpa. (24)

Prognosis of Visarpa
sidhyanti vātakaphapittakṛtā visarpāḥ sarvātmakaḥ kṣatakṛtaśca na siddhimeti |
pittātmako'ñjanavapuśca bhavedasādhyaḥ kṛcchrāśca marmasu bhavanti hi sarva eva ||25||
(su| ni| a| 10) |
Visarpas produced by anyone dosha – i.e., vata, kapha and pitta are curable. The tridoshaja and ksataja visarpas do not respond to the treatment.
Visarpa produced by pitta and that in which the body becomes black like anjana (eye salve, collyrium) are incurable. Visarpa which occurs on the vital spots / organs are difficult to cure. (25)

iti śrīmādhavakaraviracite mādhavanidāne visarpanidānaṃ samāptam ||52||
Thus ends the chapter on Visarpa.

CHAPTER FIFTY-THREE

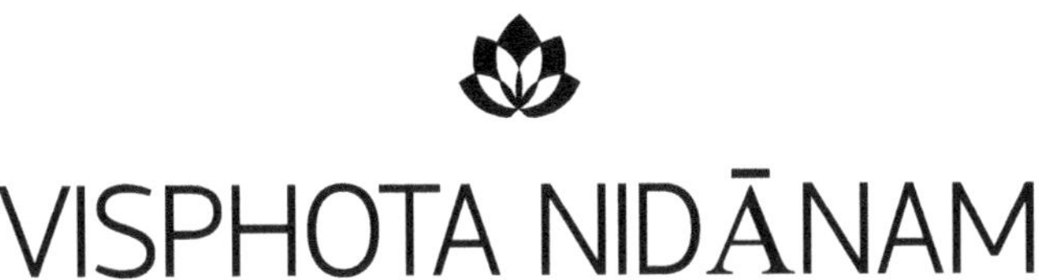

VISPHOTA NIDĀNAM

Nidana, Samprapti – Etiological factors and pathogenesis of Visphota

kaṭvamlatīkṣṇoṣṇavidāhirūkṣakṣārairajīrṇādhyaśanātapaiśca |
tathartudoṣeṇa viparyayeṇa kupyanti doṣāḥ pavanādayastu ||1||
tvacamāśritya te raktamāṃsāsthīni pradūṣya ca |
ghorān kurvanti visphoṭān sarvān jvarapuraḥsarān ||2||
Etiological Factors – excessive indulgence in foods which are pungent and sour in taste, penetrating, hot, those producing burning sensation (corrosive), dry, alkaline, uncooked and in excessive quantity, exposure to sun-light, bad effects of seasons (due to exposure to excessive heat, wind, cold etc) and abnormal seasons (excessive cold in summer, excessive cold in summer etc) are the etiological factors of visphota.
Pathogenesis – The above said etiological factors cause aggravation of vata and other doshas (pitta, kapha). These doshas in turn get lodged in the skin and contaminate blood, muscles and bones and produce many dreadful vesicles on the skin preceded by fever. (This condition is called visphota). (1-2)

Nature of Visarpa

agnidagdhanibhāḥ sphoṭāḥ sajvarā raktapittajāḥ |
kvacit sarvatra vā dehe visphoṭā iti te smṛtāḥ ||3|| (su| ni| a| 13) |
Vesicles resembling boils formed by the touch of fire (boils which occur due to fire burns), caused by aggravation of blood and pitta, associated with fever, occurring in some or all the parts of the body is known as Visphota. (3)

Symptoms of doshaja visarpa

śiroruk śūlabhūyiṣṭhaṃ jvarastṛṭ parvabhedanam |
sakṛṣṇavarṇatā ceti vātavisphoṭalakṣaṇam ||4||
jvaradāharujāsrāvapākatṛṣṇābhiranvitam |
pītalohitavarṇaṃ ca pittavisphoṭalakṣaṇam ||5||
chardyarocakajāḍyāni kaṇḍūkāṭhinyapāṇḍutāḥ |
avedanaściratpākī sa visphoṭaḥ kaphātmakaḥ ||6||
vātapittakṛto yastu kurute tīvravedanām |
kaṇḍūstaimityagurubhirjānīyāt kaphavātikam ||7||
kaṇḍūrdāho jvaraśchardiretaistu kaphapaittikaḥ |8|
Vataja Visphota – The symptoms of visphota caused by predominance of vata are headache, severe pain, fever, thirst, splitting pain in the small joints of the hands and feet and the manifestation of vesicles which are black in colour.
Pittaja Visphota – The symptoms of visphota caused by predominance of pitta are – fever, burning sensation, pain, discharges (exudates), suppuration (formation of pus), thirst and formation of vesicles which are yellow or red in colour.
Kaphaja Visphota – The symptoms of visphota caused by predominance of kapha are – vomiting, loss of taste, lassitude, itching, hardness, pallor, lack of pain and formation of vesicles which undergo slow suppuration.
Vata-pittaja Visphota – presents with severe pain.
Vata-kaphaja Visphota – presents with itching, feeling of being covered with wet leather or cloth and heaviness.
Kapha-pittaja Visphota – presents with itching, burning sensation, fever and vomiting. (4-7)

Sannipataja Visphota

madhye nimnonnato'nte ca kaṭhino'lpaprapākavān ||8||
dāharāgatṛṣāmohacchardimūrchārujājvarāḥ |
pralāpo vepathustandrā so'sādhyaḥ syāttridoṣajaḥ ||9||
The visphota (vesicles) caused by simultaneous aggravation of all the three doshas will have depression in the centre and are elevated at the edges, are hard and undergo less suppuration (with little quantity of pus in them). This condition is associated with burning sensation, redness, thirst, delusion, vomiting, fainting, pain, fever, delirium, tremors, and stupor. This

condition is incurable. (8-9)

Raktaja Visphota

raktā raktasamutthānā guñjāvidrumasannibhāḥ |
veditavyāstu raktena paittikena ca hetunā ||10||
na te siddhiṃ samāyānti siddhairyogaśatairapi |
Visphota caused by rakta (vitiated blood) will have vesicles which are red in colour resembling guñjā seed (Abrus precatorius) or coral bead. They are caused by blood vitiated by pitta aggravating etiological factors. They do not respond to any kinds of treatments even by administering hundreds of efficient recipes. (10)

Prognosis of Visphota

ekadoṣotthitaḥ sādhyaḥ kṛcchrasādhyo dvidoṣajaḥ |
sarvadoṣotthito ghorastvasādhyo bhūryupadravaḥ ||11||
Visphota caused by single dosha is curable.
Visphota caused by simultaneous aggravation of two doshas is curable with difficulty.
Visphota caused by simultaneous aggravation of all the three doshas and that which is associated with complications is incurable. (11)

iti śrīmādhavakaraviracite mādhavanidāne visphoṭanidānaṃ samāptam ||53||
Thus ends the chapter on Visphota.

CHAPTER FIFTY-FOUR

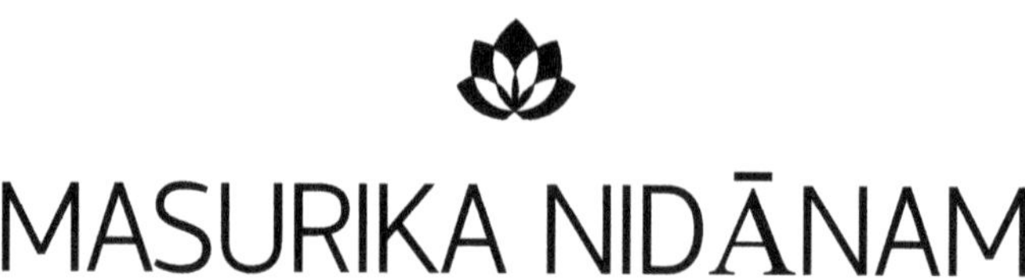

MASURIKA NIDĀNAM

Masurika Nidana – Etiological factors of Masurika

kaṭvamlalavaṇakṣāraviruddhādhyaśanāśanaiḥ |
duṣṭaniṣpāvaśākādyaiḥ praduṣṭapavanodakaiḥ ||1||
krūragrahekṣaṇāccāpi deśe doṣāḥ samuddhatāḥ |
janayanti śarīre'smin duṣṭaraktena saṅgatāḥ ||2||
masūrākṛtisaṃsthānāḥ piḍakāḥ syurmasūrikāḥ |
Below mentioned are the causative factors of masurika –

- excessive indulgence in foods which are pungent, sour, salty, alkaline and of incompatible nature (mutually opposite / antagonist foods)
- intake of foods in large quantities too frequently
- excessive consumption of contaminated foods, beans, and leafy vegetables
- excessive and repeated exposure to contaminated air and water
- influence of bad planetary positions (seeing bad planets which influences on certain areas of the country (in community of people)

Pathogenesis – Due to the above said etiological factors the doshas get aggravated in the entire body. These doshas get associated with the contaminated blood and produce eruptions on the body which resemble masura – lentils in shape and size and hence the name masurika. (1-2)

Masurika Purvarupa – Premonitory symptoms of Masurika

tāsāṃ pūrvaṃ jvaraḥ kaṇḍūrgātrabhaṅgo'ratirbhramaḥ ||3||

tvaci śothaḥ savaivarṇyo netrarāgaśca jāyate |4|
The premonitory symptoms of masurika include fever, itching, breaking pain all over the body, restlessness, giddiness, swelling in the skin, discolouration of skin and redness of the eyes. (3)

Vataja Masurika

sphoṭāḥ śyāvāruṇā rūkṣāstīvravedanayā'nvitāḥ ||4||
kaṭhināścirapākāśca bhavantyanilasambhavāḥ |
sandhyasthiparvaṇāṃ bhedaḥ kāsaḥ kampo'ratiḥ klamaḥ ||5||
śoṣastālvoṣṭhajihvānāṃ tṛṣṇā cārucisaṃyutā |6|
The symptoms of masurika caused by predominant vitiation of vata are – manifestation of eruptions which are black or crimson in colour, dry, severely painful, hard and undergo slow suppuration. This condition is also associated with splitting pain in the joints, bones and small joints of the hands and feet, cough, tremors, restlessness, exhaustion, dryness of the palate, lips and tongue, thirst and loss of taste. (4-5)

Pittaja Masurika

raktāḥ pītāsitāḥ sphoṭāḥ sadāhāstīvravedanāḥ ||6||
bhavantyacirapākāśca pittakopasamudbhavāḥ |
viḍbhedaścāṅgamardaśca dāhastṛṣṇā'rucistathā ||7||
mukhapāko'kṣirāgaśca jvarastīvraḥ sudāruṇaḥ |8|
The symptoms of masurika caused by predominant vitiation of pitta are – manifestation of eruptions which are red or yellowish white in colour associated with severe burning sensation and pain. These eruptions will undergo suppuration quickly. The patient would also have diarrhoea, pain as if someone has beaten all over the body, burning sensation, thirst, loss of taste, stomatitis (ulcerations in the mouth), redness of the eyes, very high fever and great distress. (6-7)

Raktaja Masurika

raktajāyāṃ bhavantyete vikārāḥ pittalakṣaṇāḥ ||8||
The symptoms of masurika caused by predominant vitiation of rakta (blood) are similar to those of pittaja masurika. (8)

Kaphaja Masurika

kaphaprasekaḥ staimityaṃ śirorug gātragauravam |
hṛllāsaḥ sārucirnidrā tandrālasyasamanvitāḥ ||9||
śvetāḥ snigdhā bhṛśaṃ sthūlāḥ kaṇḍūrā mandavedanāḥ ||
masūrikāḥ kaphotthāśca cirapākāḥ prakīrtitāḥ ||10||
The symptoms of masurika caused by predominant vitiation of kapha are – excessive salivation (watery discharges from the mouth), feeling as though the body has been covered by wet leather or cloth, headache, heaviness of the body, nausea, loss of taste, excessive sleep, stupor and lassitude. The eruptions are white in colour, are unctuous, big in size, and are associated with itching and mild pain. In these eruptions the suppuration is slow. (9-10)

Sannipataja Masurika

nīlāścipiṭavistīrṇā madhye nimnā mahārujāḥ |
cirapākāḥ pūtisrāvāḥ prabhūtāḥ sarvadoṣajāḥ ||11||
kaṇṭharodhārucistambhapralāpāratisaṃyutāḥ |
duścikitsyāḥ samuddiṣṭāḥ piḍakāścarmasañjñitāḥ ||12||
The symptoms of masurika caused by predominant vitiation of all three doshas together are – manifestation of eruptions which are blue in colour, flat, broad, depressed in the centre (and elevated at its edges) and severely painful. There is slow suppuration in these eruptions. Large quantities of foul-smelling discharges come out of the eruptions (pus with offensive smell). There is also obstruction in the throat, loss of taste, stiffness of the body, delirium and restlessness. This condition is also called Carmapidaka. This condition caused by aggravation of all the three doshas together is difficult to treat. (11-12)

Romantika

romakūponnatisamā rāgiṇyaḥ kaphapittajāḥ |
kāsārocakasaṃyuktā romāntyo jvarapūrvikāḥ ||13||
Small, red eruptions occurring at the roots of the hairs making slight elevations which appear like raised sweat glands / pores, caused by

abnormal increase of kapha and pitta are called Romantika (measles). This condition is associated with cough, loss of taste and preceded by fever. (13)

Dhatugata Masurika

toyabudbudasaṅkāśāstvaggatāstu masūrikāḥ |
svalpadoṣāḥ prajāyante bhinnāstoyaṃ sravanti ca ||14||
raktasthā lohitākārāḥ śīghrapākāstanutvacaḥ |
sādhyā nātyarthaduṣṭāśca bhinnā raktaṃ sravanti ca ||15||
māṃsasthāḥ kaṭhināḥ snigdhāścirapākā ghanatvacaḥ |
gātraśūlatṛṣākaṇḍūjvarāratisamanvitāḥ ||16||
medojā maṇḍalākārā mṛdavaḥ kiñcidunnatāḥ |
ghorajvaraparītāśca sthūlāḥ snigdhāḥ savedanāḥ ||17||
sammohāratisantāpāḥ kaścidābhyo vinistaret |
kṣudrā gātrasamā rūkṣāścipiṭāḥ kiñcidunnatāḥ ||18||
majjotthā bhṛśasammohavedanāratisaṃyutāḥ |
chindanti marmadhāmāni prāṇānāśu haranti hi ||19||
bhramareṇeva viddhāni kurvantyasthīni sarvataḥ |
pakvābhāḥ piḍakāḥ snigdhāḥ sūkṣmāścātyarthavedanāḥ ||20||
staimityāratisammohadāhonmādasamanvitāḥ |
śukrajāyāṃ masūryāṃ tu lakṣaṇāni bhavanti hi ||21||
nirdiṣṭaṃ kevalaṃ cihnaṃ dṛśyate na tu jīvitam |
doṣamiśrāstu saptaitā draṣṭavyā doṣalakṣaṇaiḥ ||22||
tvaggatā raktajāścaiva pittajāḥ śleṣmajāstathā |
śleṣmapittakṛtāścaiva sukhasādhyā masūrikāḥ ||23||
Twak-gata Masurika – When masurika is localised in the skin (affecting the rasa tissue), the eruptions would appear like water bubbles, discharge thin watery fluid on pricking and will have mild aggravation of doshas.
Raktagata Masurika - If Masurika is localized in the blood tissue, the eruptions would be red in colour, suppurates quickly, with thin skin. These are curable when they do not have severe vitiation of doshas. When these eruptions are pricked, they discharge blood.
Mamsagata Masurika – When the disease is localized in the muscle tissue, the eruptions are hard, unctuous, undergo suppuration slowly, and are covered with a thick layer of skin. This condition is associated with pain all over the body, thirst, itching, fever and restlessness.
Medogata Masurika – If the disease masurika invades and gets localized in

the fat tissue there is manifestation of eruptions which are in the form of round patches, soft and slightly elevated, large, unctuous (greasy), painful and accompanied with very high fever, delusion, restlessness and distress (raised heat in the body and mind). Few people would get over these conditions.

Majjagata Masurika – If masurika is localized in the bone marrow there is manifestation of eruptions which are small in size, have the same colour as that of the skin, dry, flat or slightly elevated. It is associated with severe delusion, pain, and restlessness.

Asthigata Masurika - If masurika is localized in the bones, there will be cutting pain in the marmas i.e., vital organs which would pose threat to life. The bones would appear as though many bees have made many holes (perforations) in the bones (pain in the bones as though stung by bees).

Shukragata Masurika – When masurika gets lodged in the semen, there is a manifestation of eruptions which are ripened, unctuous (greasy, waxy), small in size, severely painful. The person would feel as if covered by wet leather or cloth and will also experience restlessness, delusion, burning sensation and insanity (intoxication). The symptoms of this condition are formally explained. In any case, the patient would lose his life quickly.

These (above said) seven types of masurika located in the tissues are always associated with vata and other (pitta, kapha) doshas. Therefore, they might have symptoms of one or more of the increased doshas. They should be understood on the basis of the symptoms of increased doshas associated with masurika located in the tissues.

Masurika resides in the skin and blood, and those caused by vitiated pitta, kapha and kapha-pitta are easy to cure. (14-23)

Prognosis of Masurika

vātajā vātapittotthāḥ śleṣmavātakṛtāśca yāḥ |
kṛcchrasādhyatamāstasmādyatnādetā upācaret ||24||
asādhyāḥ sannipātotthāstāsāṃ vakṣyāmi lakṣaṇam |
pravālasadṛśāḥ kāścit kāścijjambūphalopamāḥ ||25||
lohajālasamāḥ kāścidatasīphalasannibhāḥ |
āsāṃ bahuvidhā varṇā jāyante doṣabhedataḥ ||26||

Masurika caused by vata, vāta-pitta, kapha-vata are very difficult to cure. Therefore, they shall be treated with great care and effort.

Masurika caused by sannipata i.e., all the vitiated doshas combined together is incurable. Their symptoms are hereby explained. The eruptions resemble coral beads in colour, and some resemble fruits of jambu (Eugenia jambolana) and some others appear like an iron sieve. Some others resemble fruits of atasi (linseed).
The eruptions of masurika will also have many other colours depending on the type of dosha or doshas involved therein. (24-26)

Other symptoms of incurability of masurika

kāso hikkā pramehaśca jvarastīvraḥ sudāruṇaḥ |
pralāpaścāratirmūrchā tṛṣṇā dāho'tighūrṇatā ||27||
mukhena prasravedraktaṃ tathā ghrāṇena cakṣuṣā |
kaṇṭhe ghurghurakaṃ kṛtvā śvasityatyarthavedanam ||28||
masūrikābhibhūtasya yasyaitāni bhiṣagvaraiḥ |
lakṣaṇāni ca dṛśyante na dadyādatra bheṣajam ||29||
When the below mentioned symptoms are found in a patient suffering from masurika he should not be administered with medicines and should be refused treatment (since it indicates that masurika associated with these symptoms is incurable) –

- cough,
- hiccough,
- diabetes,
- high fever,
- severe delirium,
- restlessness,
- fainting,
- thirst,
- burning sensation,
- excessive curvature of the body (cramps, excessive yawning)
- bleeding from the mouth, nose and eyes
- patient breathes with severe pain and difficulty while making cooing sounds in the throat (27-29)

Other symptoms of incurability

masūrikābhibhūto yo bhṛśaṃ ghrāṇena niḥśvaset |
sa bhṛśaṃ tyajati prāṇāṃstṛṣārto vāyudūṣitaḥ ||30||
The patient of masurika who is breathing only through his nose (very shallow breathing), has severe thirst and whose vata is severely aggravated, is definitely going to die soon. (30)

Upadrava – complications of masurika

masūrikānte śothaḥ syāt kūrpare maṇibandhake |
tathāṃ'saphalake cāpi duścikitsyaḥ sudāruṇaḥ ||31||
When at the end of masurika (last stages of masurika), if the patient develops profound swelling in the elbow, wrist and shoulder joints (shoulder blades, scapulae), the disease should be considered as incurable. (31)

iti śrīmādhavakaraviracite mādhavanidāne masūrikānidānaṃ samāptam ||54||
Thus ends the chapter on Masūrikā.

CHAPTER FIFTY-FIVE

KṢUDRA ROGA NIDĀNAM

Ajagallika

snigdhāḥ savarṇā granthitā nīrujo mudgasannibhāḥ |
kaphavātotthitā jñeyā bālānāmajagallikāḥ ||1||
(su| ni| a| 13) |
A disease characterised by appearance of papules which are unctuous (waxy, oily), having the same colour of the skin (not discoloured), having cystic appearance (nodular), devoid of pain and resemble green gram (in size and appearance), caused by abnormal increase of kapha and vata together, especially occurring in children, is called by the name ajagallika. (1)

Yavaprakhya

yavākārā sukaṭhinā grathitā māṃsasaṃśritā |
piḍakā kaphavātābhyāṃ yavaprakhyeti socyate ||2||
(su| ni| a| 13) |
Papules of the size of barley, hard, nodular, localized in the muscles and caused by combined vitiation of kapha and vata is known as Yavaprakhya. (2)

Antralaji

ghanāmavaktrāṃ piḍakāmunnatāṃ parimaṇḍalām |
antrālajīmalpapūyāṃ tāṃ vidyāt kaphavātajām ||3||
(su| ni| a| 13) |
A big (stout) papule without an opening, raised, round in shape, having less

quantity of pus in it and caused by simultaneous aggravation of kapha and vata is known as Antralaji (or Andhalaji). (3)

Vivruta

vivṛtāsyāṃ mahādāhāṃ pakvodumbarasannibhām |
vivṛtāmiti tāṃ vidyāt pittotthāṃ parimaṇḍalām ||4||
(su| ni| a| 13) |
That which has a wide opening, is associated with severe burning sensation, is of the colour (size) of a ripened udumbara fruit
(Ficus glomerata), round in shape, and produced by increased pitta is known as Vivrta. (4)

Kacchapika

grathitāḥ pañca vā ṣaḍvā dāruṇāḥ kacchapopamāḥ |
kaphānilābhyāṃ piḍakā jñeyāḥ kacchapikā budhaiḥ ||5||
(su| ni| a| 13) |
Five or six piḍakās (papules), nodular (hard), resembling the shell of a tortoise caused by increased kapha and vāta together is named as Kacchapikā by the wise. (5)

Valmika

grīvāṃsakakṣākarapādadeśe sandhau gale vā tribhireva doṣaiḥ |
granthiḥ sa valmīkavadakriyāṇāṃ jātaḥ krameṇaiva gataḥ pravṛddhim ||6||
mukhairanekaiḥ srutitodavadbhirvisarpavat sarpati connatāgraiḥ |
valmīkamāhurbhiṣajo vikāraṃ niṣpratyanīkaṃ cirajaṃ viśeṣāt ||7||
A granthi (tumour / cystic swelling) caused by increase of all the three doshas together, resembling an ants' hill, appear in the neck, shoulder (shoulder blade, scapular region), axilla (arm pits), hands, feet, bony joints or throat regions. If this is not treated properly on time, it gradually increases in size. It will have many mouths (openings) discharging fluids, with pricking pain, spreading to other parts of the body like visarpa (erysipelas), with pointed sprouts. Such a chronic disease (which has not been treated for a long time) is incurable and has been named as Valmika by the wise physicians. (6-7)

Indraviddha

padmakarṇikavanmadhye piḍakābhiḥ samācitām |
indraviddhāṃ tu tāṃ vidyādvātapittotthitāṃ bhiṣak ||8||
(su| ni| a| 13) |
Small pidakās (papules) spread out in the centre, resembling the central part of a lotus flower – which consists of seeds of lotus centred in a capsule, caused by increased väta and pitta together is known to physicians as Indraviddhā. (8)

Gardhabhika

maṇḍalaṃ vṛttamutsannaṃ saraktaṃ piḍakācitam |
rujākarīṃ gardabhikāṃ tāṃ vidyādvātapittajām ||9||
Round, elevated, red mandalas (patches), studded with small pidakas (papules) causing pain is known as Gardhabhika. This condition is caused by vatapitta – vata and pitta increased together. (9)

Pasanagardabha

vātaśleṣmasamudbhūtaḥ śvayathurhanusandhijaḥ |
sthiro mandarujaḥ snigdho jñeyaḥ pāṣāṇagardabhaḥ ||10||
A sotha (swelling) which is caused due to simultaneous vitiation of vata and kapha, manifesting in the joint of the lower jaw, which is fixed (hard), has mild pain and is unctuous (greasy, oily appearance) is known as Pāsanagardabha (10)"

Panasika

karṇasyābhyantare jātāṃ piḍakāmugravedanām |
sthirāṃ panasikāṃ tāṃ tu vidyādvātakaphotthitām ||11||
A pidakā (papule) occurring inside the ear, associated with severe pain, is fixed (hard) and caused by increased vata and kapha together is known as Panasika. (11)

Jalagardabha

visarpavat sarpati yaḥ śothastanurapākavān |
dāhajvarakaraḥ pittāt sa jñeyo jālagardabhaḥ ||12||
(su| ni| a| 13) |
A thin swelling which spreads quickly like visarpa (herpes, erysipelas), without undergoing suppuration (without pus being formed) and associated with burning sensation and fever, caused by increased pitta is known as Jalagardabha. (12)

Irivellika

piḍakāmuttamāṅgasthāṃ vṛttāmugrarujājvarām |
sarvātmikāṃ sarvaliṅgāṃ jānīyādirivellikām ||13||
A pidaka (papule) which occurs on the head, round, associated with severe pain, fever, caused by all the three doshas and having symptoms of increase of all the three doshas together, is known as Irivellika. (13)

Kaksa

bāhupārśvāṃsakakṣeṣu kṛṣṇasphoṭāṃ savedanām |
pittaprakopasambhūtāṃ kakṣāmityabhinirdiśet ||14||
(su| ni| a| 13) |
Black coloured painful sphota (vesicle) appearing on arms, flanks, or sides of the arms, shoulders (shoulder blade, scapular region), or axillae, caused due to increase of pitta is known as Kaksa. (14)

Gandhamala

ekāmetādṛśīṃ dṛṣṭvā piḍakāṃ sphoṭasannibhām |
tvaggatāṃ pittakopena gandhamālāṃ pracakṣate ||15||
(su| ni| a| 13) |
A single papule which is similar to the above-mentioned vesicle (which is similar to that explained in Kaksa – in the above context) manifesting superficially on the skin, which bursts out and is caused by increased pitta is called Gandhamala. (15)

Agnirohini

kakṣabhāgeṣu ye sphoṭā jāyante māṃsadāraṇāḥ |
antardāhajvarakarā dīptapāvakasannibhāḥ ||16||
saptāhādvā daśāhādvā pakṣādvā hanti mānavam |
tāmagnirohiṇīṃ vidyādasādhyāṃ sarvadoṣajām ||17||
(su| ni| a| 13) |
Sphotas (vesicles) developing in the axillae, which tears or bursts (burrow) deep into the muscles (and destroy them), associated with severe burning sensation inside the body and fever as if being enveloped by burning fire (being burnt by fire), which kills the patient within seven, ten or fifteen days is known as Agnirohini. It is caused by all the three doshas (aggravated together) and is said to be incurable. (16-17)

Cippa

nakhamāṃsamadhiṣṭhāya vāyuḥ pittaḥ ca dehinām |
kurvate dāhapākau ca taṃ vyādhiṃ cippamādiśet ||18||
tadevālpatarairdoṣaiḥ paruṣaṃ kunakhaṃ vadet ||19||
(su| ni| a| 13) |
Vata and pitta which have undergone increase together get lodged in the muscles in and around the nails and produce burning sensation and suppuration (formation of pus) therein. This disease is called as Cippa. Kunakha is a similar condition caused by mild increase of doshas. (18-19)

Anusayi

gambhīrāmalpasaṃrambhāṃ savarṇāmuparisthitām |
pādasyānuśayīṃ tāṃ tu vidyādantaḥprapākinīm ||20||
(su| ni| a| 13) |
A mild swelling which occurs on the upper portion of the foot and suppurates (produces pus) from deep inside and thus deep seated, has same colour of the skin (no discolouration), is known as Anusayi. (20)

Vidarika

vidārīkandavadvṛttā kakṣāvaṅkṣaṇasandhiṣu |
vidārikā bhavedraktā sarvajā sarvalakṣaṇā ||21||

(su| ni| a| 13) |
A round papule resembling vidarikanda (tuber of Pueraria tuberosa), manifesting in the joints around axillae or groins, red in colour, caused by and presenting the symptoms of all the three doshas together is known as Vidarika. (21)

Sarkararbudam

prāpya māṃsasirāsnāyūḥ śleṣmā medastathā'nilaḥ |
granthiṃ karotyasau bhinno madhusarpirvasānibham ||22||
sravatyāsrāvamanilastatra vṛddhiṃ gataḥ punaḥ |
māṃsaṃ saṃśoṣya grathitāṃ śarkarāṃ janayettataḥ ||23||
durgandhi klinnamatyarthaṃ nānāvarṇaṃ tataḥ sirāḥ |
sravanti raktaṃ sahasā taṃ vidyāccharkarārbudam ||24||
(su| ni| a| 13) |
Kapha, medas and vata undergoing increase invade the muscles, veins and ligaments (tendons, nerves), and produce a granthi (cystic swelling, tumour). When it bursts open discharges (exudates) resembling honey, ghee or muscle fat flow out of it. In due course of time, the vata aggravated (as an effect of destruction of tissues) dries up the muscles and produces small nodules which appear like sand particles in the muscles. Due to this, the veins instantly discharge excessive foul-smelling blood, containing watery content and of different colours. This condition is called as Sarkararbuda. (22-24)

Padadari

parikramaṇaśīlasya vāyuratyartharūkṣayoḥ |
pādayoḥ kurute dārīṃ pādadārīṃ tamādiśet ||25||
(su| ni| a| 13) |
In persons who are in the habit of walking too much (on rough ground without footwear), the vata gets aggravated and produces fissures in the extremely dried (soles of the) feet. This condition is known as Padadari. (25)

Kadara

śarkaronmathite pāde kṣate vā kaṇṭakādibhiḥ |
granthiḥ kolavadutsanno jāyate kadaraṃ hi tat ||26||
(su| ni| a| 13) |
When the foot gets pressed by (due to walking on) gravel or rough stones (without footwear) or gets injured (due to prick by) thorns etc, small (cystic) raised swelling of the size of a jujube fruit (Ziziphus jujuba) develop on (the sole) them. This condition is known as Kadara. (26)

Alasa

klinnāṅgulyantarau pādau kaṇḍūdāharujānvitau |
duṣṭakardamasaṃsparśādalasaṃ taṃ vibhāvayet ||27||
(su| ni| a| 13) |
Alasa is a disease characterized by ulcers formed between the toes from which discharges (exudation) occur (dampness between the toes), associated with itching, burning sensation and pain. This is caused by contact with contaminated slush. (27)

Indralupta

romakūpānugaṃ pittaṃ vātena saha mūrchitam |
pracyāvayati romāṇi tataḥ śleṣmā saśoṇitaḥ ||28||
ruṇaddhi romakūpāṃstu tato'nyeṣāmasambhavaḥ |
tadindraluptaṃ khālityaṃ ruhyeti ca vibhāvyate ||29||
(su| ni| a| 13) |
Increased pitta (Bhrajaka subtype) presents at the root of the body hairs, on getting association with (increased) vata, causes the hairs to fall off. Following this, increased kapha and blood together block the hair follicles (pores). This will not allow the new hairs to grow. This condition is known as Indralupta, Khalitya or Ruhya. (28-29)

Darunaka

dāruṇā kaṇḍurā rūkṣā keśabhūmiḥ prapāṭyate |
kaphamārutakopena vidyāddāruṇakaṃ tu tam ||30||
(su| ni| a| 13) |
The skin on the scalp gets cracked, becomes hard (rough) and dry and will

itch due to increase of kapha and vata together. This is known as Darunaka. (30)

Arumshika

arūṃṣi bahuvaktrāṇi bahukledīni mūrdhni tu |
kaphāsṛkkrimikopena nṛṇāṃ vidyādarūṃṣikām ||31||
(su| ni| a| 13) |
Small ulcers with many openings manifesting on the skin of the scalp, having discharges, caused due to aggravation of kapha, blood and worms (bacteria, infection) are called as Arumsika. (31)

Palita

krodhaśokaśramakṛtaḥ śarīroṣmā śirogataḥ |
pittaṃ ca keśān pacati palitaṃ tena jāyate ||32||
(su| ni| a| 13) |
The heat of the body produced by frequent bouts of anger, grief and physical strain (fatigue) reach the head along with increased pitta and make the hairs grey. This condition in which there is greying of hairs is known as palita. (32)

Yuvanapidaka

śālmalīkaṇṭakaprakhyāḥ kaphamārutaraktajāḥ |
yuvānapiḍakā yūnāṃ vijñeyā mukhadūṣikāḥ ||33||
(su| ni| a| 13) |34|
Papules resembling the sprouts (thorns, spikes) on the bark of salmali tree (Bombax malabaricum) appear on the face of adolescents caused by increase of kapha, vata and blood together is known as yuvanapidaka or mukhsdusika. (33)

Padminikantaka

kaṇṭakairācitaṃ vṛttaṃ maṇḍalaṃ pāṇḍukaṇḍuram |
padminīkaṇṭakaprakhyaistadākhyaṃ kaphavātajam ||34||
(su| ni| a| 13) |

Circular, pale (white) and itchy patches, studded with papules resembling thorn like projections of lotus flower, caused by increased kapha and vata together is called as Padminikantaka. (34)

Jatumani

samamutsannamarujaṃ maṇḍalaṃ kapharaktajam |
sahajaṃ lakṣma caikeṣāṃ lakṣyo jatumaṇistu saḥ ||35||
(su| ni| a| 13) |
A congenital, even or slightly elevated, painless patch on the skin caused by increased kapha and rakta (blood) together is known as jatumani. According to the opinion of other experts it is called Laksma / Janmajata Lakshana. (35)

Masaka

avedanaṃ sthiraṃ caiva yasmin gātre pradṛśyate |
māṣavatkṛṣṇamutsannamanilānmaṣakaṃ tu tat ||36|| (su| ni| a| 13) |
Painless, fixed (immovable), elevated patches (nodules), black like a black-gram, appearing on the body and caused by increased vata are called as Masaka. (36)

Tilakalaka

kṛṣṇāni tilamātrāṇi nīrujāni samāni ca |
vātapittakaphocchoṣāttān vidyāttilakālakān ||37||
(su| ni| a| 13) |
Black, painless, even (not raised above the level of the skin) spots resembling sesame seeds, is known as Tilakälaka. They are caused when kapha is dried by increased vata and pittta in the skin. (37)

Nyaccha

mahadvā yadi vā cālpaṃ śyāvaṃ vā yadi vā'sitam |
nīrujaṃ maṇḍalaṃ gātre nyacchamityabhidhīyate ||38||
(su| ni| a| 13) |
Broad (big) or small, blue or black, painless patches manifested on the skin

is known as Nycha. (38)

Vyanga

krodhāyāsaprakupito vāyuḥ pittena saṃyutaḥ |
mukhamāgatya sahasā maṇḍalaṃ visṛjatyataḥ ||39||
nīrujaṃ tanukaṃ śyāvaṃ mukhe vyaṅgaṃ tamādiśet |
(su| ni| a| 13) |
Vata undergoes increase due to anger and physical exertion, associated with pitta gets localized in the face and would suddenly produce painless, thin, black (blackish blue) patches on the skin. This condition is known as Vyanga. (39)

Nilika

kṛṣṇamevaṅguṇaṃ gātre mukhe vā nīlikāṃ viduḥ ||40||
Similar black patches appearing on the face as well as on other parts of the body are known as Nilika. (40)

Parivartika

mardanāt pīḍanādvā'ti tathaivāpyabhighātataḥ |
meḍhracarma yadā vāyurbhajate sarvataścaran ||41||
tadā vātopasṛṣṭatvāttaccarma parivartate |
maṇeradhastāt kośaśca granthirūpeṇa lambate ||42||
sarujāṃ vātasambhūtāṃ tāṃ vidyāt parivartikām |
sakaṇḍūḥ kaṭhinā vāpi saiva śleṣmasamutthitā ||43||
(su| ni| a| 13) |
Due to too much indulgence in rubbing (hard friction) or squeezing (the penis) or by injury (to the penis or its skin), the vayu which is travelling throughout the body gets aggravated and reaches the skin on the penis and gets lodged therein. Being affected by the vitiated vata, the skin of the penis becomes upturned. The sac of the skin (prepuce) hangs under the glans penis in the form of a knot (appears like a cystic swelling). This condition is called parivartika. It causes pain if vata is predominant. If kapha is predominant in the same condition, it causes itching and hardness. (41-43)

Avapatika

alpīyaḥkhāṃ yadā harṣādbalādgacchet striyaṃ naraḥ |
hastābhighātādapi vā carmaṇyudvartite balāt ||44||
yasyāvapāṭyate carma tāṃ vidyādavapāṭikām |
(su| ni| a| 13) |
When the man has forcible (aggressive, violent) coitus with a woman who has narrow vaginal opening due to extreme excitation or when he masturbates hard, forcibly with his hand, the skin of the glans penis forcibly gets upturned and eventually gets torn. This condition is known as Avapatika. (44-45)

Niruddhaprakasa

vātopasṛṣṭe meḍhre vai carma saṃśrayate maṇim ||45||
maṇiścarmopanaddhastu mūtrasroto ruṇaddhi ca |
niruddhaprakaśe tasmin mandadhāramavedanam ||46||
mūtraṃ pravartate jantormaṇirvivriyate na ca |
niruddhaprakaśaṃ vidyāt sarujaṃ vātasambhavam ||47||
(su| ni| a| 13) |
Due to the effect of abnormally increased vata, the skin over the glans penis covers the glans tightly. The glans thus covered tightly by the skin will block the passage of urine. In this condition the urine flows out in slow streams and without any pain. The glans is always covered by the skin. This painful condition caused by increased vata is known as Niruddhaprakasa. (46-47)

Sanniruddhaguda

vegasandhāraṇādvāyurvihato gudasaṃśritaḥ |
niruṇaddhi mahāsrotaḥ sūkṣmadvāraṃ karoti ca ||48||
mārgasya saukṣmyāt kṛcchreṇa purīṣaṃ tasya gacchati |
sanniruddhagudaṃ vyādhimetaṃ vidyāt sudāruṇam ||49||
(su| ni| a| 13) |
The vata which has got aggravated due to constant indulgence in suppression of the urge for defecation and fart (flatus) would reach the anal region (rectum) and causes blockage of the mahasrotas (rectal passage,

colon) and causes narrowing of its opening (lumen). Due to the narrowing of the outlet (opening), the faeces is eliminated with difficulty. This highly distressing condition is known by the name sanniruddhaguda. (48-49)

Ahiputanaka

śakṛnmūtrasamāyukte'dhaute'pāne śiśorbhavet |
svinne vā'snāpyamāne vā kaṇḍū raktakaphodbhavā ||50||
kaṇḍūyanāttataḥ kṣipraṃ sphoṭaḥ srāvaśca jāyate |
ekībhūtaṃ vraṇairghoraṃ taṃ vidyādahipūtanam ||51||
(su| ni| a| 13) |
When the faeces and urine in and around the anal region of the infants are not cleansed (washed) properly or when the anal region is not washed in spite of sweating in that area there develops itching in that region caused due to increased blood and kapha. When scratched due to itching, it quickly produces pustules and discharges (exuding pustules). (The ulcers of) these pustules join together to form an intractable ulcer. This condition is known as Ahiputana. (50-51)

Vrsanakacchu

snānotsādanahīnasya malo vṛṣaṇasaṃsthitaḥ |
yadā praklidyate svedāt kaṇḍūṃ janayate tadā ||52||
kaṇḍūyanāttataḥ kṣipraṃ sphoṭaḥ srāvaśca jāyate |
prāhurvṛṣaṇakacchūṃ tāṃ śleṣmaraktaprakopajām ||53||
(su| ni| a| 13) |
In persons who do not take bath or oil massage regularly every day, the dirt accumulated on the skin of the scrotum gets wet on getting into contact (mixed with) with the sweat therein and produces itching. This condition is known as Vrsanakacchu. It is caused by simultaneous aggravation of kapha and rakta (blood). (52-53)

Gudabhramsa

pravāhaṇātīsārābhyāṃ nirgacchati gudaṃ bahiḥ |
rūkṣadurbaladehasya gudabhraṃśaṃ tamādiśet ||54||
(su| ni| a| 13) |

In persons who are dry (emaciated) and weak, the anus (muscles of anus) comes out due to (indulgence in) straining at defecation or due to (frequent episodes of) diarrhoea. This condition is known as Gudabhramsa. (54)

Varahadamstra / Sukaradamstra

sadāho raktaparyantastvakpākī tīvravedanaḥ |
kaṇḍūmāñjvarakārī ca sa syācchūkaradaṃṣṭrakaḥ ||55||
The disease characterized by manifestation of skin ulcer with red edge, associated with severe burning sensation, suppuration, severe pain, itching and fever is known as Sakaradamstraka. (55)

iti śrīmādhavakaraviracite mādhavanidāne kṣudraroganidānaṃ samāptam ||55||
Thus ends the chapter on Kşudrarogas.

CHAPTER FIFTY-SIX

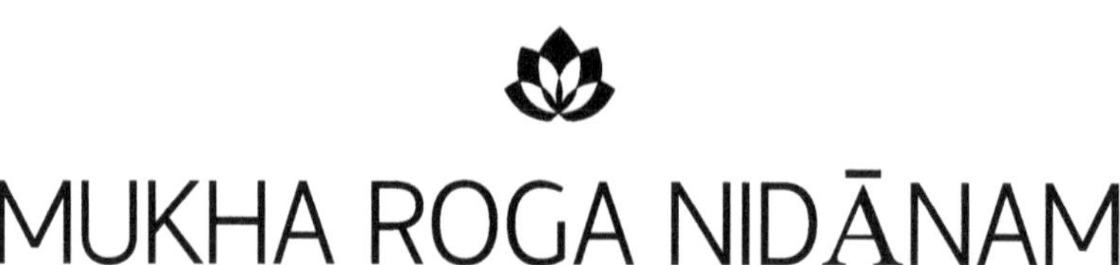

MUKHA ROGA NIDĀNAM

Mukharoga Samanya Hetu – General Etiological Factors of 'Diseases of the Mouth

ānūpapiśitakṣīradadhimatsyātisevanāt |
mukhamadhye gadān kuryuḥ kruddhā doṣāḥ kaphottarāḥ ||1||
Due to excessive indulgence in the foods prepared with meat of animals and birds of aquatic regions, milk, curds and fish, the doshas with the predominance of kapha would undergo abnormal increase and produce diseases of the mouth. (1)

Vataja Oshta Roga

karkaśau paruṣau stabdhau samprāptānilavedanau |
dālyete paripāṭyate oṣṭhau mārutakopataḥ ||2||
(su| ni| a| 16) |
When vata gets increased in the lips, the lips become rough, hard, and immobile. There would be pain of vata nature (vata type of pain). Cracks and fissures appear on the lips. (2)

Pittaja Oshta Roga

cīyete piḍakābhiśca sarujābhiḥ samantataḥ |
sadāhapākapiḍakau pītābhāsau ca pittataḥ ||3||
(su| ni| a| 16) |
In the disease of the lips caused by increase of pitta (in the lips), the lips are covered with painful papules along with burning sensation and suppuration. There is yellowish discolouration of the lips. (3)

Kaphaja Oshta Roga

savarṇābhiśca cīyete piḍakābhiravedanau |
bhavatastu kaphādoṣṭhau picchilau śītalau gurū ||4||
(su| ni| a| 16) |
When kapha gets abnormally increased in the lips, papules having colour of the skin (no discolouration) and are devoid of pain (slightly painful) develop on the lips. The lips are sticky, cold and heavy. (4)

Sannipataja Oshta Roga

sakṛtkṛṣṇau sakṛtpītau sakṛcchvetau tathaiva ca |
sannipātena vijñeyāvanekapiḍakācitau ||5||
(su| ni| a| 16) |
In the disease of the lips caused by simultaneous aggravation of all the three doshas the lips sometimes appear black, sometimes yellow and white at other times. Many types of pidakas (papules) will also appear on the lips. (5)

Raktaja Oshta Roga

kharjūraphalavarṇābhiḥ piḍakābhirnipīḍitau |
raktopasṛṣṭau rudhiraṃ sravataḥ śoṇitaprabhau ||6||
(su| ni| a| 16) |
When the lips are affected by vitiated blood, papules resembling the fruits of date-palm (Phoenix sylvestris) in appearance, which discharge blood and are red in colour, develop on the lips. (6)

Mamsaja Oshta Roga

gurū sthūlau māṃsaduṣṭau māṃsapiṇḍavadudgatau |
jantavaścātra mūrchanti narasyobhayato mukhāt ||7||
(su| ni| a| 16) |
When the lips are contaminated by the muscles, they become heavy and thick and raised like lumps of muscles. Worms are formed on both sides of the mouth. (7)

Medoja Oshta Roga

sarpirmaṇḍapratīkāśau medasā kaṇḍurau gurū |
acchaṃ sphaṭikasaṅkāśamāsrāvaṃ sravato bhṛśam ||8||
(su| ni| a| 16) |
tayorvraṇo na saṃrohenmṛdutvaṃ ca na gacchati |9|
If the lips are contaminated by vitiated medas (fat), the lips appear like the fluid portion of the ghee, develop itching and heaviness, discharges fluids which are clear like spatika and are colourless in large quantities. The ulcers formed from this neither heal easily nor become soft. (8)

Abhighataja Oshta Roga

kṣatajābhau vidīryete pāṭyete cābhighātataḥ ||9||
grathitau ca tathā syātāmoṣṭhau kaṇḍūsamanvitau |10|
(su| ni| a| 16) |
When the disease of the lips has occurred due to the injury (to the lips), the lips will be cut and become reddish as occurs in case of injury. They are cut or torn, will have lumps and will have itching. (9)

Dantamulagata Rogas – Diseases of the gums

Sitada

śoṇitaṃ dantaveṣṭebhyo yasyākasmāt pravartate |
durgandhīni sakṛṣṇāni prakledīni mṛdūni ca ||10||
dantamāṃsāni śīryante pacanti ca parasparam |
śītādo nāma sa vyādhiḥ kaphaśoṇitasambhavaḥ ||11||
(su| ni| a| 16) |
The disease in which bleeding occurs suddenly from the gums without any reason, the gums become foul smelling, black, wet (with discharges) and smooth, the muscles tear off (detach) and start suppurating each other, and is produced by abnormal increase of kapha and rakta (blood) is known as Sitada. (10-11)

Dantapupputaka

dantayostriṣu vā yasya śvayathurjāyate mahān |
dantapupputako nāma sa vyādhiḥ kapharaktajaḥ ||12||
(su| ni| a| 16) |
When severe swelling occurs in the gums surrounding two or three gums, caused by abnormal increase of kapha and blood together is known by the name dantapupputaka. (12)

Dantavesta

sravanti pūyarudhiraṃ calā dantā bhavanti ca |
dantaveṣṭaḥ sa vijñeyo duṣṭaśoṇitasambhavaḥ ||13||
(su| ni| a| 16) |
The disease in which pus and blood (pus mixed blood) is discharged from the gums and the teeth begin to shake is known as dantavesta. This condition is caused by bad (contaminated) blood. (13)

Saushira

śvayathurdantamūleṣu rujāvān kapharaktajaḥ |
lālāsrāvī sa vijñeyaḥ śauṣiro nāma nāmataḥ ||14||
(su| ni| a| 16) |
A swelling which occurs at the root of the tooth caused by increased kapha and blood together is painful and causes free flow of saliva is known as sausira.

Mahasausira

dantāścalanti veṣṭebhyastālu cāpyavadīryate |
yasmin sa sarvajo vyādhirmahāśauṣirasañjñitaḥ ||15||
(su| ni| a| 16) |
When in sausira (above explained condition), the teeth start getting loose from the gums and shaking, fissures occur in the palate (apart from the other symptoms of sausira), which is known as Mahasausira. This condition is caused by simultaneous increase of all the three doshas (together). (15)

Paridara

dantamāṃsāni śīryante yasmin ṣṭhīvati cāpyasṛk |
pittāsṛkkaphajo vyādhirjñeyaḥ paridaro hi saḥ ||16||
(su| ni| a| 16) |
The disease in which the gums undergo decomposition and causes frequent spitting of blood is called paridara. It is caused by an increase of pitta, blood and kapha together. (16)

Upakusa

veṣṭeṣu dāhaḥ pākaśca tābhyāṃ dantāścalanti ca |
yasmin sopakuśo nāma pittaraktakṛto gadaḥ ||17||
(su| ni| a| 16) |
The disease in which there is burning sensation and suppuration in the gums and due to these the teeth become loose and shaking. This disease caused due to the abnormal increase in pitta and blood together is known by the name upakusa. (17)

Vaidarbha

ghṛṣṭeṣu dantamāṃseṣu saṃrambho jāyate mahān |
calā bhavanti dantāśca sa vaidarbho'bhighātajaḥ ||18||
(su| ni| a| 16) |
The disease in which the gums get frayed (grazed or rubbed) develop severe swelling, pain and burning sensation and the teeth become loose and shaky is called vaidarbha. This condition is caused due to trauma. (18)

Khalivardhana

mārutenādhiko danto jāyate tīvravedanaḥ |
khalivardhanasañjño'sau jāte ruk ca praśāmyati ||19||
(su| ni| a| 16) |
Due to the aggravation of vata an extra tooth erupts causing severe pain during its eruption. Once the extra tooth erupts, the pain subsides. This condition is known by the name khalivardhana. (19)

Karala

śanaiḥ śanaiḥ prakurute vāyurdantasamāśritaḥ |
karālān vikaṭān dantān karālo na sa sidhyati ||20||
The vata located in the teeth undergoes an increase and gradually (over a period of time) makes the teeth irregular and ugly. This condition is known as Karala. It is incurable and does not respond to any treatment. (20)

Adhimamsa

hānavye paścime dante mahāñchotho mahārujaḥ |
lālāsrāvī kaphakṛto vijñeyaḥ so'dhimāṃsakaḥ |21|
(su| ni| a| 16) |
The condition in which a severe swelling appears in the gums surrounding the last molar tooth, which is highly painful and causes dribbling of saliva is known as adhimamsaka. It is caused by increased kapha. (21)

Dantanadi

dantamūlagatā nāḍyaḥ pañca jñeyā yatheritāḥ ||21||
(su| ni| a| 16) |
There are five kinds of nadis (sinus) which would manifest in the root of the teeth (gums). These are similar to those described previously (Nadivrana – sinus ulcers). (21)

Note - The five types of dantanadis are – vataja, pittaja, kaphaja, sannipataja and shalyaja.

Dantagata Rogas – Diseases of the teeth

Dalana

dīryamāṇeṣviva rujā yasya danteṣu jāyate |
dālano nāma sa vyādhiḥ sadāgatinimittajaḥ ||22||
(su| ni| a| 16) |
A condition of the teeth in which there is severe pain in the tooth as if they are breaking open or bursting is called Dalana. It is caused by increased vata. (22)

Krimidantaka

kṛṣṇacchidraścalaḥ srāvī sasaṃrambho mahārujaḥ |
animittarujo vātādvijñeyaḥ krimidantakaḥ ||23||
(su| ni| a| 16) |
The condition in which the tooth which has black holes in them and are shaky (loose), which have discharges, swelling and severe pain which comes on without any apparent cause and caused by vitiated vata is called as krimidanta / krimidantaka. (23)

Bhanjanaka

vaktraṃ vakraṃ bhavedyasya dantabhaṅgaśca jāyate |
kaphavātakṛto vyādhiḥ sa bhañjanakasañjñitaḥ ||24||
(su| ni| a| 16) |
A condition, in which the face assumes an irregular shape and the teeth get broken, is caused by increased kapha and vata together is called as Bhanjanaka. (24)

Dantaharsa

śītarūkṣapravātāmlasparśānāmasahā dvijāḥ |
pittamārutakopena dantaharṣaḥ sa nāmataḥ ||25||
A condition wherein due to the increased pitta and vata the teeth become incapable of tolerating the touch (contact of) of cold and dry foods, swift cold breeze and sour things (foods and drinks) is called by the name dantaharsa. (25)

Dantasarkara

malo dantagato yastu pittamārutaśoṣitaḥ |
śarkareva kharasparśā sā jñeyā dantaśarkarā ||26||
The dirt accumulated on the teeth gets dried up by the action of increased vata and pitta (together). This dried up dirt becomes hard, assumes the form of gravel and accumulates on the teeth. This condition is called as Dantasarkara. (26)

Kapalika

kapāleṣviva dīryatsu dantānāṃ saiva śarkarā |
kapāliketi vijñeyā sadā dantavināśinī ||27||
Kapalika is a more complicated version of dantasarkara (discussed above). Here the pieces of teeth along with solidified and accumulated hard dirt (as in sarkara) on them, which appear like pieces of earthen vessel (big flakes of accretions) peel off along with parts of the tooth, and finally destroy the teeth. This condition is known as Kapalika. (27)

Syavadantaka

yo'sṛṅmiśreṇa pittena dagdho dantastvaśeṣataḥ |
śyāvatāṃ nīlatāṃ vā'pi gataḥ sa śyāvadantakaḥ ||28||
(su| ni| a| 16) |
A condition in which the tooth becomes black of blue in colour, being burnt by the increased pitta combined with the vitiated blood is known as syavadantaka. (28)

Danta Vidradhi

dantamāṃse malaiḥ sāsrairbāhyāntaḥ śvayathurguruḥ |
sadāharuk sravedbhinnaḥ pūyāsraṃ dantavidradhiḥ ||29||
A severe (big) swelling occurs inside and outside the gums caused by the vitiated blood and all the three increased doshas. It is associated with burning sensation and pain. On bursting open it discharges pus mixed with blood. This is called as Danta Vidradhi. (29)

Jihvagata Rogas – Diseases of the tongue

Jihvakantaka

jihvā'nilena sphuṭitā prasuptā bhavecca śākacchadanaprakāśā |
pittena dahyatyupacīyate ca dīrghaiḥ saraktairapi kaṇṭakaiśca |
kaphena gurvī bahulā citā ca māṃsocchrayaiḥ śālmalikaṇṭakābhaiḥ ||30||
(su| ni| a| 16) |

Vataja Jihvakantaka – When increased vata affects the tongue it would become fissured, numb (loss of sensation) – loss of taste perception, and would resemble a leaf of a tree (rough, coarse).
Pittaja Jihvakantaka – When increased pitta affects the tongue there would be burning sensation in the tongue. The tongue would become studded with red coloured long thorny projections.
Kaphaja Jihvakantaka – When increased kapha affects the tongue, the tongue would become heavy, thick, and will be studded with muscular sprouts resembling those of Shalmali tree (Bombax malabaricum). (30)

Alasa

jihvātale yaḥ śvayathuḥ pragāḍhaḥ so'lāsasañjñaḥ kapharaktamūrtiḥ |
jihvāṃ sa tu stambhayati pravṛddho mūle ca jihvā bhṛśameti pākam ||31||
(su| ni| a| 16) |
A condition in which a profound swelling occurs beneath the tongue caused by combined aggravation of kapha and rakta (blood) is called Alasa. This swelling would increase in size and cause stiffness (incapable of movement) of the tongue and also would cause severe suppuration at the root of the tongue. (31)

Upajihvika

jihvāgrarūpaḥ śvayathurhi jihvāmunnamya jātaḥ kapharaktamūlaḥ |
lālākaraḥ kaṇḍuyutaḥ sacoṣaḥ sā tūpajihvā paṭhitā bhiṣagbhiḥ ||32||
(su| ni| a| 16) |
A condition in which a severe swelling caused by increased kapha and blood together, having the appearance of the tip of the tongue, is formed beneath the tongue and lifts up the tongue. This disease is called as upajihvika. This is associated with excessive salivation, itching and burning as if the tongue is in direct contact with the fire. (32)

Talugata Rogas – diseases of the palate

Kantasundi

śleṣmāsṛgbhyāṃ tālumūle pravṛddho dīrghaḥ śotho dhmātabastiprakāśaḥ |

tṛṣṇākāsaśvāsakṛttaṃ vadanti vyādhiṃ vaidyāḥ kaṇṭhaśuṇḍīti nāmnā ||33||
(su| ni| a| 16) |
An elongated swelling resembling a bag inflated with air gets manifested at the root of the palate, caused by kapha and blood getting increased together, associated with thirst, cough and dyspnoea (breathing difficulty). This disease of the palate is called by the name Kanthasundi. (33)

Tundikeri

śothaḥ sthūlastodadāhaprapākī prāguktābhyāṃ tuṇḍikerī matā tu |34|
(su| ni| a| 16) |
The swelling which is caused by kapha and blood just like the condition explained above (kanthasundi) will be known as Tundikeri if it becomes thicker and is associated with pricking pain, burning sensation and suppuration. (34)

Adhrusa

mṛduḥ śotho lohitaḥ śoṇitottho jñeyo'dhruṣaḥ sajvarastīvraruk ca ||34||
(su| ni| a| 16) |
A condition, in which a soft, red swelling is caused by increased blood, is accompanied with fever and severe pain is known by the name adhrusa. (34)

Kacchapa

kūrmonnato'vedano'śīghrajanmā rogo jñeyaḥ kacchapaḥ śleṣmaṇā tu |35|
(su| ni| a| 16) |
Kachchapa manifests in the form of a rounded big swelling resembling the upper surface of the shell of a tortoise. This condition is painless and develops slowly and is caused by increased kapha. (35)

Talvarbuda and Mamsa sanghata

padmākāraṃ tālumadhye tu śothaṃ vidyādraktādarbudaṃ proktaliṅgam ||35||
duṣṭaṃ māṃsaṃ nīrujaṃ tālumadhye kaphācchūnaṃ māṃsasaṅghātamāhuḥ |

(su| ni| a| 16) |

Talvarbuda – It is a swelling which resembles a lotus flower and manifests at the centre of the palate and has symptoms similar to that of raktarbuda.

Mamsa sanghata – It is a similar swelling (same as talvarbuda) manifesting at the centre of the palate involving mamsa – contaminated muscle tissue (it is a muscular swelling or lump at the centre of the palate), caused by increased kapha and is painless. (35)

Talupupputa, Talushosha and Talupaka

nīruk sthāyī kolamātraḥ kaphāt syānmedoyuktāt pupputastāludeśe ||36||
śoṣo'tyarthaṃ dīryate cāpi tāluḥ śvāsaścograstāluśoṣo'nilācca |
pittaṃ kuryāt pākamatyarthaghoraṃ tālunyenaṃ tālupākaṃ vadanti ||37||
(su| ni| a| 16) |

Talupupputa – A swelling (papule) of the size of a jujube fruit (Ziziphus jujuba) which is painless, fixed (immobile), caused by combination of abnormally increased kapha and medas (fat) together, developing in the palate is called by the name talupupputa.

Talushosha – Excessive dryness and fissures occurring in the palate, caused by aggravated vata and associated with severe dyspnoea (difficulty in breathing) is known as Talusosa.

Talupaka – Pitta aggravated in the palate causes severe and dreadful suppuration (in the palate). This is known as Talupaka. (36-37)

Galagata Rogas – diseases of the throat

Rohini and its types, symptoms

gale'nilaḥ pittakaphau ca mūrchitau pradūṣya māṃsaṃ ca tathaiva śoṇitam |
galopasaṃrodhakaraistathā'ṅkurairnihantyasūn vyādhiriyaṃ hi rohiṇī ||38||
(su| ni| a| 16) |
jihvāsamantādbhṛśavedanāstu māṃsāṅkurāḥ kaṇṭhanirodhino ye |
sā rohiṇī vātakṛtā pradiṣṭā vātātmakopadravagāḍhayuktā ||39||
kṣiprodgamā kṣipravidāhapākā tīvrajvarā pittanimittajā tu |
srotovirodhinyacalodgatā ca sthirāṅkurā yā kaphasambhavā sā ||40||
gambhīrapākinyanivāryavīryā tridoṣaliṅgā tritayotthitā ca |
sphoṭaiścitā pittasamānaliṅgā sādhyā pradiṣṭā rudhirātmikā tu ||41||

(su| ni| a| 16) |
Vata, pitta and kapha getting increased in the throat (either individually or all together) would invade mamsa (muscle) and rakta (blood) and produce sprouts inside the throat subsequently causing obstruction of the throat passage and death. This disease is called Rohini. \
Vataja Rohini – In vata predominant rohini there will be severe pain all over the tongue, muscular sprouts which cause obstruction to the throat, and severe complications (and other symptoms) of vata increase.
Pittaja Rohini – In pitta predominant rohini, there is quick appearance of sprouts, burning sensation and suppuration, and is associated with high fever.
Kaphaja Rohini – In kapha predominant rohini, the sprouts are immobile, big in size and fixed. They cause total obstruction of the throat.
Sannipataja Rohini – In Rohini caused by simultaneous aggravation of all the three doshas, suppuration occurs in the deeper tissues. It will not respond to any treatment (is incurable) and presents with symptoms of aggravation of all the three doshas.
Raktaja Rohini – In rohini caused by abnormally increased blood, there will be widespread red papules and will present with symptoms of pitta increase. This condition is curable. (39-41)

Kanthasaluka

kolāsthimātraḥ kaphasambhavo yo granthirgale kaṇṭakaśūkabhūtaḥ |
kharaḥ sthiraḥ śastranipātasādhyastaṃ kaṇṭhaśālūkamiti bruvanti ||42||
(su| ni| a| 16) |
A cystic swelling (tumour) of the size of seed of jujube fruit, produced by increased kapha, occurring in the throat, appearing like thorns or spikes, rough, fixed (immobile), and curable only by surgical methods is called by the name Kanthasaluka. (42)

Adhijihva

jihvāgrarūpaḥ śvayathuḥ kaphāttu jihvopariṣṭādapi raktamiśrāt |
jñeyo'dhijihvaḥ khalu roga eṣa vivarjayedāgatapākamenam ||43||
(su| ni| a| 16) |
A swelling which occurs above the level of (top of) the root of the tongue, resembling the tip of the tongue, caused by kapha along with blood is known

as adhijihva. If the swelling is found along with suppuration, it should be refused treatment (because it is incurable). (43)

Valaya

balāśa evāyatamunnataṃ ca śothaṃ karotyannagatiṃ nivārya |
taṃ sarvathaivāprativāryavīryaṃ vivarjanīyaṃ valayaṃ vadanti ||44||
(su| ni| a| 16) |
Kapha undergoing abnormal increase produces large sized swelling in the throat causing obstruction to the passage of food. This condition is called by the name valaya. It is an intractable disease which doesn't respond to any type of treatment and hence should be refused treatment. (44)

Balasa

gale tu śothaṃ kurutaḥ pravṛddhau śleṣmānilau śvāsarujopapannam |
marmacchidaṃ dustaramenamāhurbalāśasañjñaṃ nipuṇā vikāram ||45||
(su| ni| a| 16) |
Kapha and vata having aggravated together produces a swelling in the throat which causes difficulty in breathing and pain, which tends to destroy (damage) the marmas (vital organs or spots in the body). This disease is identified as Balasa by the experts and is difficult to treat. (45)

Ekavrnda

vṛttonnato'ntaḥ śvayathuḥ sadāhaḥ sakaṇḍuro'pākyamṛdurguruśca |
nāmnaikavṛndaḥ parikīrtito'sau vyādhirbalāśakṣatajaprasūtaḥ ||46||
(su| ni| a| 16) |
A swelling developing inside the throat, which is round, elevated, accompanied with burning sensation, itching, not suppurating, not too smooth (little hard) and heavy is known as Ekavrnda. This condition is caused by kapha and blood together. (46)

Vrnda

samunnataṃ vṛttamamandadāhaṃ tīvrajvaraṃ vṛndamudāharanti |
taccāpi pittakṣatajaprakopājjñeyaṃ satodaṃ pavanātmakaṃ tu ||47||

(su| ni| a| 16) |
A condition in which an elevated and rounded swelling occurs in the throat being associated with severe burning sensation and high fever is called Vrnda. This is caused by combined vitiation of pitta and blood. If vata is involved in this condition there will also be pricking pain. (47)

Shataghni

vartirghanā kaṇṭhanirodhinī yā citā'timātraṃ piśitaprarohaiḥ |
anekaruk prāṇaharī tridoṣājjñeyā śataghnī ca śataghnirūpā ||48||
(su| ni| a| 16) |
A swelling obstructing the throat studded all over with multiple muscular sprouts resembling a Sataghni (a weapon in the form of an iron ball with sharp spikes), presenting with many kinds of pain and cause death is called as Sataghni. This condition is caused by simultaneous vitiation of all the three doshas together. (48)

Galayu

granthirgale tvāmalakāsthimātraḥ sthiro'tirugyaḥ kapharaktamūrtiḥ |
saṃlakṣyate saktamivāśanaṃ ca sa śastrasādhyastu galāyusañjñaḥ ||49||
(su| ni| a| 16) |
A cystic swelling occurring in the throat which is of the size of seed of Amalaka (Phyllanthus emblica), is immobile, very painful, and caused by combined aggravation of kapha and blood is known as Galayu. Due to this, the food remains obstructed in the throat (difficulty in swallowing the food) and can be treated by surgical methods (requires surgical treatment to cure this disease). (49)

Galavidradhi

sarvaṃ galaṃ vyāpya samutthito yaḥ śotho rujaḥ santi ca yatra sarvāḥ |
sa sarvadoṣairgalavidradhistu tasyaiva tulyaḥ khalu sarvajasya ||50||
(su| ni| a| 16) |
The condition in which a swelling which involves all the areas of (entire) the throat develop, which presents with different kinds of pains caused by all the doshas, is called as galavidradhi. It is caused due to simultaneous

aggravation of all the three doshas and is similar to tridoshaja vidradhi. (50)

Galaugha

śotho mahānannajalāvarodhī tīvrajvaro vāyugaternihantā |
kaphena jāto rudhirānvitena gale galaughaḥ parikīrtyate tu ||51||
(su| ni| a| 16) |
A profound swelling in the throat, caused by increased kapha associated with vitiated blood, which causes obstruction to swallowing of food and water, associated with severe fever and causing the movements of vata (aeration, respiration) is called by the name Galaugha. (51)

Svaraghna

yastāmyamānaḥ śvasiti prasaktaṃ bhinnasvaraḥ śuṣkavimuktakaṇṭhaḥ |
kaphopadigdheṣvanilāyaneṣu jñeyaḥ sa rogaḥ śvasanāt svaraghnaḥ ||52||
(su| ni| a| 16) |
A condition in which due to the coating and subsequent obstruction of the air passages by kapha (sputum, phlegm), the patient finds difficulty in breathing along with darkness before the eyes, has broken voice, dryness of the throat and loss of movement of the throat, is known as Svaraghna. This condition is caused by vitiated vata. (52)

Mamsatana

pratānavān yaḥ śvayathuḥ sukaṣṭo galoparodhaṃ kurute krameṇa |
sa māṃsatānaḥ kathito'valambī prāṇapraṇut sarvakṛto vikāraḥ ||53||
(su| ni| a| 16) |
A broad swelling which has spread out in the throat, which is troublesome (with severe painful symptoms) and gradually obstructs the throat by hanging down and eventually causes death is known as Mamsatana. This condition is caused by simultaneous increase of all the three doshas together. (53)

Vidari

sadāhatodaṃ śvayathuṃ sutāmramantargale pūtiviśīrṇamāṃsam |

pittena vidyādvadane vidārīṃ pārśve viśeṣāt sa tu yena śete ||54||
(su| ni| a| 16) |
A swelling which occurs inside the throat and in the mouth, having burning sensation and pricking pain, has coppery colour, the muscles surrounding which has foul smell and fall off getting detached, is caused by predominant vitiation of pita is called by the name vidari. This occurs in the side of the face and throat on which the patient usually sleeps. (54)

Sarvasara Roga / Mukhapaka

sphoṭaiḥ satodairvadanaṃ samantādyasyācitaṃ sarvasaraḥ sa vātāt |
raktaiḥ sadāhaistanubhiḥ sapītairyasyācitaṃ cāpi sa pittakopāt |
avedanaiḥ kaṇḍuyutaiḥ savarṇairyasyācitaṃ cāpi sa vai kaphena ||55||
(su| ni| a| 16) |
Vataja Sarvasara / Mukhapaka – In this condition the inside of the mouth is covered by papules (sores) having pricking pain.
Pittaja Sarvasara / Mukhapaka – In this condition the inside of the mouth is covered by papules which are red or yellow in colour, thin and have a burning sensation.
Kaphaja Sarvasara / Mukhapaka – In this condition the inside of the mouth is covered by papules which are painless, have itching and are of the same colour as that of the skin (surrounding area). (54-55)

Prognosis of Oshta kopa and other conditions

oṣṭhaprakope varjyāḥ syurmāṃsaraktatridoṣajāḥ |
dantamūleṣu varjyau ca triliṅgagatiśauṣirau ||56||
danteṣu ca na sidhyanti śyāvadālanabhañjanāḥ |
jihvāroge balāśastu tālavyeṣvarbudaṃ tathā ||57||
svaraghno valayo vṛndo balāśaśca vidārikā |
galaugho māṃsatānaśca śataghnī rohiṇī gale ||58||
asādhyāḥ kīrtitā hyete rogā nava daśaiva tu |
teṣu cāpi kriyāṃ vaidyaḥ pratyākhyāya samācaret ||59||
(su| ni| a| 16) |
Among the diseases of the lips – ostha prakopa produced by mamsa – muscle, rakta – blood, rakta – blood and all the three doshas should be rejected and should not be treated.

Among the diseases of the gums – tridoshaja nadivrana and saushira are considered as incurable and hence should be rejected.
Among the diseases of the teeth – Syavadanta, Dalana and Bhanjanaka are incurable.
Among the diseases of the tongue – Balasha is incurable.
Among the diseases of the palate – Arbuda is incurable.
Among the diseases of the throar – Svaraghna, Valaya, vrnda, Balasha, Vidarika, Galaudha, Mamsatana, Shataghni and Rohini are considered incurable.

These nineteen diseases are incurable and the physician should consider them as unfit for treatment and reject them. (56-59)

iti śrīmādhavakaraviracite mādhavanidāne mukharoganidānaṃ samāptam ||56||
Thus ends the chapter on Mukharogas.

CHAPTER FIFTY-SEVEN

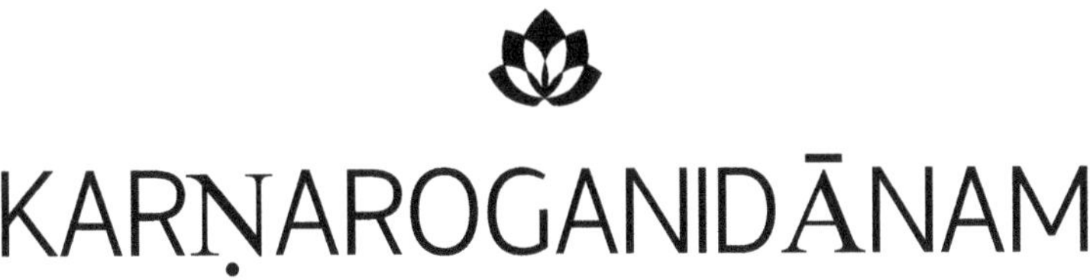

KARṆAROGANIDĀNAM

Karnasula

samīraṇaḥ śrotragato'nyathācaran samantataḥ śūlamatīva karṇayoḥ |
karoti doṣaiśca yathāsvamāvṛtaḥ sa karṇaśūlaḥ kathito durācaraḥ ||1||
(su| u| taṃ| a| 20) |
Vāta which has been enveloped by the doshas (pitta and kapha) which have undergone abnormal increase due to their own etiological factors (etiological factors causing aggravation of pitta and kapha respectively) and has moved in upward direction (abnormal movement for vata) on reaching (and getting lodged in) the ears and produces pain in the ears. This condition is called Karnasula and is difficult to treat. (1)

Karnanada

karṇasrotaḥ sthite vāte śṛṇoti vividhān svarān |
bherīmṛdaṅgaśaṅkhānāṃ karṇanādaḥ sa ucyate ||2||
When aggravated vata gets lodged in the canals of the ears the patient would hear many kinds of abnormal sounds similar to those produced by kettle drum, cymbal or conch etc. This condition is known as Karnanada. (2)

Badhirya

yadā śabdavahaṃ vāyuḥ srota āvṛtya tiṣṭhati |
śuddhaḥ śleṣmānvito vā'pi bādhiryaṃ tena jāyate ||3||
When vata either alone or in association with kapha (vata enveloped by kapha) blocks the passages of sound, the patient develops deafness. This is known as Bādhirya. (3)

Karna Ksveda

vāyuḥ pittādibhiryukto veṇughoṣopamaṃ svanam |
karoti karṇayoḥ kṣveḍaṃ karṇakṣveḍaḥ sa ucyate ||4||
A condition in which increased vata in association with pitta and other dosha (kapha) produces constant sound in the ear resembling the sound produced by a bamboo (when air is blown in hollow bamboo shoot) or flute. This is known as Karna Ksveda. (4)

Karnasrava

śiro'bhighātādathavā nimajjato jale prapākādathavā'pi vidradheḥ |
sraveddhi pūyaṃ śravaṇo'nilārditaḥ sa karṇasaṃsrāva iti prakīrtitaḥ ||5||
(su| u| taṃ| a| 20) |
Injury to the head, drowning in water (remaining underwater for long time) or ripening of an abscess in the ears causes discharge of pus from the ears. This is associated with pains and other symptoms of vata increase. This condition is known as Karnasrava. (5)

Karnakandu and Karnaguthaka

mārutaḥ kaphasaṃyuktaḥ karṇakaṇḍūṃ karoti ca |
pittoṣmaśoṣitaḥ śleṣmā kurute karṇagūthakam ||6||
Karnakandu - Vata in association with kapha produces Karnakandū (itching inside the ears).
Karnaguthaka - Kapha getting dried (and solidified) by the heat of pitta produces Karṇaguthaka (hardness of the wax). (6)

Karnapratinaha

sa karṇagūtho dravatāṃ gato yadā vilāyito ghrāṇamukhaṃ prapadyate |
tadā sa karṇapratināhasañjñito bhavedvikāraḥ śiraso'rdhabhedakṛt ||7||
(su| u| taṃ| a| 20) |
The condition in which this wax of the ears (explained above in karnaguthaka) gets liquefied (becoming watery), and reaches the nose and mouth (and gets discharged from there) is called Karnapratinaha. The

patient also suffers from a headache in one half of the head. (7)

Krimikarnaka

yadā tu mūrchantyathavā'pi jantavaḥ sṛjantyapatyānyathavā'pi makṣikāḥ |
tadvyañjanatvācchravaṇo nirucyate bhiṣagbhirādyaiḥ krimikarṇako gadaḥ ||8||
(su| u| taṃ| a| 20) |
When insects or small worms forming (entering) in the ears (due to decaying of muscles and blood), or flies producing their larva inside the ears (in the decomposed or putrefied muscles of the ears), the physicians call this disease having symptoms similar to krimiroga (worm infestation disease) as krimikarnaka. (8)

pataṅgāḥ śatapadyaśca karṇasrotaḥ praviśya hi |
aratiṃ vyākulatvaṃ ca bhṛśaṃ kurvanti vedanām ||9||
karṇo nistudyate tasya tathā pharapharāyate |
kīṭe carati ruk tīvrā niṣpande mandavedanā ||10||
If winged insects, centipedes or other insects have entered into the canals of the ears, they produce restlessness, a sense of fear or worry and severe pain. If these insects are alive and move around in the canals of the ear, they will produce pricking pain, sounds of movement of insects (movement of insects is felt), and severe pain. The pain will be mild if the insects are not moving inside the ear canals (if insects are dead). (9-10)

Karna Vidradhi

kṣatābhighātaprabhavastu vidradhirbhavettathā doṣakṛto'paraḥ punaḥ |
saraktapītāruṇamasramāsravet pratodadhūmāyanadāhacoṣavān ||11||
(su| u| taṃ| a| 20) |
One type of abscess develops due to injury or trauma to (inside) the ear and the other type develops due to aggravation of doshas inside the ear. This will cause discharge of fluids (pus) of red, yellow or crimson colour accompanied with pricking pain, feeling of hot fumes (smoke) being eliminated from the ears, burning sensation and feeling of sucking like pain. This disease is called as Karna Vidradhi. (11)

Karnapaka

karṇapākastu pittena kothavikledakṛdbhavet |
karṇavidradhipākādvā jāyate cāmbupūraṇāt ||12||
Due to aggravation of pitta or due to ripening of ear abscess or due to water entering the ears a disease called karnapaka is produced. It causes putrefaction and foul discharges from the ears. (12)

Putikarnaka

pūyaṃ sravati pūti vā sa jñeyaḥ pūtikarṇakaḥ |13|
A condition in which very foul-smelling pus is discharged from the ears is called Putikarnaka.

Karnasotha, Karnarbuda and Karnarsha

karṇaśothārbudārśāṃsi jānīyāduktalakṣaṇaiḥ ||13||
The symptoms of karnasotha, karnarbuda and karnarsha are similar to sotha (swelling, oedema), arbuda (tumour) and arsha (piles) which occur elsewhere in the body. (13)

Karnarogas based on dosha predominance

nādo'tiruk karṇamalasya śoṣaḥ srāvastanuścāśravaṇaṃ ca vātāt |
śothaḥ sarāgo daraṇaṃ vidāhaḥ sapītapūtisravaṇaṃ ca pittāt ||14||
vaiśrutyakaṇḍūsthiraśothaśuklasnigdhasrutiḥ svalparujaḥ kaphācca |
sarvāṇi rūpāṇi ca sannipātāt srāvaśca tatrādhikadoṣavarṇaḥ ||15||
(ca| ci| a| 26) |
Vataja Karnaroga – In the ear diseases caused due to predominant aggravation of vata, there will be noise in the ears, severe pain, drying (and hardening) of the dirt in the ears, less discharges (discharge of thin fluids), and loss of hearing (deafness).
Pittaja Karnaroga - In the ear diseases caused due to predominant aggravation of pitta, there will be reddish swelling, tearing / blasting pain, burning sensation, and yellowish offensive discharges from the ears.
Kaphaja Karnaroga – In the ear diseases caused due to predominant aggravation of kapha, there will be hearing of abnormal sounds, itching in

the ears, hard and immobile (fixed) swelling, white and unctuous discharges and mild pain.
Sannipataja Karnaroga – In the ear diseases caused due to simultaneous aggravation of all the three doshas there will be symptoms of all the three doshas and the discharges will have the colour of the predominantly aggravated dosha. (14-15)

Paripotaka

saukumāryāccirotsṛṣṭe sahasā'tipravardhite |
karṇaśotho bhavet pālyāṃ sarujaḥ paripoṭavān |
kṛṣṇāruṇanibhaḥ stabdhaḥ sa vātāt paripoṭakaḥ ||16||
(su| ci| a| 25) |
Due to the delicate / tender nature (of the child) if the hole punctured on the earlobe (as a part of childhood rituals) is left unattended for a long time and in later period if one tries to dilate the orifice all of a sudden, it would cause serious swelling along with pain in the ear (earlobe) which will have black or crimson colour. This hard swelling caused by increased vata is known as Paripotaka. (16)

Utpata

gurvābharaṇasaṃyogāttāḍanādgharṣaṇādapi |
śothaḥ pālyāṃ bhavecchyāvo dāhapākarujānvitaḥ ||17||
rakto vā raktapittābhyāmutpātaḥ sa gado mataḥ |
(su| ci| a| 25) |
Wearing of excessively heavy ornaments in the ears, blow (injury) or friction on the ears leads to the manifestation of swelling, black or red in colour, caused by aggravation of blood and pitta together, associated with burning sensation, suppuration and pain. This condition is known as Utpata. (17)

Unmanthaka

karṇaṃ balādvardhayataḥ pālyāṃ vāyuḥ prakupyati ||18||
kaphaṃ saṅgṛhya kurute śothaṃ stabdhamavedanam |
unmanthakaḥ sakaṇḍūko vikāraḥ kaphavātajaḥ ||19||

By forcibly attempting to pierce the pinna of the ears and trying to enhance the orifice, vata gets aggravated in the ears (earlobe). This vata getting associated with kapha produces stiff (hard) swelling without pain. This condition is called by the name Unmanthaka. It is caused by increased kapha and vata together and is associated with itching. (18-19)

Dukhavardhana

saṃvardhyamāne durviddhe kaṇḍūpākarujānvitaḥ |
śotho bhavati pākaśca tridoṣo duḥkhavardhanaḥ ||20||
(su| ci| a| 25) |
When the pinna of the ear is pierced at the wrong place and when that orifice becomes bigger, it leads to the development of swelling and ripening accompanied with itching, suppuration and pain. This condition is called Dukhavardhana and is caused by increase of all the three doshas together. (20)

Parilehina

kaphāsṛkkrimayaḥ kruddhāḥ sarṣapābhā visarpiṇaḥ |
kurvanti pālyāṃ piḍakāḥ kaṇḍūdāharujānvitāḥ ||21||
kaphāsṛkkrimisambhūtaḥ sa visarpannitastataḥ |
lihet saśaṣkulīṃ pālīṃ parilehīti sa smṛtaḥ ||22||
(su| ci| a| 25)
Increase of kapha and blood and presence of bacteria together produce pustules on the pinna of the ear, of the size of mustard seeds, spreading in nature, accompanied with itching, burning sensation, pain causing a disease called as Parilehi. This disease caused by increased kapha, blood and worms (bacteria) will spread all through the ears and eat off (destroy) the entire pinna and lobes. (21-22)

iti śrīmādhavakaraviracite mādhavanidāne karṇaroganidānaṃ samāptam ||57||
Thus ends the chapter on Karnarogas.

CHAPTER FIFTY-EIGHT

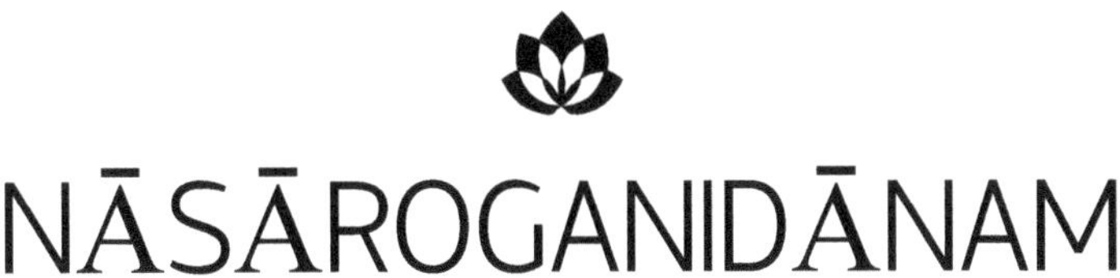

NĀSĀROGANIDĀNAM

Apinasa

ānahyate yasya viśuṣyate ca praklidyate dhūpyati cāpi nāsā |
na vetti yo gandharasāṃśca janturjuṣṭaṃ vyavasyediha pīnasena |
taṃ cānilaśleṣmabhavaṃ vikāraṃ brūyāt pratiśyāyasamānaliṅgam ||1||
(su| u| taṃ| a| 22) |
The condition in which the nasal passage of the person is obstructed (being stuffed with kapha dried by vata), dried up or moist and feeling of raised warmth (feeling of smoke being eliminated from the nose) and the person not understand (appreciate) the smell or taste of materials shall be considered as suffering from the disease Apinasa. It will have symptoms similar to that of pratisyaya and is caused by the increase of vata and kapha together. (1)

Putinasya

doṣairvidagdhairgalatālumūle sammūrchito yasya samīraṇastu |
nireti pūtirmukhanāsikābhyāṃ taṃ pūtinasyaṃ pravadanti rogam ||2||
(su| u| taṃ| a| 22) |
Vāta getting associated with the other (pitta and kapha) morbid (severely increased, burnt and accumulated) doshas localized at the roots of the throat and palate gets eliminated producing foul smell from the mouth and nose. This disease is called as putinasya. (2)

Nasikapaka

ghrāṇāśritaṃ pittamarūṃṣi kuryādyasmin vikāre balavāṃśca pākaḥ |

taṃ nāsikāpākamiti vyavasyedvikledakothāvathavā'pi yatra ||3||
(su| u| taṃ| a| 22) |
The disease in which the pitta located in the nose undergoing abnormal increase produce ulcerations inside the nose or causes severe suppuration or produces moistness and putrefaction inside the nose is known as Nasikapaka. (3)

Puyarakta

doṣairvidagdhairathavā'pi jantorlalāṭadeśe'bhihatasya taistaiḥ |
nāsā sravet pūyamasṛgvimiśraṃ taṃ pūyaraktaṃ pravadanti rogam ||4||
(su| u| taṃ| a| 22) |
A condition in which due to abnormal increase of doshas or different kinds of injuries occurring on the forehead, there is continuous discharge of blood mixed pus from the nose is known as Puyarakta. (4)

Ksavathu

ghrāṇāśrite marmaṇi sampraduṣṭo yasyānilo nāsikayā nireti |
kaphānujāto bahuśo'tiśabdastaṃ rogamāhuḥ kṣavathuṃ vidhijñāḥ ||5||
(su| u| taṃ| a| 22) |
The disease in which vata getting aggravated in the vital spots located inside the nose comes out of the nose frequently getting associated with kapha, with great force, making great (loud) sounds is named as Ksavathu by the learned people. (5)

Agantuja Ksavathu

tīkṣṇopayogādabhijighrato vā bhāvān kaṭūnarkanirīkṣaṇādvā |
sūtrādibhirvā taruṇāsthimarmaṇyudghāṭite'nyaḥ kṣavathurnireti ||6||
(su| u| taṃ| a| 22) |
Kşavathu (sneezing) may also arise from various other external causes like - the ingestion of pungent (deep penetrating) food substances or use of similar substances, smelling of spicy materials (irritants), looking up at the sun, or injury to the cartilage and vital spots inside the nose due to introduction of thread, grass etc things into the nose. (Such ksavathu is called as agantuja ksavathu.) (6)

Bramshathu

prabhraśyate nāsikayā tu yasya sāndro vidagdho lavaṇaḥ kaphastu |
prāksañcito mūrdhani sūryataptastaṃ bhraṃśathuṃ rogamudāharanti ||7||
(su| u| taṃ| a| 22) |
The thick, burnt (improperly formed) and salty kapha which had been previously accumulated inside the head melts and undergoes liquefaction by the heat of the sun and falls (comes) out of the nose. Such a condition is described as the disease Bhramsathu. (7)

Dipta Roga

ghrāṇe bhṛśaṃ dāhasamanvite tu viniḥsareddhūma iveha vāyuḥ |
nāsā pradīpteva ca yasya jantorvyādhiṃ tu taṃ dīptamudāharanti ||8||
(su| u| taṃ| a| 22) |
The disease of the nose in which the air comes out just like smoke (hot air) from the nose wherein severe burning sensation is already present and the person feels as if his nose is being burnt by the fire is known by the name Dipta Roga. (8)

Pratinaha

ucchvāsamārgaṃ tu kaphaḥ savāto rundhyāt pratīnāhamudāharettam |9|
(ca| ci| a| 26) |
Kapha along with Vata causes blockage of the passage of respiration. This condition is called Pratinaha.

Nasasrava

ghrāṇādghanaḥ pītasitastanurvā doṣaḥ sravet srāvamudāharettam ||9||
(ca| ci| a| 26) |
Discharge of thick or thin, yellow or white coloured dosha (kapha) from the nose is known as Nasasrava. (9)

Nasasosa / Nasaparisosa

ghrāṇāśrite srotasi mārutena gāḍhaṃ pratapte pariśoṣite ca |
kṛcchrācchvasedūrdhvamadhaśca janturyasmin sa nāsāpariśoṣa uktaḥ ||10||
(su| u| taṃ| a| 22) |
The disease in which the nasal passages become dry by the action of vata and warm due to the action of pitta and the person experiences difficulty in inspiration and expiration (breathing) is known as Nasasosa or Nasaparisosa. (10)

Pinasa, its ama and pakva stages

śirogurutvamarucirnāsāsrāvastanuḥ svaraḥ |
kṣāmaḥ ṣṭhīvatyathābhīkṣṇamāmapīnasalakṣaṇam ||11||
āmaliṅgānvitaḥ śleṣmā ghanaḥ kheṣu nimajjati |
svaravarṇaviśuddhiśca paripakvasya lakṣaṇam ||12||
Symptoms of Ama (unripe, early stage) Pinasa – include feeling of heaviness of the head, loss of taste / appetite, discharge of thin fluid from the nose, feeble voice and frequent expectoration of the sputum.
Symptoms of Pakva (ripened stage) Pinasa – include decrease of symptoms of ama pinasa, discharges becoming thick and adhering to the inside of nasal passages, restoration of normal voice (clarity of voice) and restoration of normal colour. (11-12)

Pratisyaya

sandhāraṇājīrṇarajotibhāṣyakrodhartuvaiṣamyaśirobhitāpaiḥ |
prajāgarātisvapanāmbuśītairavaśyayā maithunabāṣpadhūmaiḥ |
saṃstyānadoṣe śirasi pravṛddho vāyuḥ pratiśyāyamudīrayettu ||13||
(ca| ci| a| 26) |
cayaṃ gatā mūrdhani mārutādayaḥ pṛthak samastāśca tathaiva śoṇitam |
prakupyamāṇā vividhaiḥ prakopaṇaistataḥ pratiśyāyakarā bhavanti hi ||14||
(su| u| taṃ| a| 24) |
Causative factors of Pratisyaya include - suppression of the natural urges of the body, having indigestion (ingestion of uncooked foods), exposure to excessive dust (frequently), excessive talking, excessive anger, seasonal abnormalities, injury to head or exposure to etiological factors which cause headache (dust, fumes, smoke etc which enter the head through the nose and cause headache), habit of keeping awake at night, excessive sleep or

excessive day-sleep, excessive consumption of cold water, excessive exposure to snowfall (thin rain, frost, mist, dew), excessive indulgence in sexual act and excessive exposure to steam (vapours) and smoke.
Pathogenesis of Pratisyaya – The above-mentioned etiological factors (and similar others) lead to aggravation of vata in the head in which kapha has already solidified which in turn causes the disease pratisyaya.
Vata and the other doshas i.e., pitta and kapha and rakta (blood) accumulate in the head, suddenly get excited (and aggravated) either individually or in combination by their respective exciting causes (etiological factors) and produce pratisyaya. (13-14)

Pratisyaya Purvarupa – Premonitory Symptoms of Pratisyaya

kṣavapravṛttiḥ śiraso'tipūrṇatā stambho'ṅgamardaḥ parihṛṣṭaromatā |
upadravāścāpyapare pṛthagvidhā nṛṇāṃ pratiśyāyapuraḥsarāḥ smṛtāḥ ||15||
(su| u| taṃ| a| 24) |
The symptoms seen in the premonitory stage of pratisyaya include – frequent bouts of sneezing, feeling of fullness of the head, stiffness / inactivity, pain all over the body, horripilation and many other complications. (15)

Symptoms of Vataja, Pittaja and Kaphaja Pratisyaya

ānaddhā pihitā nāsā tanusrāvaprasekinī |
galatālvoṣṭhaśoṣaśca nistodaḥ śaṅkhayostathā ||16||
(su| u| taṃ| a| 24) |
kṣavapravṛttiratyarthaṃ vaktravairasyameva ca |
bhavet svaropaghātaśca pratiśyāye'nilātmake ||17||
Symptoms of Vataja Pratisyaya – In this condition there is obstruction or covering inside the nose (full or partial blockage of nose), dripping out of thin fluid from the nose, dryness of the throat, palate and lips, pricking pain in the temples, excessive sneezing, distaste in the mouth and destruction of voice (broken voice). (16-17)

uṣṇaḥ sapītakaḥ srāvo ghrāṇāt sravati paittike |
kṛśo'tipāṇḍuḥ santapto bhaveduṣṇābhipīḍitaḥ ||18||
sadhūmamagniṃ sahasā vamatīva sa mānavaḥ |

Symptoms of Pittaja Pratisyaya – In this condition there will be feeling of warmth inside the nose, yellowish discharges from the nose, emaciation, severe pallor, raised temperature (worried, restless), and exhaustion by heat (of pittta). The person feels as if he is vomiting fire along with the smoke (excessive hot air is eliminated from the mouth). (18)

ghrāṇāt kaphaḥ kaphakṛte śītaḥ pāṇḍuḥ sravedbahuḥ |
śuklāvabhāsaḥ śuklākṣo bhavedguruśirā naraḥ ||19||
kaṇṭhatālvoṣṭhaśirasāṃ kaṇḍūbhirabhipīḍitaḥ |
(su| u| taṃ| a| 24) |
Symptoms of Kaphaja Pratisyaya – In this condition there will be excessive discharge of cold, pale (whitish yellow), thick mucus (phlegm) from the nose, the body and eyes would become (appear) white in colour. The person would also experience heaviness of the head, and excessive itching in the throat, palate, lips and head. (19-20)

Sannipataja Pratisyaya

bhūtvā bhūtvā pratiśyāyo yasyākasmānnivartate ||20||
sampakvo vā'pyapakvo vā sa sarvaprabhavaḥ smṛtaḥ |
(su| u| taṃ| a| 24) |
Symptoms of Sannipataja Pratisyaya - Partisyaya appearing and disappearing frequently without any apparent reason and is either in ripened or unripe state should be understood as being caused by all the three doshas together i.e., sannipataja pratisyaya. (20)

Dushta Pratisyaya

praklidyate punarnāsā punaśca pariśuṣyati ||21||
punarānahyate vā'pi punarvivriyate tathā |
niḥśvāso vā'tidurgandho naro gandhān na vetti ca ||22||
evaṃ duṣṭapratiśyāyaṃ jānīyāt kṛcchrasādhanam |
(su| u| taṃ| a| 24) |
In this condition, the inside of the nose will become too wet (due to too much fluid) or too dry alternatively (and repeatedly). Similarly, the nose gets blocked and gets cleared (of blockage) on its own accord (repeatedly). There will be foul smell in the breath and the person would not appreciate

smell (loss of sense of smell). This condition is called Dusta Pratisyaya and is difficult to treat. (21-22)

Raktaja Pratisyaya

raktaje tu pratiśyāye raktasrāvaḥ pravartate ||23||
tāmrākṣaśca bhavejjantururoghātaprapīḍitaḥ |
durgandhocchvāsavadano gandhānapi na vetti saḥ ||24||
(su| u| taṃ| a| 24) |
In pratishyaya caused due to increase of rakta (blood) there will be bleeding from the nose, coppery colour of the eyes, and severe pain in the chest, foul smell in the breath and mouth and the person will not appreciate smell (loss of sense of smell). (23-24)

Transformation of all Pratisyayas into Dusta Pratisyaya

sarva eva pratiśyāyā narasyāpratikāriṇaḥ |
duṣṭatāṃ yānti kālena tadā'sādhyā bhavanti hi ||25||
mūrchanti cātra krimayaḥ śvetāḥ snigdhāstathā'ṇavaḥ |
krimito yaḥ śirorogastulyaṃ tenāsya lakṣaṇam ||26||
(su| u| taṃ| a| 24) |
If not treated properly at proper time, all kinds of pratisyaya would ultimately get converted into dusta pratisyaya and become incurable in due course of time. Following this, there will be the appearance of worms which are white, unctuous (oily) and minute and the patient will develop symptoms similar to those of krimija siroroga (headache caused due to worms, bacteria). (25-26)

Pratisyaya Upadrava – Complications of Pratishyaya|

bādhiryamāndhyamaghratvaṃ ghorāṃśca nayanāmayān |
śothāgnisādakāsāṃśca vṛddhāḥ kurvanti pīnasāḥ ||27||
(su| u| taṃ| a| 24) |
All varieties of peenasa when become progressive (neglected) will, in due course of time, produce deafness, blindness, loss of sense of smell, severe kinds of eye diseases, swelling of the body, poor digestion and cough. (27)

Other diseases manifesting in the nose

arbudaṃ saptadhā śothāścatvāro’rśaścaturvidham |
caturvidhaṃ raktapittamuktaṃ ghrāṇe'pi tadviduḥ ||28||
The seven kinds of abruda, four kinds of sotha, four kinds of arsas and four kinds of raktapitta described previously might also manifest in the nose (or these may also develop as complications / sequelae of diseases of the nose).

iti śrīmādhavakaraviracite mādhavanidāne nāsāroganidānaṃ samāptam ||58||
Thus ends the chapter on Nasaroga.

CHAPTER FIFTY-NINE

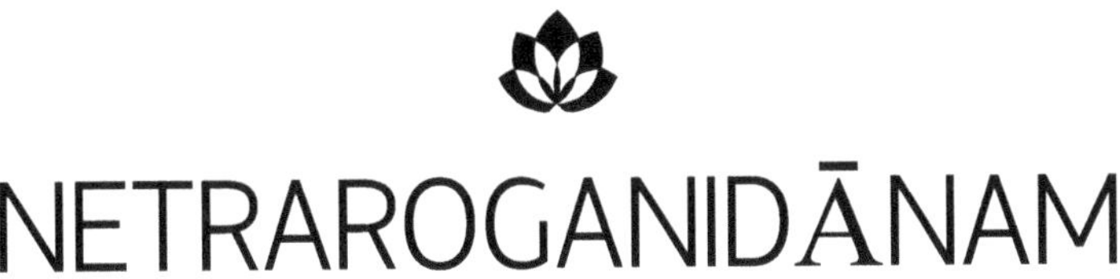

NETRAROGANIDĀNAM

Netra Roga Samanya Hetu – General Causes of Eye Diseases

uṣṇābhitaptasya jale praveśāddūrekṣaṇāt svapnaviparyayācca |
svedādrajodhūmaniṣevaṇācca chardervighātādvamanātiyogāt ||1||
dravāttathā'nnānniśi sevitācca viṇmūtravātakramanigrahācca |
prasaktasaṃrodanakopaśokācchiro'bhighātādatimadyapānāt ||2||
tathā ṛtūnāṃ ca viparyayeṇa kleśābhighātādatimaithunācca |
bāṣpagrahāt sūkṣmanirīkṣaṇācca netre vikārāñjanayanti doṣāḥ ||3||
(su| u| taṃ| a| 1) |
Entering into the water (taking bath in cold water) immediately after exposure to heat, seeing objects which are far away (by straining one's eyes), abnormal sleeping habits (like not sleeping at proper time, keeping awake during night time, sleeping in excess during day time etc), sudation or fumigation to the eyes, excessive contact / exposure of the eyes to dust and smoke, forcibly withholding the urge for vomiting or vomiting in excess (too much vomiting, too much of emesis therapy), taking watery foods (liquid foods) at night in excess, habitually suppressing the natural urges of faeces, urine and flatus, constantly weeping, getting angry and grieving, injury to the head, excessive consumption of alcoholic drinks, abnormal seasonal changes, physical and mental exhaustion, excessive indulgence in sexual act, controlling tears, seeing minute objects (microscopic objects) for prolonged periods of time, etc are the etiological factors of eye disorders. The above-mentioned etiological factors cause abnormal increase of doshas which in turn produce various diseases of the eyes. (1-3)

Types of Abhisyanda

vātāt pittāt kaphādraktādabhiṣyandaścaturvidhaḥ |
prāyeṇa jāyate ghoraḥ sarvanetrāmayākaraḥ ||4||
Abhsyanda is of four types - vātaja, pittaja, kaphaja and raktaja. It is a very dreadful disease which probably is the main cause for all other (almost) eye diseases. (4)

Vataja Abisyanda

nistodanastambhanaromaharṣasaṅgharṣapāruṣyaśiro'bhitāpāḥ |
viśuṣkabhāvaḥ śiśirāśrutā ca vātābhipanne nayane bhavanti ||5||
(su| u| taṃ| a| 6) |
Symptoms of Abisyanda caused by increased vata include pricking pain, stiffness (loss of movements or restricted movements), horripilation, irritation and roughness (friction) in the eyes, headache, absence of excretions in the eyes (dryness of eyes) and cold tears flowing out of the eyes. (5)

Pittaja Abhisyanda

dāhaprapākau śiśirābhinandā dhūmāyanaṃ bāṣpasamucchrayaśca |
uṣṇāśrutā pītakanetratā ca pittābhipanne nayane bhavanti ||6||
(su| u| taṃ| a| 6) |
Symptoms of Abisyanda caused by increased pitta include feeling of burning sensation, suppuration, desire for cold things and comforts, feeling as if hot smoke is being eliminated from the eyes, excessive flow of tears, hot tears coming from the eyes and yellowish discolouration of the eyes. (6)

Kaphaja Abhisyanda

uṣṇābhinandā gurutā'kṣiśothaḥ kaṇḍūpadehāvatiśītatā ca |
srāvo muhuḥ picchila eva cāpi kaphābhipanne nayane bhavanti ||7||
(su| u| taṃ| a| 6) |
Symptoms of Abhisyanda caused by increased kapha include desire for warm things and comforts, feeling of heaviness in the eyes, swelling, itching, accumulation of dirty excretions, excessive coldness, excessive and frequent discharge of sticky secretions (discharges, tears) from the eyes. (7)

Raktaja Abhisyanda

tāmrāśrutā lohitanetratā ca nāḍyaḥ samantādatilohitāśca |
pittasya liṅgāni ca yāni tāni raktābhipanne nayane bhavanti ||8||
(su| u| taṃ| a| 6) |
Symptoms of Abhisyanda caused by increased rakta (blood) include discharge of copper-coloured tears, redness of the eyes, redness of the capillaries in all corners of the eyes and presence of other symptoms of pittaja abhisyanda (explained above). (8)

Adhimantha

vṛddhairetairabhiṣyandairnarāṇāmakriyāvatām |
tāvantastvadhimanthāḥ syurnayane tīvravedanāḥ ||9||
(su| u| taṃ| a| 6) |
Any of the above types of abhiṣyanda, if not treated at the proper time, will undergo abnormal increase and lead to another condition called as adhimantha which causes severe pain in the eyes. (9)

Adhimantha Samanya Lakshana – General symptoms of Adhimantha

utpāṭyata ivātyarthaṃ netraṃ nirmathyate tathā |
śiraso'rdhaṃ ca taṃ vidyādadhimanthaṃ svalakṣaṇaiḥ ||10||
(su| u| taṃ| a| 6) |
A condition of the eye in which the person feels as though someone is pulling out or churning (squeezing) his eyes and half portion of his head with force is known as adhimantha. In addition to this the other symptoms of predominant doshas (as explained in dosha types of abhisyanda above) are also seen in this condition. (10)

Effect of Adhimantha

hanyāddṛṣṭiṃ ślaiṣmikaḥ saptarātrādadhimantho raktajaḥ pañcarātrāt |
ṣaḍrātrādvātiko vai nihanyānmithyācārāt paittikaḥ sadya eva ||11||
(su| u| taṃ| a| 6) |
When improperly managed and not treated properly at proper time – Kaphaja Adhimantha will destroy the vision within seven days.

Raktaja Adhimantha will destroy the vision within five days.
Vataja Adhimantha will destroy the vision within six days.
Pittaja Adhimantha will destroy the vision immediately / very soon (within three days). (11)

Sama Lakshanas of Netra Roga – Symptoms of eye diseases associated with ama (unripe stage)

udīrṇavedanaṃ netraṃ rāgaśothasamanvitam |
gharṣanistodaśūlāśruyuktamāmānvitaṃ viduḥ ||12||
The symptoms of ama (unripe) stage of eye diseases include progressively increasing severe pain, redness, swelling and rubbing pain (friction, irritation), pricking pain, pain, and discharges (excessive flow of tears) from the eyes. (12)

Pakva Lakshanas of Netra Roga – Symptoms of eye diseases devoid of ama association (ripe stage)

mandavedanatā kaṇḍūḥ saṃrambhāśrupraśāntatā |
praśastavarṇatā cākṣṇoḥ sampakvadoṣamādiśet ||13||
The symptoms of pakva (ripe) stage of eye diseases include mild pain (reduction in severity of pain) in the eyes, itching, swelling, reduction of discharges (tears) from the eyes, colour of the eyes (discolouration) returning to normal. (13)

Sothaja and Asothaja Netrapaka

kaṇḍūpadehāśruyutaḥ pakvodumbarasannibhaḥ |
saṃrambhī pacyate yastu netrapākaḥ sa śothajaḥ |
śothahīnāni liṅgāni netrapāke tvaśothaje ||14||
(su| u| taṃ| a| 6) |
Shothaja Netrapaka – In this condition the eyes will have itching, accumulation of excretion / dirt (in the eyes), excessive tearing, and will resemble the ripe Udumbara fruit. Suppuration will occur following the appearance of swelling.
Ashotha Netrapaka – In this condition all symptoms mentioned above (in sothaja netrapaka) will be found except the appearance of swelling

(suppuration of eyes occur even without the appearance of swelling). (14)

Hatadimantha

upekṣaṇādakṣi yadā'dhimantho vātātmakaḥ sādayati prasahya |
rujābhirugrābhirasādhya eṣa hatādhimanthaḥ khalu nāma rogaḥ ||15||
(su| u| taṃ| a| 6) |
When neglected (not properly treated at proper time), the Vataja Adhimantha forcefully causes severe pain in the eyes and leads to destruction of vision. This incurable disease is known as Hatadhimantha. (15)

Vataparyaya

vāraṃvāraṃ ca paryeti bhruvau netre ca mārutaḥ |
rujaśca vividhāstīvrāḥ sa jñeyo vātaparyayaḥ ||16|
A condition in which vata which has abnormally increased repeatedly causes different kinds of pain in the eyebrows and eyes (areas surrounding the eyes) is called as Vataparyaya. (16)

Suskaksipaka

yat kūṇitaṃ dāruṇarūkṣavartma sandahyate cāviladarśanaṃ yat |
sudāruṇaṃ yat pratibodhane ca śuṣkākṣipākopahataṃ tadakṣi ||17||
(su| u| taṃ| a| 6) |
The condition in which the eyelids become closed, hard and dry to touch, has burning sensation, is cloudy and unclear vision, and it becomes difficult to open the eyelids and on opening the eyes look dry is known as Suska Aksipaka. (17)

Anyatovata

yasyāvaṭukarṇaśirohanustho manyāgato vā'pyanilo'nyato vā |
kuryādrujaṃ vai bhruvi locane ca tamanyatovātamudāharanti ||18||
(su| u| taṃ| a| 6) |
A condition in which vata aggravating in the posterior part of the neck, ears, head, jaw (lower) and sides of the neck causes severe pain in the eyebrows

and eye is known as Anyatovata. (18)

Amladhyusita

śyāvaṃ lohitaparyantaṃ sarvaṃ cākṣi prapacyate |
sadāhaśothaṃ sāsrāvamamlādhyuṣitamamlataḥ ||19||
The condition in which the pitta undergoing abnormal increase due to excessive consumption of sour foods would cause bluish discolouration of the eyes with reddish borders and suppuration in the entire eye is known as Amladhyusita. This condition is also associated with burning sensation, swelling and discharges (excessive flow of tears) from the eyes. (19)

Sirotpata

avedanā vā'pi savedanā vā yasyākṣirājyo hi bhavanti tāmrāḥ |
muhurvirajyanti ca yāḥ sa tādṛgvyādhiḥ sirotpāta iti pradiṣṭaḥ ||20||
(su| u| taṃ| a| 6) |
The disease in which the network of blood vessels in the eye become coppery or red in colour, is associated or not associated with pain and the eye becomes angry red repeatedly is known by the name Sirotpata. (20)

Sirapraharsa

mohāt sirotpāta upekṣitastu jāyeta rogastu [2] sirāpraharṣaḥ |
tāmrābhamasraṃ sravati pragāḍhaṃ tathā na śaknotyabhivīkṣituṃ ca ||21||
(su| u| taṃ| a| 6) |
When sirotpata disease (explained above) is neglected (not treated promptly) due to ignorance, yet another disease known as Sirapraharsa gets manifested. In this condition the person would discharge thick coppery / red coloured fluids in large quantities and will be unable to see anything. (21)

Savrana Sukla

nimagnarūpaṃ tu bhaveddhi kṛṣṇe sūcyeva viddhaṃ pratibhāti yadvai |
srāvaṃ sraveduṣṇamatīva yacca tat savraṇaṃ śukla(kra)mudāharanti ||22||
(su| u| taṃ| a| 5) |

A deep-seated spot which is difficult to identify, which appears as if pierced by a sharp needle, located in the black of the eye (cornea) is known as Savrana Sukla or Savrana Sukra. In this condition, very hot tears discharge (tears) flow out of the eyes. (22)

Savrana Sukla

dṛṣṭeḥ samīpe na bhavettu yacca na cāvagāḍhaṃ na ca saṃsraveddhi |
avedanaṃ vā na yugmaśuklaṃ tat siddhimāyāti kadācideva ||23||
(su| u| taṃ| a| 5) |
An ulcer which is not very near to the pupil, which is not deep rooted, not having too much of discharge, is painless (has mild pain) and which doesn't have two ulcers (not affecting both eyes together) and is sometimes curable (sometimes responds to treatment and sometimes will not, especially if both eyes are afflicted with ulcers) is known as Savrana Sukla or Savrana Sukra. (23)

Symptoms of Curability of Avrana Sukla

syandātmakaṃ kṛṣṇagataṃ sacoṣaṃ śaṅkhendukundapratimāvabhāsam |
vaihāyasābhrapratanuprakāśamathāvraṇaṃ sādhyatamaṃ vadanti ||24||
(su| u| taṃ| a| 5) |
Due to the effect of Abhisyanda there appears a white coloured scar resembling the colour of conch, moon or lily flower on the cornea or the cornea appears cloudy, as if it is covered by thin (waterless) cloud, and is associated with burning sensation. This condition is known as Avrana Sukla which is easily curable. (24)

Prognosis of Avrana Sukla

gambhīrajātaṃ bahulaṃ ca śuklaṃ cirotthitaṃ cāpi vadanti kṛcchram |
vicchinnamadhyaṃ piśitāvṛtaṃ vā calaṃ sirāsūkṣmamadṛṣṭikṛcca |
dvitvaggataṃ lohitamantataśca cirotthitaṃ cāpi vivarjanīyam ||25||
(su| u| taṃ| a| 5) |
uṣṇāśrupātaḥ piḍakā ca netre yasmin bhavenmudganibhaṃ ca śuklam |
tadapyasādhyaṃ pravadanti kecidanyacca yattittiripakṣatulyam ||26||
(su| u| taṃ| a| 5) |

Avranaśukla developing from deep inside (second or third layer / tunic), is thick, and has been for a long time (has become chronic) is difficult to cure. Avrana Sukla in which there is a tear in the middle or is covered by muscle, movable, and is minute / invisible (interferes with vision) because of being enveloped with a thin network of veins should be refused treatment since it is incurable.
Avrana Sukla occurring (involving) in the second layer, having reddish edges and has become chronic is also incurable.
Similarly, avrana sukla in which warm tears are eliminated from the eyes, there is appearance of white coloured nodules of the size of green gram and that which assumes the colour of feather of tittira bird (grey partridge) should also be considered as incurable. (25-26)

Akşipäkätyaya

śvetaḥ samākrāmati sarvato hi doṣeṇa yasyāsitamaṇḍalaṃ ca |
tamakṣipākātyayamakṣirogaṃ sarvātmakaṃ varjayitavyamāhuḥ ||27||
(su| u| taṃ| a| 5) |
The eye disease in which the entire cornea becomes white (in colour) by the action of all the three abnormally increased doshas, caused by all three aggravated doshas should be rejected treatment (because it is incurable). (27)

Ajakājāta

ajāpurīṣapratimo rujāvān salohito lohitapicchilāsraḥ |
vigṛhya kṛṣṇaṃ pracayo'bhyupaiti taccājakājātamiti vyavasyet ||28||
(iti kṛṣṇajāḥ) | (su| u| taṃ| a| 5) |
A growth (projection) resembling a dried pellet of goat excreta, which is painful, red in colour, discharges red sticky fluid, and projects out piercing the cornea is called as Ajakajata. (28)

Pratama Patalagata Timira

prathame paṭale doṣā yasya dṛṣṭyāṃ vyavasthitāḥ |
avyaktāni sa rūpāṇi kadācidatha paśyati ||29||
(su| u| taṃ| a| 5) |

When timira manifests due to the increased doshas localized in the first patala (layer) of the drsti (lens), the person sees things in an indistinct or unclear way (does not see the objects clearly). (29)

Dwitiya Patalagata Timira

dṛṣṭirbhṛśaṃ vihvalati dvitīyaṃ paṭalaṃ gate |
makṣikāmaśakāṃścāpi jālakāni ca paśyati ||30||
maṇḍalāni patākāṃśca marīciṃ kuṇḍalāni ca |
pariplavāṃśca vividhān varṣamabhraṃ tamāṃsi ca ||31||
dūrasthāni ca rūpāṇi manyate sa samīpataḥ |
samīpasthāni dūre ca dṛṣṭergocaravibhramāt ||32||
yatnavānapi cātyarthaṃ sūcīpāśaṃ na paśyati |
(su| u| taṃ| a| 7) |
When the timira manifests due to the increased doshas getting localized (invade the) in the second patala (layer), his vision becomes distorted. He sees flies, mosquitoes, spider webs, round things (circular objects), flags, various types of shining things like rays of light etc, rings, jumping frogs etc, rain, clouds, and darkness. He sees distant objects to be very near to him and nearby things to be very far away due to distortion and perversion of vision and visual objects. In spite of making all efforts the person will not be able to see the eye of the needle and its thread (will not be able to put the thread into the eye of the needle). (31-32)

Trtiya Patalagata Timira

ūrdhvaṃ paśyati nādhastāttṛtīyaṃ paṭalaṃ gate ||33||
mahāntyapi ca rūpāṇi chāditānīva cāmbaraiḥ |
karṇanāsākṣihīnāni vikṛtānīva paśyati ||34||
yathādoṣaṃ ca rajyeta dṛṣṭirdoṣe balīyasi |
(su| u| taṃ| a| 7) |
adhaḥsthite samīpasthaṃ dūrasthaṃ coparisthite ||35||
pārśvasthite tathā doṣe pārśvasthaṃ naiva paśyati |
samantataḥ sthite doṣe saṅkulānīva paśyati ||36||
dṛṣṭimadhyasthite doṣe mahaddhrasvaṃ ca paśyati |
dvidhā sthite dvidhā paśyedbahudhā cānavasthite ||37||
(su| u| taṃ| a| 7) |

When the timira manifests due to the increased doshas getting localized (invade the) in the third patala (layer), the person will be able to see objects which are at the top but cannot see the objects placed at the bottom. Even the larger objects appear to him as though covered by cloth. He sees the other people as being devoid of ears, nose and eyes or sees them (ears, nose and eyes) as abnormal and distorted. Depending on the doshas which become predominant in the disease, the colour corresponding to that particular predominant dosha will manifest in the drsti – lens.
When the doshas get localized in the lower portion of the drsti (lens) one cannot see the objects which are nearby. If the doshas are located in the upper portion, one cannot see the objects which are far away. When the doshas are localized at the sides, one cannot see the objects which are on the sides.
If doshas are spread all over, in all directions, the objects will be seen as mixed up in different ways. On the other hand, if the doshas are located at the centre, the big objects are seen as small by the patient. If the doshas are located in two places, all the objects appear double. If the doshas are located in many places, all objects appear to be of many types. If the doshas are located obliquely in the drsti, the person sees one object as two. (33-37)

Chaturtha Patalagata Timira

timirākhyaḥ sa vai doṣaścaturthaṃ paṭalaṃ gataḥ ||38||
ruṇaddhi sarvato dṛṣṭiṃ liṅganāśamataḥ param |
asminnapi tamobhūte nātirūḍhe mahāgade ||39||
candrādityau sanakṣatrāvantarīkṣe ca vidyutaḥ |
nirmalāni ca tejāṃsi bhrājiṣṇūnyatha paśyati ||40||
(su| u| taṃ| a| 7) |
sa eva liṅganāśastu nīlikā kācasañjñitaḥ |41|
(su| u| taṃ| a| 7) |
When the same increased doshas of (having the form of) timira located in the third patala (layer) reaches to invade the fourth patala (layer), they cause complete loss of vision. This condition is called Linganasa (loss of capacity to see and perceive the objects – total loss of vision).
If this dreadful disease which is in the form of darkness is not deep rooted or if it has not run a long course and become chronic (much time has not lapsed since the onset of blindness), the person will be able to see very

bright objects such as the moon, sun, stars and lightning in the sky and also other clear bright objects elsewhere. This linganasa is also known as Nilika or Kaca. (38-40)

Timira Symptoms based on 'predominant dosha' involved

vātena cāpi rūpāṇi bhramantīva ca paśyati ||41||
āvilānyaruṇābhāni vyāviddhānīva mānavaḥ |
pittenādityakhadyotaśakracāpataḍidguṇān ||42||
nṛtyataścaiva śikhinaḥ sarvaṃ nīlaṃ ca paśyati |
kaphena paśyedrūpāṇi snigdhāni ca sitāni ca ||43||
(gauracāmaragaurāṇi śvetābhrapratimāni ca |
paśyedasūkṣmāṇyatyarthaṃ vyabhre caivābhrasamplavam) |
salilaplāvitānīva parijāḍyāni mānavaḥ |
paśyedraktena raktāni tamāṃsi vividhāni ca ||44||
sa sitānyapi kṛṣṇāni pītānyapi ca mānavaḥ |
sannipātena citrāṇi viplutānīva paśyati ||45||
bahudhā ca dvidhā cāpi sarvāṇyeva samantataḥ |
hīnādhikāṅgānyapi tu jyotīṃṣyapi ca bhūyasā ||46||
(su| u| taṃ| a| 7) |
Vataja Timira – In timira, when vata is predominant, the patient sees the objects constantly moving in front of his eyes. The objects are perceived as being dirty, of slightly red (reddish yellow) in colour and crooked (irregular or broken).
Pittaja Timira – In timira, when pitta is predominant, the patient sees the (shapes, forms of) sun, glow-worm, rainbow, and sparks of fire and dancing peacocks – all objects blue in colour.
Kaphaja Timira – In timira, when kapha is predominant, the patient sees all objects as being unctuous and white in colour and very big in size. He sees a clear sky as if covered by clouds. He sees all the objects being drowned in the water and devoid of any movement (still and stagnant).
Raktaja Timira – In timira, when rakta (vitiated blood) is predominant, the person sees all the objects red in colour. He also would see different types of darkness (darkness of varying intensity). Even the white coloured objects are seen as being black or yellow coloured.
Sannipataja Timira – In timira caused by predominance of all the three doshas, the person sees different objects and also strange objects and in

different forms (not in their actual form) with many colours and irregularities. He sees one object as many (all objects everywhere) or one object as two or many (many mingled into one). He sees people etc with absence of some body parts or with extra parts. He also sees the stars as being deformed. (41-46)

Parimlayi Kacha

pittaṃ kuryāt parimlāyi mūrchitaṃ pittatejasā |
pītā diśastu khadyotān bhāskaraṃ cāpi paśyati ||47||
vikīryamāṇān khadyotairvṛkṣāṃstejobhireva vā |
(su| u| taṃ| a| 7) |
Pitta in association with blood produces another condition known as Parimlayi. In this condition, the patient sees yellow in everything and everywhere. He also sees glow worms and sun here and there (at any time). He sees trees surrounded by glow worms, fire or any other shining things. (47)

Types of Linganasha

vakṣyāmi ṣaḍvidhaṃ rāgairliṅganāśamataḥ param ||48||
Further on, I will describe six types of linganāśas pertaining to (based on) colours.

Manifestation of different colours in different types of doshaja linganasha

rāgo'ruṇo mārutajaḥ pradiṣṭo mlāyī ca nīlaśca tathaiva pittāt |
kaphāt sitaḥ śoṇitajaḥ saraktaḥ samastadoṣaprabhavo vicitraḥ ||49||
(su| u| taṃ| a| 7) |
aruṇaṃ maṇḍalaṃ dṛṣṭyāṃ sthūlakācāruṇaprabham |50|
(su| u| taṃ| a| 7) |
In timira / linganāśa caused by increased vata, all objects will appear crimson red in colour.
In linganasa caused by increased pitta, all the objects will appear yellowish blue or blue in colour.
In linganasa caused by increased kapha, all the objects will appear white in

colour.
In linganasa caused by increased blood, all objects will appear red in colour.
In linganasa caused by all the three doshas increased together, all objects will appear to have strangely mixed colours. (49)
The crimson red colour described (for vātaja linganāśa) will be like bright circular rings as seen coming out of a thick lens. (50)

Specific features of Parimlayi

parimlāyini roge syānmlāyi nīlaṃ ca maṇḍalam ||50||
doṣakṣayāt svayaṃ tatra kadācit syāttu darśanam |
(su| u| taṃ| a| 7) |
In parimlāyī, the lens becomes dirty and blue coloured. Sometimes when the doshas decrease on their own accord in due course of time, the person regains sight even without any treatment. (50)

Symptoms of coloured lens in accordance to dosha predominance

aruṇaṃ maṇḍalaṃ vātāccañcalaṃ paruṣaṃ tathā ||51||
pittānmaṇḍalamānīlaṃ kāṃsyābhaṃ pītameva ca |
śleṣmaṇā bahulaṃ pītaṃ śaṅkhakundendupāṇḍuram ||52||
calatpadmapalāśasthaḥ śuklo bindurivāmbhasaḥ |
mṛjyamāne ca nayane maṇḍalaṃ tadvisarpati ||53||
pravālapadmapatrābhaṃ maṇḍalaṃ śoṇitātmakam |
dṛṣṭirāgo bhaveccitro liṅganāśe tridoṣaje |
yathāsvaṃ doṣaliṅgāni sarveṣveva bhavanti hi ||54||
(su| u| taṃ| a| 7) |
In case of increase of vata, the vision / lens become crimson in colour, unsteady and rough (irregular).
In case of increase of pitta, the lens becomes blue, whitish yellow like bronze and yellow in colour.
In case of increase of kapha, the lens becomes thick, yellow or of the colour (resemblance) of conch, jasmine flower or moon, whitish yellow in colour or white in colour resembles a drop of water on a moving lotus leaf. The lens moves here and there while rubbing the eyes.
In case of increase of rakta – blood, the rings (lens) will resemble coral or leaf of red coloured lotus.

In case of increase of all the three doshas together, the rings (lens) will be of mixed colours. The other symptoms in this condition will be in accordance to the predominance of particular dosha in the combined vitiation. (51-54)

To sum up

ṣaḍ liṅganāśāḥ ṣaḍime ca rogā dṛṣṭyāśrayāḥ ṣaṭ ca ṣaḍeva vācyāḥ |55|
(su| u| taṃ| a| 7) |
Six types of Linganasas occur in the eye as explained above. Six other diseases affecting the lens (vision) will be detailed further on. (55)

Pitta Vidagdha Drsti

pittena duṣṭena sadā tu dṛṣṭiḥ pītā bhavedyasya narasya kiñcit ||55||
pītāni rūpāṇi ca tena paśyet sa vai naraḥ pittavidagdhadṛṣṭiḥ |
prāpte tṛtīyaṃ paṭalaṃ tu doṣe divā na paśyenniśi cekṣate saḥ ||56||
rātrau ca śītānugṛhītadṛṣṭiḥ pittālpabhāvādapi tāni paśyet |
(su| u| taṃ| a| 7) |
If the drsti (lens, vision) due to the influence of vitiated pitta always remains slight yellowish in colour, the person starts seeing everything in his surrounding as being yellow in colour. This condition is called as pitta vidagdha drsti (also called divandhya – day blindness). If pitta gets localized in the third patala (layer) of drsti mandala (eye, lens) the person cannot see any objects during day time. He can only see things during night time. Due to the influence of coldness prevailing at night, the pitta gets subsided and hence he can see things during night time. (55-56)

Shlesma / Kapha Vidagdha Drsti

tathā naraḥ śleṣmavidagdhadṛṣṭistānyeva śuklāni tu manyate saḥ ||57||
triṣu sthito'lpaḥ paṭaleṣu doṣo naktāndhyamāpādayati prasahya |
divā sa sūryānugṛhītadṛṣṭiḥ paśyettu rūpāṇi kaphālpabhāvāt ||58||
(su| u| taṃ| a| 7) |
Similarly, when the drsti (lens, vision) of the person is afflicted by vitiated kapha, the person sees everything (all objects) as white (in colour). When the doshas get lodged in all the three patalas (layers), the person would suffer from a condition called naktandhya (night blindness). In the day time, due to less quantity of kapha and due to the influence of (heat of)

the Sun, he can see the objects properly. This condition is called as Kaphavidagdha Drsti or Naktandya which means night blindness. (57-58)

Dhumadarsi

śokajvarāyāsaśiro'bhitāpairabhyāhatā yasya narasya dṛṣṭiḥ |
dhūmrāṃstathā paśyati sarvabhāvān sa dhūmadarśīti naraḥ pradiṣṭaḥ ||59||
(su| u| taṃ| a| 7) |
Drsti (lens, vision) getting affected by causes such as grief, fever, excessive exertion and headache etc leads to the manifestation of a disease called Dhumadarsi in which the person sees all objects as if covered by smoke. (59)

Hrsvajadya

yo hrasvajāḍyo divaseṣu kṛcchrāddhrasvāni rūpāṇi ca tena paśyet |60|
(su| u| taṃ| a| 7) |
The disease in which the person finds it very difficult to see the objects during daytime and also sees big objects as small is known as Hrasvajādya. (60)

Nakulandhya

vidyotate yasya narasya dṛṣṭirdoṣābhipannā nakulasya yadvat ||60||
citrāṇi rūpāṇi divā sa paśyet sa vai vikāro nakulāndhyasañjñaḥ |
(su| u| taṃ| a| 7) |
When all the three vitiated doshas affect the drsti (vision, lens) the eyes of the person shine like the eyes of mongoose. Such a person sees objects in different (mixed) shapes and colours. This condition is known as Nakulandhya. (60)

Gambhirika

dṛṣṭirvirūpā śvasanopasṛṣṭā saṅkocamabhyantaratastu yāti ||61||
rujāvagāḍhā ca tamakṣirogaṃ gambhīriketi pravadanti tajjñāḥ |
(su| u| taṃ| a| 7) |
The drsti (lens, vision, eyes) affected by vitiated vata makes the eye

deformed (sees things in unnatural state) and the eyeball sinks deep inside the socket of the eye. In this condition there is severe pain in the eye. This disease is called Gambhirika by experts. (61)

Agantuja Linganasa

bāhyau punardvāviha sampradiṣṭau nimittataścāpyanimittataśca ||62||
nimittatastatra śiro'bhitāpājjñeyastvabhiṣyandanidarśanaḥ saḥ |
surarṣigandharvamahoragāṇāṃ sandarśanenāpi ca bhāskarasya ||63||
hanyeta dṛṣṭirmanujasya yasya sa liṅganāśastvanimittasañjñaḥ |
tatrākṣi vispṛṣṭamivāvabhāti vaidūryavarṇā vimalā ca dṛṣṭiḥ ||64||
(iti dṛṣṭigatāḥ) | (su| u| taṃ| a| 7) |
Agantuja Linganasha (that caused by external agents) is of two types. They are – Nimittaja Linganasha and Animittaja Linganasha.
Nimittaja Linganasha – Linganasa caused due to headache (caused by etiological factors like poisons, smell of flowers, exposure to severe winds etc) is called as Nimittaja Linganasa. This will have symptoms similar to those of Abhisyanda (conjunctivitis).
Animittaja Linganasha – Loss of vision caused due to unusual (sudden) sight of gods, sages, gandharvas, divine serpents, or the Sun is known as Animittaja Linganasa. In this condition the eyes are quite normal and not deformed. The lens too will be bright and will have the colour and glitter of vaidurya (Cat's Eye) and clear (but they would have lost the capacity to see and perceive). (62-64)

Prastaryarma (Prastari Arma)

prastāryarma tanu stīrṇaṃ śyāvaṃ raktanibhaṃ site |65|
A thin, broad, black or blackish blue or red coloured mass of tissue (fleshy growth) formed on the white of the eye (sclera – sita mandala) is known as Prastaryarma. (65)

Shuklarma (Shukla Arma)

saśvetaṃ mṛdu śuklārma śukle tadvardhate cirāt ||65||
A white soft mass (fleshy strip), developing slowly (over many days) on the white portion of the eye (sclera) is known as Shuklarma (Sukla Arma). (65)

Raktarma (Rakta Arma) & Adhimamsarma (Adhimamsa Arma)

padmābhaṃ mṛdu raktārma yanmāṃsaṃ cīyate site
pṛthu mṛdvadhimāṃsārma bahulaṃ ca yakṛnnibham |66|
A soft muscular tissue / strip resembling a red lotus petal developing on the white of the eye (sclera) is known as Raktarma (Rakta Arma).
A muscular strip / fleshy strip which is soft, thick and resembling a piece of liver, developing on the white of the eye (sclera) is known as Adhimäṁsārma (Adhimamsa Arma). (66)

Snayvarma (Snayu Arma)

sthiraṃ prastāri māṃsāḍhyaṃ śuklaṃ snāyvarma pañcamam ||66||
Immovable, widespread, dry, muscular (or tendinous) tissue is the fifth kind of arma. It is known as Snayvarma (Snayu Arma). (66)

Shuktika & Arjuna

śyāvāḥ syuḥ piśitanibhāśca bindavo ye śuktyābhāḥ sitaniyatāḥ sa śuktisañjñaḥ |67|
(su| u| taṃ| a| 7) |
eko yaḥ śaśarudhiropamaśca binduḥ śuklastho bhavati tamarjunaṃ vadanti ||67||
(su| u| taṃ| a| 4) |
A spot (papule) which is blackish blue in colour, which resembles muscle tissue and oyster shell developing on the white of the eye (sclera) is known as Shuktika.
Arjuna – A single spot (papule) resembling the blood of a rabbit (deep / dark red in colour) which occurs on the white of the eye (sclera) is known as Arjuna. (67)

Pistika

śleṣmamārutakopena śukle piṣṭaṃ samunnatam |
piṣṭavat piṣṭakaṃ viddhi malāktādarśasannibham ||68||
Kapha and väta getting increased causes a raised papule resembling ground

rice flour or of the colour of a dirty mirror (dust laden mirror) on the white of the eye (sclera). This condition is called as Pistaka. (68)

Sirajala

jālābhaḥ kaṭhinasiro mahān saraktaḥ santānaḥ smṛta iha jālasañjñitastu |69|
(su| u| taṃ| a| 4) |
A big and red coloured covering having a network of hard veins developing over the white of the eye (sclera) is known as Sirajala. (68)

Siraja Pidaka

śuklasthāḥ sitapiḍakāḥ sirāvṛtā yāstā brūyādasitasamīpajāḥ sirājāḥ |69|
(su| u| taṃ| a| 4) |
White papules covered with veins, developing on the white of the eye (sclera), very near to the black of the eye (cornea, iris) is known as Siraja Pidaka.

Balasa Grathita

kāṃsyābho'mṛduratha vāribindukalpo vijñeyo nayanasite balāsasañjñaḥ ||69||
(su| u| taṃ| a| 4) |
A papule (cyst) developing on the white of the eye (sclera), having the colour of bronze, raised – resembling water bubble and hard to touch is known as Balasa or Balasagrathita. (69)

Puyalasaka

pakvaḥ śothaḥ sandhijo yaḥ satodaḥ sravet pūyaṃ pūti pūyālasākhyaḥ |70|
(su| u| taṃ| a| 2) |
A well-formed (matured) swelling (vesicle), which occurs at the inner angle (corner) of the eye, along with pain and discharge of foul-smelling pus is known as Puyalasaka.

Upanaha

granthirnālpo dṛṣṭisandhāvapākī kaṇḍūprāyo nīrujastūpanāhaḥ ||70||

(su| u| taṃ| a| 2) |
A big sized cyst (tumour) occurring at the junction of cornea and pupil, not suppurating (not forming pus) having itching and devoid of pain is known as Upanaha. (70)

Chaturvidha Srava – four types of discharges

gatvā sandhīnaśrumārgeṇa doṣāḥ kuryuḥ srāvān lakṣaṇaiḥ svairupetān |
taṃ hi srāvaṃ netranāḍīti caike tasyā liṅgaṃ kīrtayiṣye caturdhā ||71||
(su| u| taṃ| a| 2) |
The aggravated doshas reach the joints of the eyes through the asruvahi nadis i.e., channels which carry tears and cause discharges associated with their corresponding features (symptoms). This is called Netrasrava. Some experts also call it Netranadi. Four types of symptoms of these nadis shall be enumerated ahead. (71)

Symptoms of four kinds of Srava

pākāt sandhau saṃsravedyastu pūyaṃ pūyāsrāvo'sau gadaḥ sarvajastu |72|
(su| u| taṃ| a| 2) |
śvetaṃ sāndraṃ picchilaṃ yaḥ sravettu śleṣmāsrāvo'sau vikāro matastu ||72||
(su| u| taṃ| a| 2) |
raktasrāvaḥ śoṇitottho vikāraḥ sraveddusṭaṃ tatra raktaṃ prabhūtam |73|
(su| u| taṃ| a| 2) |
haridrābhaṃ pītamuṣṇaṃ jalābhaṃ pittāt srāvaḥ saṃsravet sandhimadhyāt ||73||
(su| u| taṃ| a| 2) |
Puyasrāva – Due to suppuration (formation of pus) in the angles (corners) of the eye, there will be discharge of pus caused due to simultaneous increase of all the three doshas. This condition is called Puyasrava.
Shlesmasrava – The disease in which there is white, thick and sticky discharge is called Kaphaja Puyasrava or Shlesmasrava.
Raktasrava – The disease caused by vitiated rakta (blood) in which there is excessive bleeding from the corner (inner angle) of the eye is called Raktaja Puyasrava or Raktasrava.
Pittasrava – Discharges which resemble turmeric colour, yellow, hot and watery in nature which occurs from the inner angle of the eye caused by aggravated pitta is called as Pittaja Puyasrava or Pittasrava. (72-73)

Parvani and Alaji

tāmrā tanvī dāhaśūlopapannā raktājjñeyā parvaṇī vṛttaśothā |
jātā sandhau kṛṣṇaśukle 'lajī syāt tasminneva khyāpitā pūrvaliṅgai ||74||
(su| u| taṃ| a| 2) |
Parvani - A rounded swelling of coppery (red) colour, thin (small), associated with burning sensation and pain, caused by aggravated blood, developing at the junction of sclera and cornea is known as Parvani.
Alaji – Another identical disease known as Alaji occurs at the same place i.e. at the junction of sclera and cornea, will have the symptoms of the disease alaji which has already been described (under Prameha Pidaka). (74)

Krimigranthi

krimigranthirvartmanaḥ pakṣmaṇaśca kaṇḍūṃ kuryuḥ krimayaḥ sandhijātāḥ
|
nānārūpā vartmaśuklāntasandhau carantyantarlocanaṃ dūṣayantaḥ ||75||
(su| u| taṃ| a| 2) |
The micro-organisms which are produced at the corners of the eyes (inner and outer angles of the eye) on reaching the eyelids and eyelashes produce itching therein. These organisms are of different kinds. They move around and on reaching the junction between eyelids and the white of the eye (sclera), they also gain entry into and contaminate the inside of the eye. This disease is known as Krimigranthi. (75)

Utsangini / Utsanga Pidaka

abhyantaramukhī tāmrā bāhyato vartmanaśca yā |
sotsaṅgotsaṅgapiḍakā sarvajā sthūlakaṇḍurā ||76||
(su| u| taṃ| a| 2) |
A cyst is formed on the outer side of the eyelid with its opening pointed inwards into the eye, is coppery (red) in colour, covered by many small cysts (papules), elevated (big in size), with severe itching and caused by increase of all three doshas together is called as Utsangini or Utsanga Pidaka. (76)

Kumbhika

vartmānte piḍakā dhmātā bhidyante ca sravanti ca |
kumbhīkābījapratimāḥ kumbhīkāḥ sannipātajāḥ ||77||
(su. u. taṃ. a. 3) |
Multiple papules of the size of seeds of kumbhikä formed on the margins of the eyelids, which get swollen and burst open repeatedly and produce discharges, caused by increase of all the three doshas together is known as Kumbika. (77)

Pothaki

srāviṇyaḥ kaṇḍurā gurvyo raktasarṣapasannibhāḥ |
rujāvatyaśca piḍakāḥ pothakya iti kīrtitāḥ ||78||
(su. u. taṃ. a. 3) |
A disease in which many papules are formed inside the eyelids, which has discharges, itching, is heavy (hard), resembling (size of) red mustard seeds, and has pain is known as Pothaki. (78)

Vartmasarkara

piḍakā yā kharā sthūlā sūkṣmābhirabhisaṃvṛtā |
vartmasthā śarkarā nāma sa rogo vartmadūṣakaḥ ||79||
(su| u| taṃ| a| 3) |
A rough and hard papule, surrounded by many smaller ones inside the lids, is known as Vartmasarkara. This disease causes distortion of eyelids. (79)

Arsovartma

ervārubījapratimāḥ piḍakā mandavedanāḥ |
ślakṣṇāḥ kharāśca vartmasthāstadarśovartma kīrtyate ||80||
(su| u| taṃ| a| 3) |
A papule which resembles a seed of a melon, is slightly painful, unctuous (smooth), rough and is caused either inside or outside or obth sides of the eyelid is known as Arśovartma. (80)

Shuska Arshas

dīrghāṅkuraḥ kharaḥ stabdho dāruṇo'bhyantarodbhavaḥ |
vyādhireṣo'bhivikhyātaḥ śuṣkārśo nāma nāmataḥ ||81||
(su| u| taṃ| a| 3) |
A papule comprising of long sprouts, rough, stiff (hard), immovable, very troublesome (painful) and arising from deep inside the eyelid is known as Suska Arsas. (81)

Anjana Namika

dāhatodavatī tāmrā piḍakā vartmasambhavā |
mṛdvī mandarujā sūkṣmā jñeyā sā'ñjananāmikā ||82||
(su| u| taṃ| a| 3) |
A papule associated with burning sensation, pricking pain, coppery (red) coloured, occurring inside the eyelid, is soft, with mild pain, and small in size is known as Anjana Namika. (82)

Bahula Vartma

vartmopacīyate yasya piḍakābhiḥ samantataḥ |
savarṇābhiḥ sthirābhiśca vidyādbahulavartma tat ||83||
(su| u| taṃ| a| 3) |
The disease in which the eyelid becomes with numerous hard papules which are of the same colour of the surrounding skin (not discoloured) developing inside the eyelid is known as Bahulavartma or Bahalavartma. (83)

Vartma Bandhaka

kaṇḍūmatā'lpatodena vartmaśothena yo naraḥ |
na sa sañcchādayedakṣi yatrāsau vartmabandhakaḥ ||84||
(su| u| taṃ| a| 3) |
The disease in which eyelids get swollen being associated with itching and mild pricking pain and the person is unable to cover the eye (with the lids) i.e., unable to close the eyes properly is known as Vartma Bandhaka. (84)

Klista Vartma

mṛdvalpavedanaṃ tāmraṃ yadvartma samameva ca |
akasmācca bhavedraktaṃ kliṣṭavartmeti tadviduḥ ||85||
(su| u| taṃ| a| 3) |
The disease in which the eyelids become soft, slightly painful, and coppery red in colour and even and the eyelids suddenly become angry red without any apparent reason is known as Klista Vartma. (35)

Vartmakardama

kliṣṭaṃ punaḥ pittayutaṃ śoṇitaṃ vidahedyadā |
tataḥ klinnatvamāpannamucyate vartmakardamaḥ ||86||
(su| u| taṃ| a| 3) |
In the same Klista Vartma disease (mentioned above) when increased pitta associated with rakta (blood) causes burning sensation, the lids become moist. This condition is called as Vartmakardama. (86)

Syava Vartma

yadvartma bāhyato'ntaśca śyāvaṃ śūlaṃ savedanam |
tadāhuḥ śyāvavartmeti vartmarogaviśāradāḥ ||87||
(su| u| taṃ| a| 3) |
The disease in which the eyelids become blackish blue both inside and outside, gets swollen and becomes painful is called as Syavavartma by experts. (87)

Praklinna Vartma

arujaṃ bāhyataḥ śūnaṃ vartma yasya narasya hi |
praklinnavartma tadvidyāt klinnamatyarthamantataḥ ||88||
(su| u| taṃ| a| 3) |
The disease in which the eyelids are swollen and painless from outside (externally) but the inside of the lids is moist with discharges is known as Praklinna Vartma. (88)

Aklinna Vartma

yasya dhautānyadhautāni sambadhyante punaḥ punaḥ |
vartmānyaparipakvāni vidyādaklinnavartma tat ||89||
(su| u| taṃ| a| 3) |
A disease in which the lids stick (together) to each other often whether they are washed with water or not and suppuration of the eyelids do not take place (lids show signs of unripe state – pus not being formed) is known as Aklinna Vartma. (89)

Vatahara Vartma

vimuktasandhi niśceṣṭaṃ vartma yasya na mīlyate |
etadvātahataṃ vartma jānīyādakṣicintakaḥ ||90||
(su| u| taṃ| a| 3) |
The disease in which the lids get displaced from their joints (junction between the eyelids and the white of the eyes – sclera) and becomes motionless and the person unable to close or open his eyelids is known by the experts as Vatahata Vartma. (90)

Vartma Arbuda

vartmāntarasthaṃ viṣamaṃ granthibhūtamavedanam |
ācakṣītārbudamiti saraktamavilambitam ||91||
(su| u| taṃ| a| 3) |
A cystic swelling (tumour) developing from inside the eyelids, irregular in shape, having mild pain (or painless), red coloured and quickly increasing in size is known as Vartmarbuda. (91)

Nimesha

nimeṣiṇīḥ sirā vāyuḥ praviṣṭaḥ sandhisaṃśrayāḥ |
pracālayati vartmāni nimeṣaṃ nāma tadviduḥ ||92||
(su| u| taṃ| a| 3) |
A disease in which the vata which has got increased gets lodged in the siras (veins, blood vessels) responsible for winking the eyes located in the junction of the eyelid and white of the eye (sclera) and causes too much of winking (blinking) of the eyelids is known as Nimesa. (92)

Sonitarsas (Raktarsas)

yaḥ sthito vartmamạdhye tu lohito mṛduraṅkuraḥ |
tadraktajaṃ śoṇitārśaśchinnaṃ chinnaṃ pravardhate ||93||
(su| u| taṃ| a| 3) |

A disease in which red coloured soft sprouts develop at the centre of the inside of the eyelid, caused by increased rakta (blood) is known as Sonitarsa or Raktarsa. Thes sprouts continuously (again and again) keep growing even after they are excised. (93)

Lagana

apākī kaṭhinaḥ sthūlo granthirvartmabhavo'rujaḥ,
lagaṇo nāma sa vyādhirliṅgataḥ parikīrtitaḥ ||94|| (su| u| taṃ| a| 3) |

A disease in which a non-suppurating, hard, big, painless cystic swelling (tumour) develops inside the eyelid is known as Lagana. (94)

Bisa Vartma

trayo doṣā bahiḥśothaṃ kuryuśchidrāṇi vartmanoḥ |
prasravantyantarudakaṃ bisavadbisavartma tat ||95||
(vā| u| a| 8) |

A disease caused by all the three doshas increased together, wherein a swelling is produced on the exterior (outside) of the eyelid, having many small openings through which watery discharges come out from inside the lids, just like from the stalk of a lotus flower is called by the name Bisa Vartma. (95)

Kuncana

vātādyā vartmasaṅkocaṃ janayanti malā yadā |
tadā draṣṭuṃ na śaknoti kuñcanaṃ nāma tadviduḥ ||96||

A disease in which when vata and other doshas (pitta, kapha) undergo increase together and cause contractures of the eyelids leading to inability (of the person) to see things (due to inability to open the eyelids) is known as Kuncana. (96)

Paksmakopa

pracālitāni vātena pakṣmāṇyakṣi viśanti hi |
ghṛṣyantyakṣi muhustāni saṃrambhaṃ janayanti ca ||97||
asite sitabhāge ca mūlakoṣāt patantyapi |
pakṣmakopaḥ sa vijñeyo vyādhiḥ paramadāruṇaḥ ||98||
When the aggravated vata causes the eyelashes turned inwards into the eye, and causes friction on the eyeball repeatedly, and swelling of both white and black portions of the eye, and the hairs may also get dislodged from their roots and fall off. This dreadful disease is known as Paksmakopa. (97-98)

Paksmasata

vartmapakṣmāśayagataṃ pittaṃ romāṇi śātayet |
kaṇḍūṃ dāhaṃ ca kurute pakṣmaśātaṃ tamādiśet ||99||
A disease in which increased pitta located in the eyelids and lashes (junction of eyelids and eyelashes) makes the eyelashes to fall off from their roots (eyelids) and is associated with itching and burning sensation is known as Paksmasata. (99)

Compilation of all the eye diseases

nava sandhyāśrayāsteṣu vartmajāstvekaviṃśatiḥ |
śuklabhāge daśaikaśca catvāraḥ kṛṣṇabhāgajāḥ ||100||
sarvāśrayāḥ saptadaśa dṛṣṭijā dvādaśaiva tu |
bāhyajau dvau samākhyātau rogau paramadāruṇau ||101||
bhūya etān pravakṣyāmi saṅkhyārūpacikitsitaiḥ ||102||
(iti vartmagatāḥ) |
(su| u| taṃ| a| 1) |
(So far have been described nine diseases of joints of the eye, twenty-one diseases of the eyelids, eleven diseases of the white of the eye i.e. sclera, four diseases of the black portion of the eye, seventeen diseases occurring in the entire eye, twelve diseases of the vision and two external diseases of the lashes which are dreadful in nature).

iti śrīmādhavakaraviracite mādhavanidāne netraroganidānaṃ samāptam ||59||
Thus ends the chapter on Netra Roga.

CHAPTER SIXTY

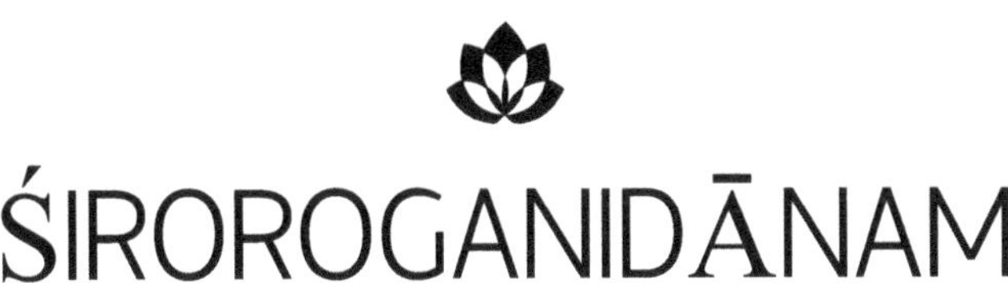

ŚIROROGANIDĀNAM

Siroroga Bheda – types of Siroroga based on the causes

śirorogāstu jāyante vātapittakaphaistribhiḥ |
sannipātena raktena kṣayeṇa krimibhistathā |
sūryāvartānantavātārdhāvabhedakaśaṅkhakaiḥ ||1||
(su| u| taṃ| a| 25) |
The diseases of the head (headache) are caused by individual doshas i.e. aggravated vata, pitta and kapha or by simultaneous vitiation of all three doshas together (sannipataja). They are also caused by rakta (vitiated blood), ksaya (loss, decrease of the tissues) or by krimis (infection from microorganisms). They also manifest by the names Suryavarta, Anantavata, Ardhavabheda and Sankhaka. (1)

Notes - Siroroga is of 11 kinds. They are –

Vataja Siroroga
Pittaja Siroroga
Kaphaja Siroroga
Sannipataja Siroroga
Raktaja Siroroga
Ksayaja Siroroga
Krimija Siroroga
Suryavarta
Anantavata
Ardhavabhedaka
Sankhaka

Vataja Siroroga

yasyānimittaṃ śiraso rujaśca bhavanti tīvrā niśi cātimātram |
bandhopatāpaiḥ praśamaśca yatra śiro'bhitāpaḥ sa samīraṇena ||2||
(su| u| taṃ| a| 25) |
The symptoms of headache caused by increased vata are –

- sudden appearance of severe headache without any apparent cause,
- headache being more severe at night (gets worse at night)
- gets reduced (relieved) by applying tight bandage and fomentation (warm comforts) (2)

Pittaja Siroroga

yasyoṣṇamaṅgāracitaṃ yathaiva bhavecchiro dhūpyati cākṣināsam |
śītena rātrau ca bhavecchamaśca śirobhitāpaḥ sa tu pittakopāt ||3||
(su| u| taṃ| a| 25) |
The symptoms of headache caused by increased pitta are –

- the head of the patient feels hot as if his head is enveloped by burning charcoal
- feeling as if smoke is coming out of the eyes and nose
- gets relieved with cold comforts and at night time (3)

Kaphaja Siroroga

śiro bhavedyasya kaphopadigdhaṃ guru pratiṣṭabdhamato himaṃ ca |
śūnākṣikūṭaṃ vadanaṃ ca yasya śiro'bhitāpaḥ sa kaphaprakopāt ||4||
(su| u| taṃ| a| 25) |
The symptoms of headache caused by increased kapha are –

- the head becomes coated with kapha (feeling as if the head is full or is coated with kapha)
- heaviness of the head

- tightness of the head
- coldness of the head
- swelling of the face and orbits (region around the eyes) (4)

Sannipataja Siroroga

śiro'bhitāpe tritayapravṛtte sarvāṇi liṅgāni samudbhavanti |5|
(su| u| taṃ| a| 25) |
In the headache caused by all the three doshas increased together, there will be presence of the symptoms of (aggravation of) all the three doshas at the same time.

Raktaja Siroroga

raktātmakaḥ pittasamānaliṅgaḥ sparśāsahatvaṃ śiraso bhavecca ||5||
(su| u| taṃ| a| 25) |
In the headache caused by (abnormally) increased blood the symptoms will be similar to those of pittaja siroroga. In addition, there will be intolerance to touch / tenderness of the head (the person cannot tolerate if his head is touched / will not allow the head to be touched). (5)

Ksayaja Siroroga

asṛgvasāśleṣmasamīraṇānāṃ śirogatānāmiha saṅkṣayeṇa |
kṣayapravṛttaḥ śiraso'bhitāpaḥ kaṣṭo bhavedugrarujo'timātram |
saṃsvedanacchardanadhūmanasyairasṛgvimokṣaiśca vivṛddhimeti ||6||
(su| u| taṃ| a| 25) |
When there is loss or abnormal decrease of blood, muscle-fat, kapha and vata residing normally in the head a severe form of headache which is difficult to cure manifests with severe pain in the head. This type of headache is called Ksayaja Siroroga. The headache increases by administering of therapies like sudation, emesis, herbal (medicated) smoking, instillation of nasal drops and bloodletting. (6)

Krimija Siroroga

nistudyate yasya śiro'timātraṃ sambhakṣyamāṇaṃ sphuratīva cāntaḥ |
ghrāṇācca gacchet salilaṃ sapūyaṃ śirobhitāpaḥ krimibhiḥ sa ghoraḥ ||7||
(su| u| taṃ| a| 25) |
The symptoms of headache caused by krimis (infection by microorganisms) are –

- excessive and constant pricking pain in the head,
- a feeling as if the head is being eaten away from inside
- feeling of pulsations or movements within the head
- watery discharges mixed with pus flowing out of the nose

This headache is said to be dreadful in nature. (7)

Suryavarta

sūryodayaṃ yā prati mandamandamakṣibhruvaṃ ruk samupaiti gāḍhā |
vivardhate cāṃśumatā sahaiva sūryāpavṛttau vinivartate ca |
sarvātmakaṃ kaṣṭatamaṃ vikāraṃ sūryāpavartaṃ tamudāharanti ||8||
(su| u| taṃ| a| 25) |
The headache which starts at sunrise and the pain gradually increases and spreads to involve the eyes and eyebrows, which gradually increases in severity as the sun reaches its peak (ascent - upward movement of the sun, towards noon) and gradually decreases with the descent of the sun i.e. sunset is called as Suryavarta or Suryapavarta. It is a troublesome (dreadful) disease and is caused by all the three doshas (undergoing increase together). (8)

Anantavata

doṣāstu duṣṭāstraya eva manyāṃ sampīḍya ghāṭāsu rujāṃ sutīvrām |
kurvanti yo'kṣibhruvi śaṅkhadeśe sthitiṃ karotyāśu viśeṣatastu ||9||
gaṇḍasya pārśve tu karoti kampaṃ hanugrahaṃ locanajāṃśca rogān |
anantavātaṃ tamudāharanti doṣatrayotthaṃ śiraso vikāram ||10||
(su| u| taṃ| a| 25) |
All the three doshas (vata, pitta and kapha) which have undergone excessive

increase together get lodged (invade) and troubles (pain) in the nape of the neck and produce severe pain at the back of the neck. This pain quickly spreads to the eyes, eyebrows and temples and gets localized therein. This will lead to throbbing (pulsation) on the sides of the cheek bones, stiffness of the lower jaw and many diseases of the eyes. This disease of the head caused by simultaneous vitiation of all the three doshas is known as Anantavata. (9-10)

Ardhavabheda

rūkṣāśanātyadhyaśanaprāgvātāvaśyamaithunaiḥ |
vegasandhāraṇāyāsavyāyāmaiḥ kupito'nilaḥ ||11||
kevalaḥ sakapho vā'rdhaṃ gṛhītvā śiraso balī |
manyābhrūśaṅkhakarṇākṣilalāṭārdhe'tivedanām ||12||
śastrāraṇinibhāṃ kuryāttīvrāṃ so'rdhāvabhedakaḥ |
nayanaṃ vā'thavā śrotramativṛddho vināśayet ||13||
Causes of Ardhavabheda – Excessive indulgence in (eating) dry foods, too much food frequently, habit of eating food before the previously consumed food is properly digested (eating in presence of indigestion), exposure to heavy breeze coming from the east direction, excessive exposure to snowfall, excessive indulgence in sexual intercourse, habit of suppressing the natural urges, excessive physical exertion and excessive indulgence in physical exercises are the causative factors which cause increase of vata and subsequent manifestation of Ardhavabhedaka.
Pathogenesis – The above said etiological factors would cause abnormal increase of vata. This vata, either alone or gaining strength due to its association with kapha, would invade half the portion of the head and cause the disease Ardhavabhedaka.
Symptoms of Ardhavabhedaka – Ardhavabhedaka is marked by severe pain in the sides of the neck, eyebrows, temples, ears, eyes and forehead of any one side i.e. left or right side. The pain of Ardhavabhedaka is very severe. The person feels as if his head is being cut by a sharp weapon or being burnt by fire or being churned by a churner. If the disease progresses, it will also cause destruction of the functions of eyes or ears.
This disease is called as Ardhavabhedaka. (11-13)

Shankhaka

raktapittānilā duṣṭāḥ śaṅkhadeśe vimūrchitāḥ |
tīvrarugdāharāgaṃ hi śothaṃ kurvanti dāruṇam ||14||
sa śiro viṣavadvegī nirundhyāśu galaṃ tathā |
trirātrājjīvitaṃ hanti śaṅkhako nāmataḥ param |
tryahājjīvati bhaiṣajyaṃ pratyākhyāya samācaret ||15||
Abnormally increased rakta (blood), pitta and vata get lodged and mixed with each other in the temples and would cause severe pain, burning sensation and reddish swelling therein (in the temples). This swelling having the intensity and velocity (as powerful as) of a life-threatening poison quickly causes obstruction in the head and neck and takes away the life of the person within three days. This disease is known as Sankhaka.
By chance if the patient survives even after three days (many times the patient will not survive after three days), it should be treated by considering (announcing) that it is incurable (treating in refusal). According to Master Videha, the treatment of Sankhaka should be done in refusal (announcing that it is difficult to cure or incurable) within three days. After three days this disease becomes incurable. (14-15)

iti śrīmādhavakaravicite mādhavanidāne śiroroganidānaṃ samāptam ||60||
Thus ends the chapter on SiroRogas.

CHAPTER SIXTY-ONE

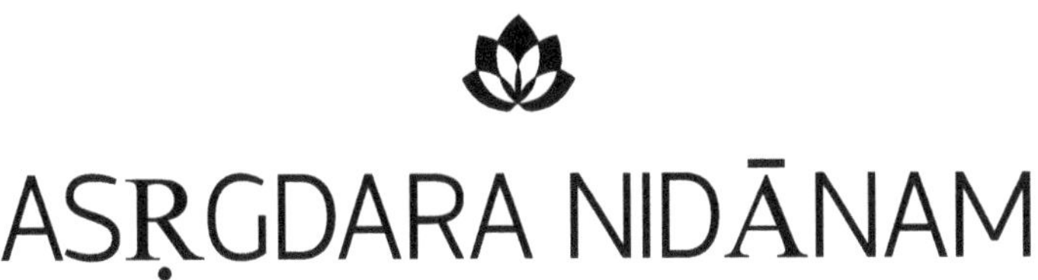

ASṚGDARA NIDĀNAM

Asrgdara Nidana, Bheda – Causative factors and types of Menorrhagia

viruddhamadyādhyaśanādajīrṇādgarbhaprapātādatimaithunācca |
yānādhvaśokādatikarṣaṇācca bhārābhighātācchayanāddivā ca |
taṃ śleṣmapittānilasannipātaiścatuṣprakāraṃ pradaraṃ vadanti ||1||
Causative factors –

- excessive indulgence (by the woman) in incompatible foods (foods mutually opposite / antagonistic in nature), alcoholic beverages and over-eating,
- eating (in excess) uncooked foods / having indigestion
- frequent abortions
- indulgence in excessive sexual intercourse
- excessive riding on animals
- walking long distances
- excessive grief
- emaciation – excessive loss of tissues due to excessive starvation / fasting and similar other causes
- carrying heavy loads
- trauma
- excessive sleeping during day time

Types of Pradara / Asrgdara – The above-mentioned etiological factors lead to manifestation of four kinds of pradara (excessive menstruation). The four types of pradara are – kaphaja, pittaja, vataja and sannipataja (caused by all doshas together. (1)

Asrgdara Samanya Lakshana – General symptoms of Asrgdara

asṛgdaraṃ bhavet sarvaṃ sāṅgamardaṃ savedanam |2|
(su| śā| a| 2) |
General symptoms of Asrgdara are – aches all over the body and abdominal pain during menstrual periods.

Complications of excessive menstrual bleeding

tasyātivṛttau daurbalyaṃ bhramo mūrchā madastṛṣā |
dāhaḥ pralāpaḥ pāṇḍutvaṃ tandrā rogāśca vātajāḥ ||2||
(su| śā| a| 2) |
Excessive bleeding during menstruation leads to many complications like debility, giddiness, fainting, intoxication, excessive thirst, burning sensation, delirium, pallor, stupor and some diseases of vata origin. (2)

Symptoms of types of Asrgdara

āmaṃ sapicchāpratimaṃ sapāṇḍu pulākatoyapratimaṃ kaphāttu |
sapītanīlāsitaraktamuṣṇaṃ pittārtiyuktaṃ bhṛśavegi pittāt ||3||
rūkṣāruṇaṃ phenilamalpamalpaṃ vātārti vātāt piśitodakābham |
sakṣaudrasarpirharitālavarṇaṃ majjaprakāśaṃ kuṇapaṃ tridoṣāt ||4||
Kaphaja Asrgdara – In this type of pradara caused by increased kapha, the menstrual discharge will be ill-processed (ama), is sticky (mixed with mucus), is pale (yellowish-white) coloured, resembles ground sesamum (or some bad grain) or meat or mallow plant washed water.
Pittaja Asrgdara – In this type of pradara caused by increased pitta, the menstrual discharge will be yellow, blue, black or red in colour, hot (warm), will have pitta type of pains and comes out with great force (in gushes).
Vataja Asrgdara – In this type of pradara caused by increased vata, the menstrual blood will be dry (viscid), of crimson colour, frothy, scanty, will have vata type of pains, and resembles meat (mutton) washed water.
Tridoshaja / Sannipataja Asrgdara – In this type of pradara caused by all the three doshas together, the flow / discharges will appear like honey, ghee, orpiment or bone marrow in colour, and will emit cadaveric smell.

Asrgdara Asadhyata – prognosis of Asrgdara

taṃ cāpyasādhyaṃ pravadanti tajjñā, na tatra kurvīta bhiṣak cikitsām |
śaśvat sravantīmāsrāvaṃ tṛṣṇādāhajvarānvitām |
kṣīṇaraktāṃ durbalāṃ ca tāmasādhyāṃ vinirdiśet ||5||
The expert physicians consider tridoshaja type of asrgdara as incurable and hence shall not be treated.
Similarly, the asrgdara in which there is continuous menstrual bleeding for long time, and the woman develops thirst, burning sensation, fever, severe loss of blood and debility should also be considered as incurable. (3-5)

Vishuddha Artava Lakshana – Signs / symptoms of normal or clean (uncontaminated) menstrual blood

māsānniṣpicchadāhārti pañcarātrānubandhi ca |
naivātibahulātyalpamārtavaṃ śuddhamādiśet ||6||
śaśāsṛkpratimaṃ yacca yadvā lākṣārasopamam |
tadārtavaṃ praśaṃsanti yaccāpsu na virajyate ||7||
(su| śā| a| 2) |
Menstrual blood (Menstruation) is considered to be normal if it occurs regularly every month, for a period of five days, the fluid not being sticky (not having mucus), and not associated with burning sensation and pain and the flow being neither too much in quantity or too less.
The menstrual fluid (blood) which resembles the blood of a rabbit or a solution of lac and the cloth soaked in such fluid when washed in water does not retain any blood stains (can be washed off easily) is considered to be healthy. (6-7)

iti śrīmādhavakaraviracite mādhavanidāne asṛgdaranidānaṃ samāptam ||61||
Thus ends the chapter on Asṛgdara.

CHAPTER SIXTY-TWO

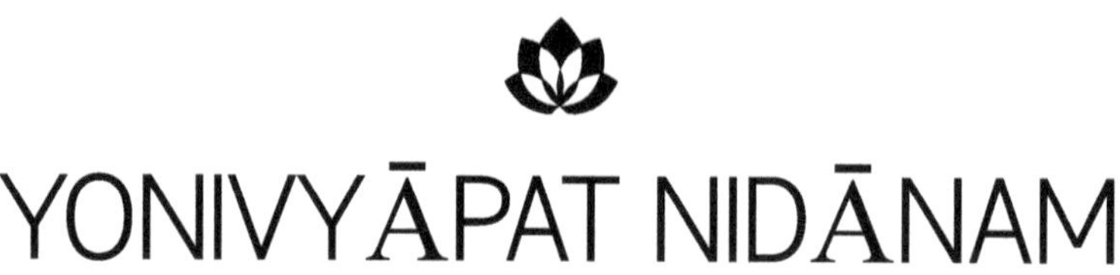

YONIVYĀPAT NIDĀNAM

Yonivyapat Samkhya, Samanya Nidana – Number and general causes of diseases of the vaginal tract

viṃśatirvyāpado yonau nirdiṣṭā rogasaṅgrahe |
mithyācāreṇa tāḥ strīṇāṃ praduṣṭenārtavena ca ||1||
jāyante bījadoṣācca daivācca śṛṇu tāḥ pṛthak |
(ca| ci| a| 30) |
viṃśatirvyāpado yonau nirdiṣṭā rogasaṅgrahe |
mithyācāreṇa tāḥ strīṇāṃ praduṣṭenārtavena ca ||1||
jāyante bījadoṣācca daivācca śṛṇu tāḥ pṛthak |
(ca| ci| a| 30) |
Number of Yonivyapat - Twenty diseases of the vaginal tract have been enumerated in the rogasangraha (Ashtodariya chapter – chapter 19 of sutrasthana section of Charaka Samhita).
Etiological Factors of Yonivyapat - These diseases occur in women who indulge in unhealthy foods and habits, due to contamination of menstrual blood or disorders of menstruation, due to bijadosha (disease of the ovary and ovum) and by influence of gods. (1)

Vataja Yoni Vyapad (5 in number) – caused due to predominance of vata – Udavarta, Vandhya, Vipluta, Paripluta, Vatala yoni

sā phenilamudāvartā rajaḥ kṛcchreṇa muñcati ||2||
vandhyāṃ naṣṭārtavāṃ vidyādviplutāṃ nityavedanām |
pariplutāyāṃ bhavati grāmyadharmeṇa rugbhṛśam ||3||
vātalā karkaśā stabdhā śūlanistodapīḍitā |
catasṛṣvapi cādyāsu bhavantyanilavedanāḥ ||4||

(su| u| taṃ| a| 38) |

Udavarta Yonivyapat – In this condition the woman discharges frothy menstrual blood with difficulty (pain).

Vandhya Yonivyapat - the woman in whom the menstrual blood has been destroyed (who has stopped menstruating and is sterile) is known as Vandhyā. Such a condition is known as Vandhya Yonivyapat.

Vipluta Yonivyapat – In this condition the woman always has pain (constant pain).

Paripluta Yonivyapat – In this condition the woman experiences severe pain during sexual intercourse.

Vatala Yonivyapat – It is a condition in which the vagina afflicted by aggravated vata is rough and stiff and is associated with pain and pricking pain.

In the first four conditions (explained above) also there will be vataja types of pains (and other symptoms of vata increase). (2-4)

Pittaja Yoni Vyapad (5 in number) – caused due to predominance of pitta – Lohitaksaya, Vamini, Prasramsini, Putraghni, Pittala yoni

sadāhaṃ kṣīyate raktaṃ yasyāṃ sā lohitakṣayā |
savātamudgiredbījaṃ vāminī rajasā yutam ||5||
prasraṃsinī sraṃsate ca kṣobhitā duṣprajāyinī |
sthitaṃ sthitaṃ hanti garbhaṃ putraghnī raktasaṅkṣayāt ||6||
atyarthaṃ pittalā yonirdāhapākajvarānvitā |
catasṛṣvapi cādyāsu pittaliṅgocchrayo bhavet ||7||
(su| u| taṃ| a| 38) |

Lohitaksaya Yonivyapat – It is a condition in which the woman has large quantities of menstrual flow along with burning sensation. There is severe loss of blood and hence this condition is known as Lohitaksaya.

Vamini Yonivyapat – In this condition both the ovum and menstrual fluid (blood) are expelled out from the vagina along with vata.

Prasramsini Yonivyapat – It is a condition in which the vagina is displaced from its place repeatedly due to irritation. This woman gives birth to a child with great difficulty.

Putraghni Yonivyapat – The woman who repeatedly undergoes abortion after having conceived the embryo due to severe loss of blood is said to be suffering from Putraghni Yonivyapat.

Pittala Yonivyapat – In this condition there will be severe burning sensation and suppuration in the vaginal tract and is accompanied with fever.
In the first four conditions (explained above) also there will be pittaja types of pains (and other symptoms of pitta increase). (5-7)

Kaphaja Yoni Vyapad (5 in number) – caused due to predominance of kapha – Atyananda, Karnini, Acarana, Aticarana, Shleshmala yoni

atyānandā na santoṣaṃ grāmyadharmeṇa gacchati |
karṇinyāṃ karṇikā yonau śleṣmāsṛgbhyāṃ prajāyate ||8||
maithune'caraṇā pūrvaṃ puruṣādatiricyate |
bahuśaścāticaraṇā tayorbījaṃ na vindati ||9||
śleṣmalā picchilā yoniḥ kaṇḍūgrastā'tiśītalā |
catasṛṣvapi cādyāsu śleṣmaliṅgocchrayo bhavet ||10||
(su| u| taṃ| a| 38) |
Atyananda Yonivyapat – In this condition the woman does not experience pleasure during coitus.
Karnini Yonivyapat – In this condition a ring-like muscular mass is produced by vitiated kapha and blood inside the vaginal passage.
Acarana Yonivyapat – In this condition the woman (uterus) discharges much earlier than the man (ejaculates the semen) during coitus.
Aticarana Yonivyapat – In this condition the woman (uterus) discharges only after excessive and prolonged coitus. Both these conditions (acarana and aticarana) will not retain the seed / sperm (i.e., women having these two conditions do not conceive).
Shlesmala Yonivyapat – In this condition the vaginal passage of the woman will be sticky; will have severe itching and coldness.
In the first four conditions (explained above) also there will be kaphaja types of pains / symptoms (and other symptoms of kapha increase). (8-10)

Sannipataja Yoni Vyapad (5 in number) – caused due to predominance of all three doshas – Sandi, Andali, Vivrta, Sucimukhi, Tridoshaja yoni

anārtavā'stanī ṣaṇḍī kharasparśā ca maithune |
atikāyagṛhītāyāstaruṇyāstvaṇḍalī bhavet ||11||
vivṛtā ca mahāyoniḥ sūcīvaktrā'tisaṃvṛtā |
sarvaliṅgasamutthānā sarvadoṣaprakopajā ||12||

catasṛṣvapi cādyāsu sarvaliṅgocchrayo bhavet |
pañcāsādhyā bhavantīha yonayaḥ sarvadoṣajāḥ ||13||
(su| u| taṃ| a| 38) |

Sandi Yonivyapat – It is a condition in which the woman would not menstruate (not menstruating), not have breasts or have small and underdeveloped breasts and will have roughness of the vagina during coitus.

Andali Yonivyapat – In this condition the young woman would have a prolapsed vagina (uterus) caused due to coitus with a person having a big or stout penis.

Vivrta Yonivyapat – In this condition the vaginal passage (opening) of the woman would be very wide.

Sucivaktra / Sucimukhi Yonivyapat – It is a condition in which the woman would have a very narrow vaginal (uterine) passage.

Tridoshaja Yonivyapat – In this condition caused due to simultaneous vitiation of all three doshas, the causative factors and symptoms of all the three doshas will be found together.

In the first four conditions (explained above) also there will be tridoshaja types of pains / symptoms (and other symptoms of tridosha increase).

All these five kinds of tridoshaja yonivyapat are said to be incurable.
(11-13)

iti śrīmādhavakaraviracite mādhavanidāne yonivyāpannidānaṃ samāptam ||62||

Thus ends the chapter on Yonivyāpat.

CHAPTER SIXTY-THREE

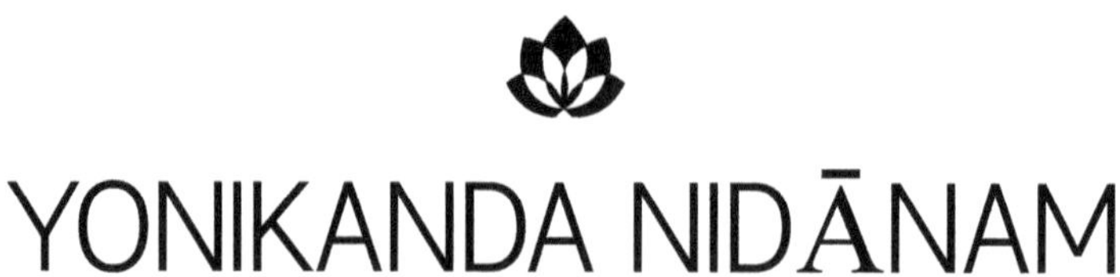

YONIKANDA NIDĀNAM

Yonikanda Hetu – Etiological factors of Yonikanda

divāsvapnādatikrodhādvyāyāmādatimaithunāt |
kṣatācca nakhadantādyairvātādyāḥ kupitā yadā ||1||
pūyaśoṇitasaṅkāśaṃ nikucākṛtisannibham |
janayanti yadā yonau nāmnā kandaḥ sa yonijaḥ ||2||
Etiological factors - excessive sleeping during the daytime, excessive (frequent episodes) of anger, indulgence in excessive exercises (physical strain) and sexual intercourse, injury (to the vagina) by nails, teeth and other foreign bodies
Pathogenesis, nature and form of yonikanda – the above-mentioned etiological factors cause excessive (abnormal) increase of vata and other doshas (pitta and kapha). These doshas produce a mass in the vagina which has the size and shape of a jujube fruit, round, having the colour of pus mixed blood. This is known as Yonikanda. (1-2)

Yonikanda Bheda, Lakshana – Types and symptoms of Yonikanda

rūkṣaṃ vivarṇaṃ sphuṭitaṃ vātikaṃ taṃ vinirdiśet |
dāharāgajvarayutaṃ vidyāt pittātmakaṃ tu tam ||3||
nīlapuṣpapratīkāśaṃ kaṇḍūmantaṃ kaphātmakam |
sarvaliṅgasamāyuktaṃ sannipātātmakaṃ viduḥ ||4||
Vataja Yonikanda – Yonikanda caused by increased vata is dry, discoloured and fissured.
Pittaja Yonikanda – Yonikanda caused by increased pitta presents with burning sensation, redness and fever.
Kaphaja Yonikanda – Yonikanda caused by increased kapha has colour of

nilapuspa i.e. flower of atasi (linseed) and has itching.
Sannipataja Yonikanda – In Yonikanda caused by the increase of all the three doshas together, the symptoms of all the three doshas are seen together. (3-4)

iti śrīmādhavakaraviracite mādhavanidāne yonikandanidānaṃ samāptam ||63||
Thus ends the chapter on Yoni Kanda.

CHAPTER SIXTY-FOUR

MŪḌHAGARBHA NIDĀNAM

Definition of Mudha Garbha

sarvāvayavasampūrṇo manobuddhyādisaṃyuta: |
viguṇāpānasaṃmūḍho mūḍhagarbho'bhidhīyate || 1||
The condition in which the foetus whose body parts have been properly and completely formed (matured), and has been endowed (associated) with mind, intellect etc, gets obstructed in the birth passage due to the influence of aggravated apana vata is called as mudhagarbha.

Garbhapata

bhayābhighātāttīkṣṇoṣṇapānāśananiṣevaṇāt |
garbhe patati raktasya saśūlaṃ darśanaṃ bhavet ||1||
Sudden fear, injury (assault), excessive consumption of foods and drinks which are sharp and hot in nature causes falling off (abortion) of the embryo accompanied with pain and heavy bleeding. (This condition is known as garbhapata – miscarriage or abortion). (1)

Types of Garbhapata

ācaturthāttato māsāt prasravedgarbhavidravaḥ |
tataḥ sthiraśarīrasya pātaḥ pañcamaṣaṣṭhayoḥ ||2||
(su| ni| a| 8) |
Garbhasrava - If this (premature falling off of the embryo) happens within the first four months of pregnancy when the uterine contents are still in fluid state (embryo is in fluid state) it is known as Garbhasrava (abortion).
Garbhapata - If the premature embryo is expelled from the uterus in the

fifth or sixth month when the embryo has been developed and the body parts are stable (hard parts), it is known as Garbhapata (miscarriage). (2)

Garbhapata hetu – Causative factors for miscarriage

garbho'bhighātaviṣamāśanapīḍanādyaiḥ pakvaṃ drumādiva phalaṃ patati kṣaṇena |3|
Just as a ripe fruit fall from a tree, the embryo too falls off suddenly (garbhpat takes place) by trauma on the abdomen, consumption of unhealthy foods, and unnecessary massage or pressure over abdomen.

Nature and symptoms of Mudhagarbha

mūḍhaḥ karoti pavanaḥ khalu mūḍhagarbhaṃ śūlaṃ ca yonijaṭharādiṣu mūtrasaṅgam ||3||
If vata (apana vata) gets increased (goes out of balance), it causes difficulty in delivery. This condition is accompanied with pain in the vagina (uterine passages), abdomen etc and urinary obstruction. (3)

Mudhagarbha Ashta Vidha – Eight kinds of Mudhagarbha

bhugno'nilena viguṇena tataḥ sa garbhaḥ saṅkhyāmatītya bahudhā samupaiti yonim |
dvāraṃ nirudhya śirasā jaṭhareṇa kaścit kaściccharīraparivartitakubjadehaḥ ||4||
ekena kaścidaparastu bhujadvayena tiryaggato bhavati kaścidavāṅmukho'nyaḥ |
pārśvāpavṛttagatireti tathaiva kaściddityaṣṭadhā gatiriyaṃ hyaparā caturdhā ||5||
Väta undergoing increase affects the foetus and creates many kinds of abnormal presentations of the foetus inside the vagina (in the vaginal tract). Among such abnormal presentations of the foetus, eight main presentations are mentioned here. They are –

1. obstruction of the mouth (opening) of the uterus by the face of the foetus
2. obstruction of the opening of the uterus by the abdomen of the foetus

3. obstruction of the mouth of the uterus by the back of the foetus, curved and shortened
4. obstruction of the mouth of the uterus by one shoulder of the foetus
5. obstruction of the mouth of the uterus by both the shoulders of the foetus
6. obstruction of the mouth of the uterus by the body of the foetus placed in transverse position
7. obstruction of the mouth of the uterus by the face of the foetus bent down (foetus faces downwards)
8. obstruction of the mouth of the uterus by the flanks of the foetus (3-5)

Four special types of presentations of the foetus

saṅkīlakaḥ pratikhuraḥ parigho'tha bījasteṣūrdhvabāhucaraṇaiḥ śirasā ca yonim |
saṅgī ca yo bhavati kīlakavat sa kīlo dṛśyaiḥ khuraiḥ pratikhuraṃ sa hi kāyasaṅgī |
gacchedbhujadvayaśirāḥ sa ca bījakākhyo yonau sthitaḥ sa parighaḥ parigheṇa tulyaḥ ||6||
Some other authorities enumerate four other kinds of presentations of foetus. They are named as Kilaka, Pratikhura, Parigha and Bijaka.
Kilaka / sankilaka – It is the presentation in which the foetus blocks the mouth of the uterus / vagina, like a wedge, by raising its hands, feet and head upwards.
Pratikhura – In this presentation we can see the bending of the body of the foetus like a horse's hoof with hands, feet and head of the foetus obstructing the opening of the uterus / vagina. Even in this, the body becomes obstructed.
Bijaka – It is a presentation in which both the shoulders (hands) and head cause obstruction to the opening of the uterus (which may prolapse).
Parigha – Here we can see the transverse position of the foetus, like the bolt of a door inside the uterus (obstructing the vaginal passage / uterus). (6)

Prognosis of Mudha Garbha

apaviddhaśirā yā tu śītāṅgī nirapatrapā |

nīlodgatasirā hanti sā garbhaṃ sa ca tāṃ tathā ||7||
(su| ni| a| 8) |
The woman in labour who is unable to keep / hold her head straight (in position) i.e., the head keeps falling to one or the other side, whose body has become cold, who is devoid of (natural) shyness and on whose abdomen has blue prominent veins would kill the child and that child would kill her (mother). (7)

Mrita Garbha

garbhāspandanamāvīnāṃ praṇāśaḥ śyāvapāṇḍutā |
bhaveducchvāsapūtitvaṃ śūnatā'ntarmṛte śiśau ||8||
(su| ni| a| 8) |
Absence of movements of the foetus and cessation of labour pains, blackish yellow or bluish yellow discolouration of the skin, bad smell in her breath and swelling (abnormally swollen abdomen) are the symptoms of the woman whose foetus is dead inside (the womb). (8)

Reason for the death of the foetus

mānasāgantubhirmāturupatāpaiḥ prapīḍitaḥ |
garbho vyāpadyate kukṣau vyādhibhiśca nipīḍitaḥ ||9||
(su| ni| a| 8) |
Due to mental disorders, external injury, excessive physical strain for the mother and as an effect of many diseases, the foetus would die inside the womb (uterus). (9)

Prognosis of Mudhagarbha

yonisaṃvaraṇaṃ saṅgaḥ kukṣau makkalla eva ca |
hanyuḥ striyaṃ mūḍhagarbhāṃ yathoktāścāpyupadravāḥ ||10||
Yonisamvaraṇa (total obstruction of the uterus), kukṣisanga (obstruction of the foetus inside the abdomen / womb or dead foetus staying in the uterus for long time) and makkalla (pain after delivery) developing as complications of mūḍhagarbha and other complications are going to kill the woman. (10)

Makkalla

vāyuḥ prakupitaḥ kuryāt saṃrudhya rudhiraṃ srutam |
sūtāyā hṛcchirobastiśūlaṃ makkallasañjñakam ||11||
(A condition in which abnormally increased vata causes obstruction of the blood being discharged after delivery and causes pain in the region of the heart, head and urinary bladder is called Makkalla.)

iti śrīmādhavakaraviracite mādhavanidāne mūḍhagarbhanidānaṃ samāptam ||64||
Thus ends the chapter on Mudha Garbha.

CHAPTER SIXTY-FIVE

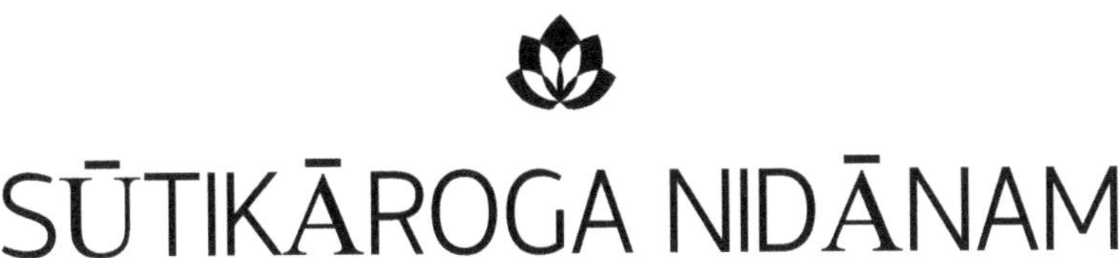

SŪTIKĀROGA NIDĀNAM

Sutikaroga Lakshana – Symptoms of disease of puerperium

aṅgamardo jvaraḥ kampaḥ pipāsā gurugātratā |
śothaḥ śūlātisārau ca sūtikārogalakṣaṇam ||1||
The symptoms of Sutikaroga (puerperal disorders) are – pain in the body parts / general malaise, fever, tremors, thirst, feeling of heaviness of the body, swelling, pain in the abdomen and diarrhoea. (1)

Sutikaroga Hetu – Etiological factors of Sutikaroga

mithyopacārāt saṅkleśādviṣamājīrṇabhojanat |
sūtikāyāśca ye rogā jāyante dāruṇāstu te ||2||
Improper management of puerperium i.e., woman indulging in unhealthy foods and activities soon after delivery, consumption of foods which would increase the doshas or mental strain, consumption of improper foods and drinks and uncooked foods (consumption of foods in the presence of indigestion) lead to the manifestation of many kinds of diseases in the woman in puerperium, which are dreadful (difficult to cure). These diseases are called as sutikaroga – puerperal diseases. (2)

Sutikaroga – Puerperal disorders

jvarātīsāraśothāśca śūlānāhabalakṣayāḥ |
tandrāruciprasekādyāḥ kaphavātāmayodbhavāḥ ||3||
Fever, diarrhoea, oedema, pain in the abdomen (colic) and flatulence (distension of the abdomen), debility, stupor, loss of taste / appetite, excessive salivation and other disorders caused by increase of kapha and

vāta manifest in the puerperal period.

Prognosis of Sutikarogas

kṛcchrasādhyā hi te rogāḥ kṣīṇamāṃsabalāgnitaḥ |
te sarve sūtikānāmnā rogāste cāpyupadravāḥ ||4||
The above-mentioned diseases become difficult to treat in those who have weak muscles, strength and digestive strength (activity). These diseases are called sutika rogas – puerperal diseases. There may also occur many complications of these diseases. These diseases will also be called by the name sutikarogas. (2-7)

iti śrīmādhavakaraviracite mādhavanidāne sūtikāroganidānaṃ samāptam ||65||
Thus ends the chapter on SūtikāRoga.

CHAPTER SIXTY-SIX

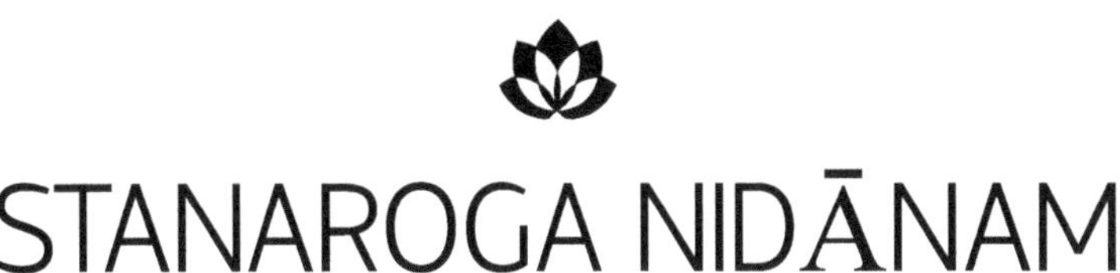

STANAROGA NIDĀNAM

Stana Roga Samprapti – Pathogenesis of diseases of the breast)

sakṣīrau vā'pyadugdhau vā prāpya doṣaḥ stanau striyāḥ |
pradūṣya māṃsarudhiraṃ stanarogāya kalpate ||1||
The doshas which have undergone abnormal increase (vitiation) get localized in the breasts filled with milk (during the period of lactation) or without milk (other than lactation period – when mother is not feeding the child), contaminate the muscles and blood therein and produce many diseases of the breasts. (1)

Stanaroga Bheda, Lakshana – Types and symptoms of breast diseases

pañcānāmapi teṣāṃ hi raktajaṃ vidradhiṃ vinā |
lakṣaṇāni samānāni bāhyavidradhilakṣaṇaiḥ ||2||
The five kinds of diseases of the breasts (produced by the increase of vata, pitta, kapha and all the three doshas together and that caused due to external agents) will have similar symptoms as those of five types of bahya vidradhi i.e. abscesses occurring outside (on the exterior) the body i.e. the symptoms of vataja, pittaja, kaphaja, sannipataja and agantuja vidradhi respectively, while excluding the raktaja vidradhi (abscess caused by the vitiated blood) i.e. there will be no raktaja stana roga as in raktaja vidradhi. (2)

iti śrīmādhavakaraviracite mādhavanidāne stanaroganidānaṃ samāptam ||66||
Thus ends the chapter on StanaRoga

CHAPTER SIXTY-SEVEN

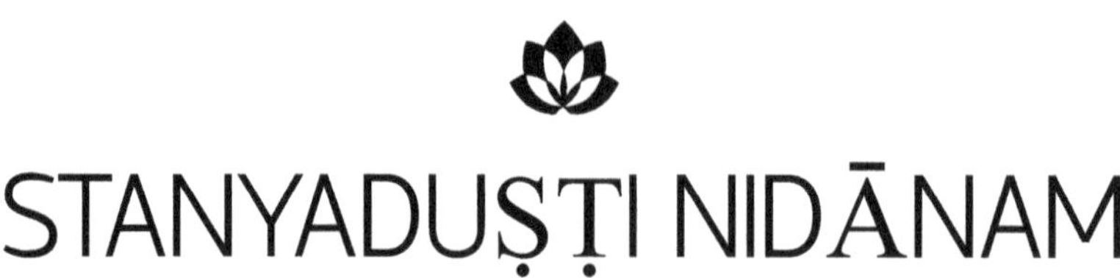

STANYADUṢṬI NIDĀNAM

Similarities between discharge of sukra (semen) in men and stanya (breast milk) in women

viśaṃsteṣvapi gātreṣu yathā śukraṃ na dṛśyate |
sarvadehāśritatvācca śukralakṣaṇamucyate ||1||
tadeva ceṣṭayuvaterdarśanāt smaraṇādapi |
śabdasaṃśravaṇāt sparśāt saṃharṣācca pravartate ||2||
suprasannaṃ manastatra harṣaṇe heturucyate |
āhārarasayonitvādevaṃ stanyamapi striyāḥ ||3||
tadevāpatyasaṃsparśāddarśanāt smaraṇādapi |
grahaṇācca śarīrasya śukravat sampravartate |
sneho nirantarastatra prasrave heturucyate ||4||
Just as sukra (semen, reproductive element of the male) though (described as) present all over the body cannot be seen even if any part of the body is cut open but comes out of the body on its own (ejaculated) by the sight, remembrance, hearing or excitement caused due to touch of the beloved woman. Sheer pleasantness (pleasure) of the mind is the cause for sexual excitation (and consequent discharge of semen).
Similar is the case with stanya (breast milk). Since stanya is the product of (produced by) the food that we consume (ahara rasa – essence or juice of the digested food) it is also (like sukra – semen) spread out all through the body. This breast milk will also flow freely out of the breasts by the touch, sight, and remembrance and fondling of the baby, just like the semen (as explained above).
The cause of continuous lactation (flow of breast milk) is the love of the mother towards her child. (3-4)

Stanya Dushti Hetu – Etiological factors for contamination of breast mil

gurubhirvividhairannairduṣṭairdoṣaiḥ pradūṣitam |
kṣīraṃ mātuḥ kumārasya nānārogāya kalpate ||5||
The doshas which undergo vitiation due to indulgence in different kinds of heavy (to digest) foods and similar other types of foods contaminate the breast milk of the mother which eventually becomes the cause for manifestation of many diseases in the child (which would consume such contaminated milk). (5)

Dushta Stanya Lakshana – symptoms of milk contaminated by the doshas

kaṣāyaṃ salilaplāvi stanyaṃ mārutadūṣitam |
kaṭvamlalavaṇaṃ pītarājīmat pittasañjñitam ||6||
kaphaduṣṭaṃ ghanaṃ toye nimajjati sapicchalam |
dviliṅgaṃ dvandvajaṃ vidyāt sarvaliṅgaṃ tridoṣajam ||7||
Vata Dusta Stanya – The breast milk vitiated by increased vata will be astringent in taste and float on the water.
Pitta Dusta Stanya – The breast milk vitiated by increased pitta will be pungent, sour or salty in taste and appears with yellowish threads (milk appears to have yellow thread like suspensions). Kapha Dusta Stanya – The breast milk vitiated by increased kapha is thick, sinks in water and is sticky.
Dwidosha and Tridosha Dusta Stanya – The breast milk vitiated by two or all three doshas which have simultaneously undergone vitiation will produce symptoms of two or three doshas together respectively. (6-7)

Shuddha Dugdha Swarupa – Features of normal / pure (not contaminated by doshas) breast milk

aduṣṭaṃ cāmbunikṣiptamekībhavati pāṇḍuram |
madhuraṃ cāvivarṇaṃ ca prasannaṃ tat praśasyate ||8||
Breast milk is said to be normal or pure (not contaminated with doshas) when it is found to mix evenly with water when put into water, is pale / slightly yellowish white in colour, is sweet in taste, doesn't have abnormal colours and is clear. (8)

iti śrīmādhavakaraviracite mādhavanidāne stanyaduṣṭinidānaṃ samāptam

||67||
Thus ends the chapter on StanyaDusti.

CHAPTER SIXTY-EIGHT

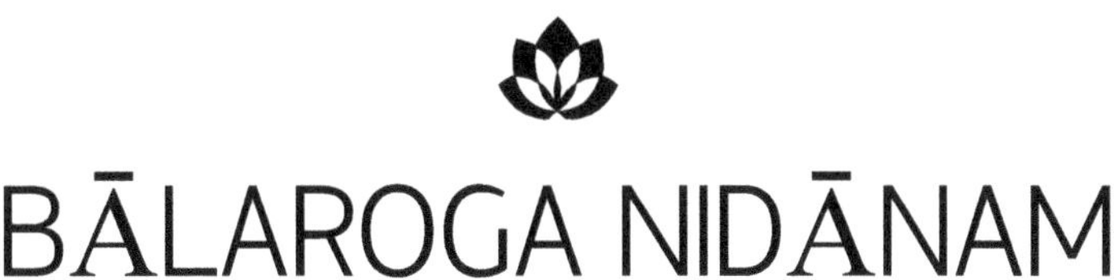

BĀLAROGA NIDĀNAM

Balarogas caused by milk vitiated by Vata

vātaduṣṭaṃ śiśuḥ stanyaṃ piban vātagadāturaḥ |
kṣāmasvaraḥ kṛśāṅgaḥ syādbaddhaviṇmūtramārutaḥ ||1||
When the child drinks milk which is vitiated by increased vata (in the lactating mother) it will become afflicted with diseases of vata origin. As a result, the child's voice becomes feeble and the child gets emaciated. The faeces, urine and flatus will not get eliminated. (1)

Balarogas caused by milk vitiated by Pitta

svinno bhinnamalo bālaḥ kāmalāpittarogavān |
tṛṣṇāluruṣṇasarvāṅgaḥ pittaduṣṭaṃ payaḥ piban ||2||
Drinking milk which is vitiated by pitta will make the child get afflicted with excessive sweating, diarrhoea, jaundice or other diseases of pitta origin. The child will suffer from severe thirst and the body will become extremely hot (increased body temperature). (2)

Balarogas caused by milk vitiated by Kapha

kaphaduṣṭaṃ piban kṣīraṃ lālāluḥ śleṣmarogavān |
nidrānvito jaḍaḥ śūnavaktrākṣaśchardanaḥ śiśuḥ ||3||
Drinking milk which is vitiated by increased kapha, will cause excessive salivation in the child. The child would be afflicted by many diseases of kapha origin. Apart from this excessive sleep, inactiveness, swelling of the face and eyes and vomiting are also present. (3)

Balarogas caused by simultaneous vitiation of milk by two or three doshas together

dvandvaje dvandvajaṃ rūpaṃ sarvaje sarvalakṣaṇam |4|
Milk vitiated by the increase of two doshas would produce symptoms of two doshas together and the milk vitiated by the increase of all three doshas together would produce symptoms of all three doshas together.

Antargata Vedana Jgnana Upaya – Methods of knowing (diagnosing) different types of pains in the child

śiśostīvrāmatīvrāṃ ca rodanāllakṣayedrujam ||4||
sa yaṃ spṛśedbhṛśaṃ deśaṃ yatra ca sparśanākṣamaḥ |
tatra vidyādrujaṃ mūrdhni rujaṃ cākṣinimīlanāt ||5||
hṛdi jihvauṣṭhadaśanaśvāsamuṣṭinipīḍanaiḥ |
koṣṭhe vibandhavamathustanadaṃśāntrakūjanaiḥ |
ādhmānapṛṣṭhanamanajaṭharonnamanairapi ||6||
bastau guhye ca viṇmūtrasaṅgatrāsadigīkṣaṇaiḥ |
srotāṃsyaṅgāni sandhīṃśca paśyedyatnānmuhurmuhuḥ ||7||
Recognizing the nature and intensity of pain - The nature of pain (or discomfort) in the child i.e., whether the pain is severe or less severe shall be recognized by the nature of crying, i.e., if the child is crying loudly, it indicates that the pain is severe and if the child is crying mildly it means to tell that the intensity of the pain is less severe.
Knowing the seat of pain - The part of the body which the child touches by its hands repeatedly or the part of the body which the child does not allow anyone to touch shall be recognized as the painful part (part affected by the disease).
Recognizing Headache or other diseases of the head – When the child keeps his eyes closed, it should be understood that the child is suffering from headache.
Recognizing pain or diseases of the abdomen – It should be inferred (understood) that the child is suffering from pain (or diseases) in the abdomen when the child has constipation, vomiting, biting of breast (of mother), gurgling noises in the intestines, distension of abdomen, bending (backward or forward) of back or abdomen.
Recognizing pain or diseases of urinary bladder and genitals / groins –

Obstruction to the passage of faeces and urine, fear and unsteady vision (seeing in either directions and getting scared / terrified) indicate pain or disease in urinary bladder / genitals in children.
This is the reason that the physician should carefully observe the channels (orifices), body parts, joints and other places of the body of the child frequently. (4-7)

Kukunaka

kukūṇakaḥ kṣīradoṣācchiśūnāmeva vartmani |
jāyate tena tannetraṃ kaṇḍūraṃ ca sravenmuhuḥ ||8||
śiśuḥ kuryāllalāṭākṣikūṭanāsāvagharṣaṇam |
śakto nārkaprabhāṃ draṣṭuṃ na vartmonmīlanakṣamaḥ ||9||
Kukūṇaka is a disease which occurs in the eyelids of the children. It is caused due to the effect of the child (infant) drinking the vitiated breast milk.
In this condition there will be itching and repeated discharges (exudates) from the eye / eyes. The child will repeatedly rub its forehead, region around the eye (orbit) and nose. The child will be incapable of seeing the sunlight and also in making movements of the eyelids (opening, closing). (8-9)

Parigarbhika

mātuḥ kumāro garbhiṇyāḥ stanyaṃ prāyaḥ pibannapi |
kāsāgnisādavamathutandrākārśyārucibhramaiḥ ||10||
yujyate koṣṭhavṛddhyā ca tamāhuḥ pārigarbhikam |
rogaṃ paribhavākhyaṃ ca yuñjyāttatrāgnidīpanam ||11||
Children drinking milk of the pregnant mother (i.e., mother of the child whom she is feeding, who has concurrently become pregnant) will develop cough, loss of digestion capacity (poor digestive capacity), vomiting, stupor, emaciation, loss of taste / appetite, giddiness and enlargement of abdomen. This disease is known by the name Parigarbhika or Paribhava. This condition shall be treated with herbs / medicines which increases digestion (power of digestion). (10-11)

Talukantaka

tālumāṃse kaphaḥ kruddhaḥ kurute tālukaṇṭakam |
tena tālupradeśasya nimnatā mūrdhni jāyate ||12||
tālupātaḥ stanadveṣaḥ kṛcchrāt pānaṃ śakṛddravam |
tṛḍakṣikaṇṭhāsyarujā grīvādurdharatā vamiḥ ||13||
Kapha undergoing increase in the muscles of the palate of the child produces a disease known as Talukaṇṭaka. In this condition, a depression appears in the upper part of the palate. The palate hangs down; the child will have aversion towards breasts and the child drinks breast milk with difficulty. The child will also have watery stools (diarrhoea), thirst, pain in the eyes, throat (neck) and mouth, instability of neck (inability to hold the neck / head upright) and vomiting. (12-13)

Mahapadma

visarpastu śiśoḥ prāṇanāśano bastiśīrṣajaḥ |
padmavarṇo mahāpadmanāmā doṣatrayodbhavaḥ ||14||
śaṅkhābhyāṃ hṛdayaṃ yāti hṛdayādvā gudaṃ vrajet |15|
Visarpa (erysipelas) developing in the urinary bladder and on the head in children is dreadful and life threatening. This condition caused by all the three doshas increased together will be red in colour resembling that of petals of red coloured lotus flower and hence called by the name Mahapadma. This disease may spread from temples to the region of the heart (chest) or from the chest to the anal / rectal region. (14)

Ajagallika and Ahiputana

kṣudraroge ca kathite tvajagallyahipūtane ||15||
The two diseases Ajagallika and Ahipūtana which have been described under ksudrarogas will also occur commonly in children. (15)

Jwara (fever) & other diseases occurring in children

jvarādyā vyādhayaḥ sarve mahatāṃ ye pureritāḥ |
bāladehe'pi te tadvadvijñeyāḥ kuśalaiḥ sadā ||16||
Jwara (fever) and all other major diseases which are explained earlier (which manifest in adults) will also affect the children. They should be

recognized by the learned physicians in the same way (as they would recognize and diagnose them in adults) by their specific symptoms. (16)

Grahajusta Laksanas – Symptoms of child affected by grahas (spirits)

kṣaṇādudvijate bālaḥ kṣaṇāttrasyati roditi |
nakhairdantairdārayati dhātrīmātmānameva vā ||17||
ūrdhvaṃ nirīkṣate dantān khādet kūjati jṛmbhate |
bhruvau kṣipati dantauṣṭhaṃ phenaṃ vamati cāsakṛt ||18||
kṣāmo'ti niśi jāgarti śūnākṣo bhinnaviṭsvaraḥ |
māṃsaśoṇitagandhiśca na cāśnāti yathā purā ||19||
sāmānyaṃ grahajuṣṭānāṃ lakṣaṇaṃ samudāhṛtam |20|
(When the child is affected by grahas – spirits) the child suddenly becomes agitated (perturbed, frightened, terrified, irritable), frightened and begins to cry without any apparent cause. The child scratches / injures self and also the wet-nurse (mother) by his nails and teeth, would stare upwards, bites/ grinds his own teeth, moans / makes indistinct sounds of helplessness and yawns frequently. He moves (throws, scatters) the brows (frown), teeth and lips here and there, vomits froth frequently. The child becomes excessively emaciated, does not sleep at night, has swelling around his eyes, diarrhoea and broken voice. The child's body emits the smell of flesh and blood and he would not take the food like before.
These are the general symptoms seen when the child is possessed by the Grahas i.e., evil spirits. (17-19)

Symptoms of child possessed by Skandagraha

ekanetrasya gātrasya srāvaḥ spandanakampanam ||20||
ūrdhvaṃ dṛṣṭyā nirīkṣeta vakrāsyo raktagandhikaḥ |
dantān khādati vitrastaḥ stanyaṃ naivābhinandati ||21||
skandagrahagṛhītānāṃ rodanaṃ cālpameva ca |22|
Below mentioned are the symptoms of child possessed by Skandagraha –

- Tearing from one eye (left or right eye)
- Excessive sweating from one side (half) of the body
- Pulsations / shivering in one side of the body
- Convulsions / tremors on one side of the body

- Gaze of the child is fixed upwards
- Deviation of one side of the face
- Smell of blood emitted from the face / skin
- Biting / grinding of the teeth
- Fretfulness
- Does not like (relish) drinking breast milk
- Crying less (crying mildly) (20-21)

Symptoms of child possessed by Skandapasmara

naṣṭasañjño vamet phenaṃ sañjñāvānatiroditi |
pūyaśoṇitagandhitvaṃ skandāpasmāralakṣaṇam ||22||
Below mentioned are the symptoms of child possessed by Skandapasmara –

- Fainting along with frothy vomiting
- Too much crying after gaining consciousness
- Smell of pus and blood emitted from the body of the child (22)

Symptoms of child possessed by Sakunigraha

srastāṅgo bhayacakito vihaṅgagandhiḥ sāsrāvavraṇaparipīḍitaḥ samantāt |
sphoṭaiśca pracitatanuḥ sadāhapākairvijñeyo bhavati śiśuḥ kṣataḥ śakunyā ||23||
(su| u| taṃ| a| 27) |
Below mentioned are the symptoms of child possessed by Sakunigraha –

- Drooping of the limbs / body parts
- Fretfulness
- Alarmed / shocked
- Smell resembling that of the aquatic birds emitted from the body of the child,
- Many ulcers / papules along with discharges spread out all over the body
- Many blisters spread out all over the body along with burning sensation and suppuration (23)

Symptoms of child possessed by Revatigraha

vraṇaiḥ sphoṭaiścitaṃ gātraṃ paṅkagandhaṃ sravedasṛk |
bhinnavarcā jvarī dāhī revatīgrahalakṣaṇam ||24||
Below mentioned are the symptoms of child possessed by Revatigraha –

- Ulcers and boils spread out all through the body
- Blood having the smell of silt is discharged from the ulcers
- Watery stools (diarrhoea)
- Fever
- Burning sensation in the body (24)

Symptoms of child possessed by Putanagraha

atīsāro jvarastṛṣṇā tiryakprekṣaṇarodanam |
naṣṭanidrastathodvigno grastaḥ pūtanayā śiśuḥ ||25||
Below mentioned are the symptoms of child possessed by Putanagraha –

- Diarrhoea
- Fever
- Thirst
- Looking side-wards
- Crying
- Loss of sleep
- Irritability (25)

Symptoms of child possessed by Andhaputana

chardiḥ kāso jvarastṛṣṇā vasāgandho'tirodanam |
stanyadveṣo'tisāraśca andhapūtanayā bhavet ||26||
Below mentioned are the symptoms of child possessed by Andhaputana graha –

- Vomiting

- Cough
- Fever
- Thirst
- Body emitting smell of muscle fat
- Excessive crying
- Aversion to breast milk
- Diarrhoea (26)

Symptoms of child possessed by Sitaputana

vepate kāsate kṣīṇo netrarogo vigandhitā |
chardyatīsārayuktaśca śītapūtanayā śiśuḥ ||27||
Below mentioned are the symptoms of child possessed by Sitaputana graha –

- Tremors / abnormal movements in the body parts
- Cough
- Emaciation
- Eye disorders
- Abnormal smell emitted from the body
- Vomiting
- Diarrhoea (27)

Symptoms of child possessed by Mukhamandika Graha

prasannavarṇavadanaḥ sirābhirabhisaṃvṛtaḥ |
mūtragandhī ca bahvāśī mukhamaṇḍikayā bhavet ||28||
Below mentioned are the symptoms of child possessed by Mukhamandika graha –

- Pleasantness of body colour
- Pleasantness / brightness of the face,
- Presence of prominent veins all over the body
- Smell of urine emitted from the body
- Eating too much food (28)

Symptoms of child possessed by Naigamesa Graha

chardispa(sya)ndanakaṇṭhāsyaśoṣamūrchāvigandhitāḥ |
ūrdhvaṃ paśyeddaśeddantān naigameyagrahaṃ vadet ||29||
Below mentioned are the symptoms of child possessed by Naigamesa graha –

- Vomiting,
- Visible pulsations
- Dryness of the throat and mouth
- Fainting
- Bad / foul smell emitted from the body
- Gaze fixed upwards
- Biting / grinding of teeth (29)

Prognosis of possession by evil spirits

prastabdhākṣaḥ stanadveṣī muhyate cāniśaṃ muhuḥ |
taṃ bālamacirāddhanti grahaḥ sampūrṇalakṣaṇaḥ |
viparītatamaṃ sādhyaṃ cikitsedacirārditam ||30||
The grahas (possession by evil spirits) will kill the child in quick time in the presence of the below mentioned symptoms (symptoms of bad prognosis) –

- Loss of movements in the eyes (and other sense organs)
- Aversion towards breast / breast milk
- Frequent fainting
- Appearance of all the symptoms of grahas (30)

iti śrīmādhavakaraviracite mādhavanidāne bālaroganidānaṃ samāptam ||68||
Thus ends the chapter on BalaRogas.

CHAPTER SIXTY-NINE

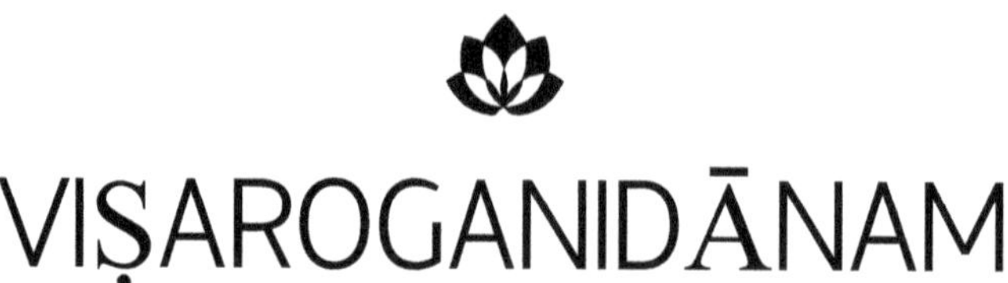

VIṢAROGANIDĀNAM

Visa Bheda - Types of Poisons

sthāvaraṃ jaṅgamaṃ caiva dvividhaṃ viṣamucyate |
mūlādyātmakamādyaṃ syāt paraṃ sarpādisambhavam ||1||
Poisons are of two kinds - Sthavara Visa and Jangama Visa.
Poisons obtained from roots and other parts of the plants (leaves, flowers etc) are known as Sthavara Visa.
Poisons of animals like snakes are called Jangama Visa. (1)

General symptoms caused by the effect of Jangama Visa

nidrāṃ tandrāṃ klamaṃ dāhamapākaṃ lomaharṣaṇam |
śothaṃ caivātisāraṃ ca jaṅgamaṃ kurute viṣam ||2||
(ca| ci| a| 23) |3|
Sleep, stupor, exhaustion, burning sensation, indigestion, horripilations, swelling and diarrhoea are the general symptoms caused by (the effect of) Jangama Viṣa (animal poison).(2)

General symptoms caused by the effect of Sthavara Visa

sthāvaraṃ ca jvaraṃ hikkāṃ dantaharṣaṃ galagraham |
phenacchardyaruciśvāsaṃ mūrchāṃ ca kurute bhṛśam ||3||
(ca| ci| a| 23) |4|
The general symptoms caused (by the effect of) Sthavara Visa include - fever, hiccough, tingling sensation in the teeth (gums), catch / stiffness / choking in the throat, vomiting of froth, loss of taste (appetite), difficulty in breathing and fainting. (3)

Visa Datara – signs of person who is habituated to administer poisons to others

iṅgitajño manuṣyāṇāṃ vākceṣṭāmukhavaikṛtaiḥ |
jānīyādviṣadātāramebhirliṅgaiśca buddhimān ||4||
na dadātyuttaraṃ pṛṣṭo vivakṣurmohameti ca |
apārthaṃ bahu saṅkīrṇaṃ bhāṣate cāpi mūḍhavat ||5||
hasatyakasmāt sphoṭayatyaṅgulīrvilikhenmahīm |
vepathuścāsya bhavati trastaścānyonyamīkṣate ||6||
vivarṇavaktro dhyāmaśca nakhaiḥ kiñcicchinattyapi |
ālabhetāsanaṃ dīnaṃ kareṇa va śiroruham ||7||
vartate viparītaṃ ca viṣadātā vicetanaḥ |
(su| ka| a| 1) |

An intelligent person (physician) who can identify the signs and expressions of anyone should also find out the characteristic features of a Visadata (person who is habituated to administer poisons to others) by his talks, actions and facial expressions and also with the help of below mentioned signs –

- When asked about anything the person (who has poisoned) will either not reply or even if he tries to reply he fumbles or gets confused (scared), acts ignorant
- Gives wrong replies, speaks too much or gives irrelevant replies (in an unclear way) just like a fool / idiot
- Laughs suddenly without any reason
- Cracks his knuckles (makes sounds from his fingers)
- Scratches the ground (earth) with his toes / fingers
- Keeps shivering, gets scared and looks at others (for help or support),
- Face becomes discoloured and unclean (bad expressions)
- Keeps cutting something or the other (grass etc) with his nails,
- Takes seat (sits) with timidity and hesitation,
- Repeatedly touches (pulls) the hairs on his head with his hands
- Keeps changing his seat and position every now and then
- Will not be in his senses (behaves in an unusual manner) (4-7)

General symptoms produced by poisons derived from roots etc

udveṣṭanaṃ mūlaviṣaiḥ pralāpo moha eva ca ||8||
jṛmbhaṇaṃ vepanaṃ śvāso mohaḥ patraviṣeṇa tu |
muṣkaśothaḥ phalaviṣairdāho'nnadveṣa eva ca ||9||
bhavet puṣpaviṣaiśchardirādhmānaṃ śvāsa eva ca |
tvaksāraniryāsaviṣairupayuktairbhavanti hi ||10||
āsyadaurgandhyapāruṣyaśirorukkaphasaṃsravāḥ |
phenāgamaḥ kṣīraviṣairviḍbhedo gurugātratā ||11||
hṛtpīḍanaṃ dhātuviṣairmūrchā dāhaśca tāluni |
prāyeṇa kālaghātīni viṣāṇyetāni nirdiśet ||12||
(su| ka| a| 2) |
Mula Visa / Poisonous roots – when consumed will produce pain all over the body as though hit by a stick, delirium and delusion.
Patra Visa / Poisonous leaves – when consumed will produce excess yawning, tremors, difficulty in breathing and delusion.
Phala Visa / Poisonous fruits – when consumed will cause swelling in the scrotum, burning sensation and aversion towards food.
Puspa Visa / Poisonous flowers – when consumed will produce vomiting, distension of the abdomen and difficulty in breathing.
Twaksara & Niryasa Visa / Poisonous bark and resin (gum) – when consumed will produce foul smell in the mouth, roughness of the body, headache and discharge of kapha from mouth.
Ksira Visa / Poisonous latex – when consumed will cause frothy discharges from the mouth, diarrhoea and feeling of heaviness in the body.
Dhatu Visa / Poisonous minerals (ores) etc – when consumed will produce pain in the region of the heart (cardiac region), fainting / loss of consciousness and burning sensation in the palate.
Probably all the above kinds of poisons are considered to be kalaghatini i.e., would kill the person in due course of time. (8-12)

Digdahata, Visa Digda & Visapita Laksana

sadyaḥkṣataṃ pacyate yasya jantoḥ sravedraktaṃ pacyate cāpyabhīkṣṇam |
kṛṣṇībhūtaṃ klinnamatyarthapūti kṣatānmāṃsaṃ śīryate cāpi yasya ||13||
tṛṣṇā mūrchā jvaradāhau ca yasya digdhāhataṃ taṃ puruṣaṃ vyavasyet |

liṅgānyetānyeva kuryādamitrairvraṇe viṣaṃ yasya dattaṃ pramādāt ||14||
sapītaṃ gṛhadhūmābhaṃ purīṣaṃ yo'tisāryate |
phenamudvamate cāpi viṣapītaṃ tamādiśet ||15||
(su| ka| a| 3) |
Digdahata (wounds caused by poison smeared weapons) - The person in whom the fresh wound undergoes immediate suppuration, discharges plenty of blood and suppuration becomes progressive (occurs repeatedly), the wound becomes black in colour, has too much of discharge, is foul smelling and the muscles surrounding the wound fall off all by themselves (after getting decomposed) are the signs of wounds caused by weapons smeared with poison. The person will also suffer from thirst, fainting, fever and burning sensation.
Visadigda (wounds poisoned by poison) – Sometimes when a person is not cautious, some enemies will poison their wounds (or even make the wounded person drink poison forcefully). Even in these conditions the signs and symptoms mentioned above (digdahata) will be found. This is called Visadigda.
Visapita (one who has drunk poison) – A person should be considered to have consumed (administered) poison when he repeatedly eliminates stools (diarrhoea) which are yellow in colour or a colour resembling soot of chimney (black), and has frothy vomiting. (13-15)

1.It is more appropriate to read 'Mukha' instead of Muska in this stanza.

Sarpa and Sarpavisa – Snakes and snake poison

vātapittakaphātmāno bhogimaṇḍalirājilāḥ |
yathākramamaṃ samākhyātā dvyantarā dvandvarūpiṇaḥ ||16||
Bhogi - snakes with a hood, Mandala – snakes with patches and Rajila – snakes with stripes are predominant in vata, pitta and kapha doshas respectively (tend to vitiate these doshas respectively). The hybrid snakes will have mixed qualities of two or more doshas. (16)

Symptoms of bites of different kinds of snakes

daṃśo bhogikṛtaḥ kṛṣṇaḥ sarvavātavikārakṛt |
pīto maṇḍalijaḥ śotho mṛduḥ pittavikāravān ||17||

rājilottho bhaveddaṃśaḥ sthiraśothaśca picchilaḥ |
pāṇḍuḥ snigdho'tisāndrasṛk sarvaśleṣmavikārakṛt ||18||
Bhogi Sarpa - The site of the bite by a hooded snake will become black. It causes all the symptoms (diseases) of vata increase.
Mandala Sarpa – The bite of the mandala snake (snake with patches) will become yellow in colour. The swelling which occurs is soft and it causes all the symptoms (diseases) of pitta to increase.
Rajila Sarpa – The site of the bite of rajila snake (striped snakes) will have an immobile (hard) swelling, is sticky, of yellowish white (pale) colour and discharges very thick blood. It causes all the symptoms (diseases) of kapha to increase. (17-18)

Prognosis of snake bite

aśvatthadevāyatanaśmaśānavalmīkasandhyāsu catuṣpatheṣu |
yāmye ca daṣṭāḥ parivarjanīyā ṛkṣe sirāmarmasu ye ca daṣṭāḥ ||19||
(su| ka| a| 3) |
Snake bite happening in the below mentioned places should be rejected treatment (because they are incurable) –

- Near / Below Aswattha tree (Ficus religiosa)
- In a temple
- In a crematorium
- In / near an anthill
- In the evening time
- At crossroads
- In Bharani constellation
- If the bite is on veins and vital spots of the body (or vital spots of the body wherein there is predominance of veins) (19)

Effect of snake bite on life

darvīkarāṇāṃ viṣamāśughāti sarvāṇi coṣṇe dviguṇībhavanti |20|
(su| ka| a| 3) |
The poison of darvikara sarpa i.e., hooded snakes kill the person immediately (quickly). The effect of the other poisons becomes twice

powerful in hot season (or when associated with heat – as in exposure to sunlight, fire, hot objects, fomentation etc). (20)

Other conditions in which the effect of poisons becomes powerful

ajīrṇapittātapapīḍiteṣu bāleṣu vṛddheṣu bubhukṣiteṣu ||20||
kṣīṇakṣate mehini kuṣṭhayukte rūkṣe'bale garbhavatīṣu cāpi |
(su| ka| a| 3) |
Likewise, the effect of poison will become doubly powerful (incurable) in persons suffering from indigestion, those afflicted by diseases caused by increased pitta, and exposed to sun. It is also true in case of children, aged people, and those hungry and wounded / emaciated due to wounds, in those suffering from diabetes and skin diseases (leprosy), in those who have dryness of the body, malnourished (weak) and in pregnant women.

Other signs and symptoms of incurability of snake bite cases

śastrakṣate yasya na raktameti rājyo latābhiśca na sambhavanti ||21||
śītābhiradbhiśca na romaharṣo viṣābhibhūtaṃ parivarjayettam |
jihmaṃ mukhaṃ yasya ca keśaśāto nāsāvasādaśca sakaṇṭhabhaṅgaḥ ||22||
kṛṣṇaḥ saraktaḥ śvayathuśca daṃśe hanvoḥ sthiratvaṃ ca vivarjanīyaḥ |
vartirghanā yasya nireti vaktrādraktaṃ sravedūrdhvamadhaśca yasya ||23||
daṃṣṭrānipātāścaturaśca yasya taṃ cāpi vaidyaḥ parivarjayecca |
unmattamatyarthamupadrutaṃ vā hīnasvaraṃ vā'pyatha vā vivarṇam ||24||
sāriṣṭamatyarthamaveginaṃ ca jñātvā naraṃ karma na tatra kuryāt |
(su| ka| a| 3) |
If in a person who has been bitten by a snake – if bleeding does not occur in spite of a cut being made by a sharp instrument, if linear marks do not appear on the skin (at the site) even if beaten or tied with a creeper / rope, horripilations does not occur in spite of sprinkling with cold water (cannot bring the person back to consciousness by sprinkling cold water), he or she should be refused treatment (because they are incurable).
Irregularity / crookedness of the face, falling of hairs (or the person pulling off his hairs by himself), displacement / deformity of the nose, inability to hold the neck straight in position (hoarseness of voice), reddish black coloured swelling at the site of bite, and stiffness of the lower jaw (lockjaw) when seen in the patient who has been bitten by the snake should be

rejected (because the presence of these symptoms indicates that the condition is incurable).

Similarly a person in whom thick wick-like saliva comes out of the mouth, bleeding occurs through both upper (nose, mouth etc) and lower (anal, urethra etc) passages, and the physician attending such person not having expertise to remove poison (impression of four fangs are found at the site of bite) should also be refused treatment considering that it is incurable.

The person who after being bitten by snake has become insane (lost the mind balance), has many complications, feeble voice, and discolouration, who has developed signs of death and who does not have urges of the body (in whom the urges of defecation, urination etc are not manifested) should be rejected, the condition being incurable. (21-24)

Dusivisa

jīrṇaṃ viṣaghnauṣadhibhirhataṃ vā dāvāgnivātātapaśoṣitaṃ vā ||25||
svabhāvato vā guṇaviprahīnaṃ viṣaṃ hi dūṣīviṣatāmupaiti |
(su| ka| a| 2) |

Dusivisa is a poison or poisonous substance which is very old, whose properties have been nullified as an effect of (after being mixed with) anti-poisonous drugs, which has been dried up by the forest fire, breeze and sunlight and by nature does not have powerful properties of poisons (having lesser properties in comparison to a strong poison). (25)

Properties of poor potency poisons

vīryālpabhāvānna nipātayettat kaphānvitaṃ varṣagaṇānubandhi ||26||
tenārdito bhinnapurīṣavarṇo vaigandhyavairasyayutaḥ pipāsī |
mūrchāṃ bhramaṃ gadgadavāgvamiṃ ca viceṣṭamāno'ratimāpnuyādvā ||27||
(su| ka| a| 2) |

Because of its poor potency and being associated with kapha (kapha dilutes the strong and intense properties of the poison), it does not kill the person (suddenly or even later). Such a poison remains inside the body for years without undergoing digestion. The person who is afflicted with such poison will have diarrhoea, discolouration, and bad smell from the body, bad smell from the mouth, thirst, fainting, giddiness, stammer, vomiting, unnatural body movements and restlessness. (26-27)

Symptoms of Dusivisa based on the place / organ in which it is located

āmāśayasthe kaphavātarogī pakvāśayasthe'nilapittarogī |
bhavet samuddhvastaśiroruhāṅgo vilūnapakṣastu yathā vihaṅgaḥ ||28||
(su| ka| a| 2) |
If Dusivisa is located in the stomach, diseases of kapha-vata origin get manifested. If Dusivisa is located in the intestines, the person would become a patient of diseases of vata-pitta origin. Apart from this, due to the loss of hairs of the head and body, he appears like a bird whose wings have been cut off. (28)

Symptoms of dusivisa lodged in different tissues

sthitaṃ rasādiṣvathavā yathoktān karoti dhātuprabhavān vikārān |
kopaṃ ca śītāniladurdineṣu yātyāśu pūrvaṃ śṛṇu tasya rūpam ||29||
(su| ka| a| 2) |
If the dusivisa is lodged in rasa and other tissues of the body, it produces the symptoms / diseases which are likely to develop in those tissues. The symptoms become severe and troublesome due to exposure to cold winds and on cloudy days. First make a note of its premonitory symptoms. (29)

Premonitory Symptoms of effect of Dusivisas

nidrāgurutvaṃ ca vijṛmbhaṇaṃ ca viśleṣaharṣāvathavā'ṅgamardam |
tataḥ karotyannamadāvipākāvarocakaṃ maṇḍalakoṭhajanma ||30||
māṃsakṣayaṃ pādakarapraśothaṃ mūrchāṃ tathā chardimathātisāram |
dūṣīviṣaṃ śvāsatṛṣājvarāṃśca kuryāt pravṛddhiṃ jaṭharasya cāpi ||31||
(su| ka| a| 2) |
Excessive sleep, feeling of heaviness of the body, yawning, looseness of the body parts, horripilations, and pains in the body parts (as if beaten), (later) feeling of intoxication after having meals, indigestion, loss of taste (tastelessness), manifestation of rashes and papules, depletion of muscles (emaciation), swelling of feet and hands, fainting, vomiting, loose motions (diarrhoea), dyspnoea (difficulty in breathing), thirst, fever and enlargement of abdomen – are the premonitory symptoms of effect of dusivisa. (30-31)

Different diseases caused by Dusivisa

unmādamanyajjanayettathā'nyadānāhamanyat kṣapayecca śukram |
gādgadyamanyajjanayecca kuṣṭhaṃ tāṃstān vikārāṃśca bahuprakārān ||32||
(su| ka| a| 2) |
Some kinds of dusivisa will produce insanity, some others would produce flatulence (enlargement of abdomen) and some other types would bring about loss of semen. Other types of dusivisa will cause stuttering / stammer and some others will cause skin disorders (leprosy) and many other kinds of diseases. (32)

Definition of Dusivisa

dūṣitaṃ deśakālānnadivāsvapnairabhīkṣṇaśaḥ |
yasmāt sandūṣayeddhātūn tasmāddūṣīviṣaṃ smṛtam ||33||
sādhyamātmavataḥ sadyo yāpyaṃ saṃvatsarotthitam |
dūṣīviṣamasādhyaṃ syāt kṣīṇasyāhitasevinaḥ ||34||
(su| ka| a| 2) |
Dūsī visa is so called because it keeps vitiating the dhātus (tissues) often, being aggravated by the influence of deśa (habitat), kāla (season), anna (food) and divāsvapana (day sleep). Dusivisa of recent origin and present in those who have self-control (strong will) is curable. It becomes manageable after one year (can be cured but it keeps recurring when favourable conditions are available, hence needs monitoring throughout life). It is incurable in those who are emaciated (weak) and are habituated to getting indulged in unhealthy foods and life activities. (33-34)

Symptoms of persons affected by Garavisa

saubhāgyārthaṃ striyaḥ svedaṃ rajo nānāṅgajān malān |
śatruprayuktāṃśca garān prayacchantyannamiśritān ||35||
taiḥ syāt pāṇḍuḥ kṛśo'lpāgnirgaraścāsyopajāyate |
marmapradhamanādhmānaṃ hastayoḥ śothalakṣaṇam ||36||
jaṭharaṃ grahaṇīdoṣo yakṣmā gulmaḥ kṣayo jvaraḥ |
evaṃvidhasya cānyasya vyādherliṅgāni darśayet ||37||

Women expecting wealth (or other benefits or to take someone under their control and influence) administer sweat, menstrual blood, excretions (waste products) produced by different body parts, or artificial poison provided by enemies mixed with food. Poisons administered in this form are called Garavisa (homicidal poison).
Effect of Garavisa (symptoms of impact of garavisa) – The person affected by garavisa becomes pale, emaciated, and would have poor digestion. These things will produce garavisa in the body of the person who has consumed them. The person will have pain in vital organs of the body, distension of the body, symptoms of swelling in their hands, abdominal disorders (abdomen enlargement), duodenal disorders, tuberculosis, abdominal tumour, emaciation (consumption), fever and symptoms of many such (allied) diseases. (35-37)

Lutavisa

yasmāllūnaṃ tṛṇaṃ prāptā muneḥ prasvedabindavaḥ |
tasmāllūtāstu bhāṣyante saṅkhyayā tāśca ṣoḍaśa ||38||
(su| ka| a| 8) |
The droplets of sweat of the sage Vaşistha (who had become angry with Viswamitra at the abduction of Kamadhenu, the cow) which fell on the grass become converted into Lūtās (spiders). Lutas are of sixteen kinds. (38)

General Symptoms of Spider bite

tābhirdaṣṭe daṃśakothaḥ pravṛttiḥ kṣatajasya ca |
varo dāho'tisāraśca gadāḥ syuśca tridoṣajāḥ ||39||
piḍakā vividhākārā maṇḍalāni mahānti ca |
śothā mahānto mṛdavo raktāḥ śyāvāścalāstathā ||40||
sāmānyaṃ sarvalūtānāmetaddaṃśasya lakṣaṇam |
(su| ka| a| 8) |42|
When bitten by these spiders, putrefaction at the site of the bite occurs. Apart from this, there will be bleeding, fever, burning sensation, diarrhoea and other symptoms (diseases) caused by the increase of all the three doshas together. Papules of different kinds, big patches, profound soft swelling, red or black in colour and movable are formed. These are the

general symptoms of spider bite. (39-40)

Symptoms of bite of Dusivisa type of spiders

daṃśamadhye tu yat kṛṣṇaṃ śyāvaṃ vā jālakācitam ||41||
ūrdhvākṛti bhṛśaṃ pākaṃ kledaśothajvarānvitam |
dūṣīviṣābhirlūtābhistaddaṣṭamiti nirdiśet ||42||
(ca| ci| a| 23) |
Below mentioned are the features (symptoms) found in person bitten by dusivisa type of spiders (spiders having slow acting poisons) –

- Blackish or blackish blue colour at the centre of the site of spider bite
- Appearance of network (like structure) at the site of bite
- Elevation of skin around the bite
- Severe suppuration
- Exudation
- Swelling
- Fever (41-42)

Symptoms of bite of sauvarnika etc spiders

śothāḥ śvetāḥ sitā raktāḥ pītā vā piḍakā jvaraḥ |
prāṇāntikāśca jāyante śvāsahikkāśirograhāḥ ||43||
(ca| ci| a| 23) |
Bite of Sauvarnika etc eight types of spiders' cause swelling, along with papules which are white, red or yellow in colour, fever, dyspnoea (difficulty in breathing), hiccough and headache. The poisons of these
types of spiders are said to be quick acting and fatal. (43)

Symptoms of Musika Dusivisa

ādaṃśācchoṇitaṃ pāṇḍumaṇḍalāni jvaro'ruciḥ |
lomaharṣaśca dāhaścāpyākhudūṣīviṣārdite ||44||
(ca| ci| a| 23) |
The symptoms of poisoning by musika (rat) dusivisa include bleeding from the site of bite, appearance of white coloured patches, fever, loss of taste, horripilation and burning sensation. (44)

Symptoms of incurability of poisonous rat bite

mūrchāṅgaśothavaivarṇyakledaśabdāśrutijvarāḥ |
śirogurutvaṃ lālāsṛkchardiścāsādhyamūṣikaiḥ ||45||
(ca| ci| a| 23) |

The symptoms of incurability when bitten by a poisonous rat include – fainting, swelling of body parts, discolouration, wetness / moistness of the body, deafness, fever, heaviness of the head, excessive salivation and blood vomiting. (45)

Symptoms of Krkalasa Damsa (bite by chameleon)

kārṣṇyaṃ śyāvatvamathavā nānāvarṇatvameva vā |
moho'tha varcaso bhedo daṣṭe syāt kṛkalāsakaiḥ ||46||
(ca| ci| a| 23) |

The symptoms caused by bite of chameleon include blackish or blackish blue discolouration or appearance of different colours on the skin (site of bite), delusion and diarrhoea. (46)

Symptoms of Vrscika damsa - Scorpion sting

dahatyagnirivādau ca bhinattīvordhvamāśu ca |
vṛścikasya viṣaṃ yāti daṃśe paścāttu tiṣṭhati ||47||
daṣṭo'sādhyaśca hṛdghrāṇarasanopahato naraḥ |
māṃsaiḥ patadbhiratyarthaṃ vedanārto jahātyasūn ||48||
(ca| ci| a| 23) |

The symptoms of scorpion sting include – Immediately after the sting by scorpion the person would experience a severe burning sensation as if burnt by fire and splitting pain at the site of sting. Following this the poison quickly ascends upwards and later once again becomes limited to (settled in) the site of sting.

If the scorpion sting has caused destruction of (diseases of) heart, loss of functions of nose and tongue, it should be considered as an incurable condition. Similarly, if the muscles (after undergoing putrefaction) around the site of scorpion sting falls off and if the person suffers from severe pain, the person will die soon. (47-48)

Symptoms of Kanabha Dasta – wasp sting

visarpaḥ śvayathuḥ śūlaṃ jvaraśchardirathāpi ca |
lakṣaṇaṃ kaṇabhairdaṣṭe daṃśaścaivāvasīdati ||49||
(ca| ci| a| 23) |
Erysipelas (or ulcer spreading from one place to the other), swelling, pain, fever and vomiting are the symptoms found in a person stung by a wasp. Apart from this, the surroundings (muscles etc) of the sting would fall off. (49)

Symptoms of Ucchitinga Damsa – bite by poisonous crab

hṛṣṭalomocciṭiṅgena stabdhaliṅgo bhṛśārtimān |
daṣṭaḥ śītodakeneva siktānyaṅgāni manyate ||50||
(ca| ci| a| 23) |

Horripilations, stiffness (sustained erection) of penis, and severe pain are the symptoms found in a person bitten by ucchitinga (poisonous crab, variety of scorpion). (50)

Symptoms of bite by Poisonous frogs, fishes and leeches

ekadaṃṣṭrārditaḥ śūnaḥ sarujaḥ pītakaḥ satṛṭ |
chardirnidrā ca saviṣairmaṇḍūkairdaṣṭalakṣaṇam ||51||
matsyāstu saviṣāḥ kuryurdāhaṃ śothaṃ rujaṃ tathā |
kaṇḍūṃ śothaṃ jvaraṃ mūrchāṃ saviṣāstu jalaukasaḥ ||52||
(ca| ci| a| 23) |
Bite by poisonous frogs – causes symptoms including swelling, pain and yellow discolouration at the site of bite, thirst, vomiting and excessive sleep.
Bite by poisonous fish – causes symptoms including burning sensation, swelling and pain.
Bite by poisonous leeches – causes symptoms including itching, swelling, and fever and fainting. (51-52)

Symptoms of bite by house lizard, centipede, mosquitoes, bees

vidāhaṃ śvayathuṃ todaṃ svedaṃ ca gṛhagodhikā |53| (ca| ci| a| 23) |
daṃśe svedaṃ rujaṃ dāhaṃ kuryācchatapadīviṣam ||53|| (ca| ci| a| 23) |
kaṇḍūmān maśakairīṣacchothaḥ smānmandavedanaḥ |

asādhyakīṭasadṛśamasādhyaṃ maśakakṣatam ||54|| (ca| ci| a| 23) |
sadyaḥprasrāviṇī śyāvā dāhamūrchājvarānvitā |
piḍakā makṣikādaṃśe tāsāṃ tu sthagikā'suhṛt ||55||
(ca| ci| a| 23) |
Bite by house lizard - will cause severe burning sensation, swelling, pricking pain and perspiration.
Bite by the centipede - will cause excessive sweating, pain and burning sensation.
Bite by ordinary mosquitoes - will cause itching, slight swelling and mild pain. Bite of poisonous mosquitoes will be incurable just like the bit of poisonous insects.
Sting by bee – will produce immediate discharge (of blood), blackish discolouration, burning sensation, fainting, fever and papules. Among all the bees, the sting of sthagika variety of bee will be fatal. (53-55)

Symptoms of bite by animals of four or two legs

catuṣpadbhirdvipadbhiśca nakhadantaviṣaṃ ca yat |
śūyate pacyate vā'pi sravati jvarayatyapi ||56||
Assault by the claws and teeth of animals of four or two legs will cause swelling, suppuration (putrefaction), discharges (exudation) and fever. (56)

Symptoms of effect of poison in tiger etc wild animals

śvaśṛgālatarakṣvarkṣavyāghrādīnāṃ yadā'nilaḥ |
śleṣmapraduṣṭo muṣṇāti sañjñāṃ sañjñāvahāśritaḥ ||57||
tadā prasrastalāṅgūlahanuskandho'tilālavān |
avyaktabadhirāndhaśca so'nyonyamabhidhāvati ||58||
pramūḍho'nyatamastveṣāṃ khādan viparidhāvati |
tenonmattena daṣṭasya daṃṣṭriṇā saviṣeṇa tu ||59||
suptatā jāyate daṃśe kṛṣṇaṃ cātisravatyasṛk |
digdhaviddhasya liṅgena prāyaśaścopalakṣitaḥ ||60||
yena cāpi bhaveddaṣṭastasya ceṣṭāṃ rutaṃ naraḥ |
bahuśaḥ pratikurvāṇaḥ kriyāhīno vipaśyati ||61||
daṃṣṭriṇā yena daṣṭaśca tadrūpaṃ yastu paśyati |
apsu cādarśabimbe vā tasya tadriṣṭamādiśet ||62||

trasyatyakasmādyo'bhīkṣṇaṃ dṛṣṭvā spṛṣṭvā'pi vā jalam |
jalatrāsaṃ tu taṃ vidyādriṣṭaṃ tadapi kīrtitam ||63||

In animals like dogs, fox, hyena, bear, tiger etc, when Vata is vitiated by increased kapha attacks and destroys the nervous system, the consciousness (intelligence) of these animals get hampered and they become rabid. In such animals the tail, lower jaw and shoulders will drop down, saliva starts dribbling from their mouth in large quantities. The animals appear blind and deaf to a certain extent and run towards each other. Among these the one which has gone excessively mad will run amuck everywhere and run to bite the others. If bitten by such rabid animals there will be loss of sensation at the site of bite, discharge of black coloured blood in excess (or there will be blackish discolouration at the site and severe bleeding). There will be symptoms of wounds caused by poisonous weapons.

The person who has been bitten by a rabid animal such as a dog etc will repeatedly keep imitating all the actions of that animal (whichever animal has bitten) and produces sounds (cries, shouts) similar to that animal. He will not be able to do any of his activities (becomes unconscious) and will face death. If one sees the image / reflection of the animal which has bitten him instead of his reflection in the water or mirror it shall be considered as a fatal sign. If the person bitten by a rabid animal becomes afraid of seeing or touching water it is known as Jalatrasa – hydrophobia. This is also a fatal sign. (57-63)

Another fatal sign

adaṣṭo vā jalatrāsī na kathañcana siddhyati |
prasupto votthito vā'pi svasthastrasto na siddhyati ||64||
(su| ka| a| 7) |

In spite of not being bitten by a rabid animal, if a person develops fear towards water, the condition should be considered as incurable. Similarly, if a healthy person develops fear towards water while sleeping or after waking up (in woken state) the condition shall be considered to be incurable. (64)

Nirvisa Purusa Laksana – symptoms of person relieved from poison

praśāntadoṣaṃ prakṛtisthadhātumannābhikāmaṃ samamūtraviṭkam |
prasannavarṇendriyacittaceṣṭaṃ vaidyo'vagacchedaviṣaṃ manuṣyam ||65||

(su| ka| a| 6) |

Aggravation of doshas coming down (all the increased dosas getting back to normal), all the tissues coming back to normal state (become pure), developing desire for food, proper and timely elimination of urine and faeces, restoration of (becoming normal and pleasant) normal colour and complexion, functioning of the senses and mind and activities and behaviour – should be considered by the physician as the symptoms of the person completely relieved of poison. (65)

iti śrīmādhavakaraviracite mādhavanidāne viṣanidānaṃ samāptam ||69||
Thus ends the chapter on Visa.

CHAPTER SEVENTY

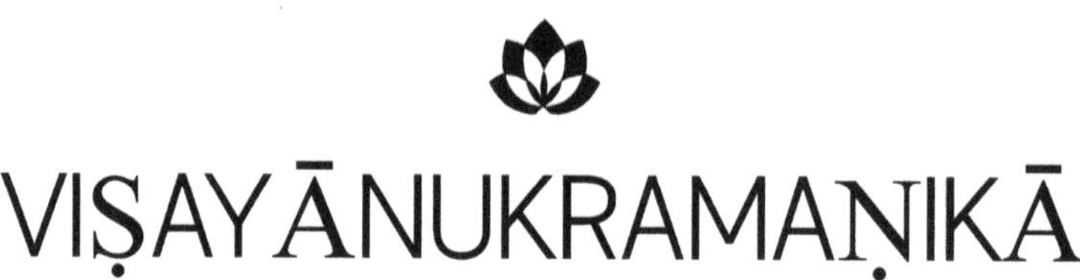

VIṢAYĀNUKRAMAṆIKĀ

Contents of Rugviniscaya treatise

jvaro'tisāro grahaṇī cārśo'jīrṇaṃ visūcikā |
alasaśca vilambī ca krimirukpāṇḍukāmalāḥ ||1||
halīmakaṃ raktapittaṃ rājayakṣmā uraḥkṣatam |
kāso hikkā saha śvāsaiḥ svarabhedastvarocakaḥ ||2||
chardistṛṣṇā ca mūrchādyā rogāḥ pānātyayādayaḥ |
dāhonmādāvapasmāraḥ kathito'thānilāmayaḥ ||3||
vātaraktamūrustambha āmavāto'tha śūlaruk |
paktijaṃ śūlamānāha udāvarto'tha gulmaruk ||4||
hṛdrogo mūtrakṛcchraṃ ca mūtrāghātastathā'śmarī |
prameho madhumehaśca piḍakāśca pramehajāḥ ||5||
medastathodaraṃ śotho vṛddhiśca galagaṇḍakaḥ |
gaṇḍamālā'pacī granthirarbudaḥ ślīpadaṃ tathā ||6||
vidradhirvraṇaśothaśca dvau vraṇau bhagnanāḍike |
bhagandaropadaṃśau ca śūkadoṣastvagāmayaḥ ||7||
śītapittamudardaśca koṭhaścaivāmlapittakam |
visarpaśca savisphoṭaḥ saromāntyo masūrikāḥ ||8||
kṣudrāsyakarṇanāsākṣiśiraḥstrībālakāmayāḥ |
viṣaṃ cetyayamuddiṣṭo rugviniścayasaṅgrahaḥ ||9||

Jwara, Atisāra, Grahani, Arśas, Ajirna, Visucikā, Alaska, Vilambikā, Krimiroga, Pāndu, Kāmalā, Halimaka, Raktapitta, Rājayaksmā, Urahksata, Kāsa, Hikkā, Swāsa, Swarabheda, Arocaka, Chardi, Trsnā, Mürchā, etc., Pānātyaya, etc., Dāha, Unmāda, Apasmāra, Vātavyādhis, Vātarakta, Urustambha, Amavāta, Sula,

PaktijaSūla, Anāha, Udāvarta, Gulmaroga, Hrdroga, Mutrakrchra, Mutrāghāta, Asmari, Prameha, Madhumeha, Prameha pidakās, Medoroga,

Udararoga, Sotha, Vrddhi, Galaganda, Gandamālā, Apacī, Granthi, Arbuda, Slīpada, Vidradhi, Vranaśotha, Two kinds of Vranas, Bhagna, Nadivrana, Bhagandara, Upadamsa, Sukadosa, Twakrogas (kustha), Sītapitta, Udarda, Kotha, Amlapitta, Visarpa, Visphota
Romāntika, Masūrika, Ksudrarogas, Asyarogas (mukharoga), Karnarogas, Nasikarogas, Aksirogas (netra rogas), Sirorogas, Strīrogas, Balarogas and Visa rogas are the contents of the treatise Rugviniscaya. (1-9)

Efforts of Madhava in compiling the contents of rugviniscaya

subhāṣitaṃ yatra yadasti kiñcittat sarvamekīkṛtamatra yatnāt |
viniścaye sarvarujāṃ narāṇāṃ śrīmādhavavenendukarātmajena ||10||
The best descriptions regarding rugviniscaya (methods for diagnosis and understanding diseases) in human beings found in different places (texts) have been compiled here with great effort, by Sri Madhava, son of Indukara, for understanding of all diseases. (10)

yat kṛtaṃ sukṛtaṃ kiñcit kṛtvaivaṃ rugviniścayam |
muñcantu jantavastena nityamātaṅkasantatim ||11||
Whatever good I have done by creating (writing) this treatise 'Rugviniscaya' with good intention, may all the living beings keep getting rid of chain of diseases permanently with its (Rugviniscaya treatise) help.

iti śrīmādhavakaraviracitaṃ mādhavanidānaṃ samāptam ||70||
Thus ends RogaViniscaya of Madhavakara.

www.ingramcontent.com/pod-product-compliance
Ingram Content Group UK Ltd.
Pitfield, Milton Keynes, MK11 3LW, UK
UKHW041632190726
13854UKWH00006B/2463